LIFE ON WHEELS

For the Active Wheelchair User

LIFE ON WHEELS

For the Active Wheelchair User

Gary Karp

O'REILLY®

Beijing · Cambridge · Farnham · Köln · Paris · Sebastopol · Taipei · Tokyo

Life on Wheels: For the Active Wheelchair User
by Gary Karp

Copyright © 1999 O'Reilly & Associates, Inc. All rights reserved.
Printed in the United States of America.

Published by O'Reilly & Associates, Inc., 101 Morris Street, Sebastopol, CA 95472.

Editor: Linda Lamb

Production Editor: Claire Cloutier

Printing History:

>   July 1999: First Edition

Library of Congress Cataloging-in-Publication Data:

Karp, Gary, 1955– .
    Life on wheels: for the active wheelchair user / Gary Karp.
        p.   cm.—(Patient-centered guides)
    Includes bibliographical references and index.
    ISBN 1-56592-253-0 (pbk.)
       1. Paraplegia—Popular works. 2. Paraplegics—Care.
3. Wheelchairs. 4. Paralysis—Popular works.   I. Title. II. Series.
RC406.P3K37   1999
362.4'3—dc21

>   99-10557
>   CIP

This book is printed on acid-free paper with 85% recycled content, 15% post-consumer waste. O'Reilly & Associates is committed to using paper with the highest recycled content available consistent with high quality.
[M]   [1/00]

For my parents
Sam and Bette

Table of Contents

Preface

The wheelchair is widely viewed as a symbol of illness and loss. Becoming a wheelchair user is thought of as failure, to be avoided at all costs, even when conditions cry out for an alternative method of mobility. People with progressive conditions such as multiple sclerosis or amyotrophic lateral sclerosis do all they can to delay using a wheelchair, feeling that to do so would be to surrender to their disability. Many people in the early months after a traumatic event such as spinal cord or brain injury resist the purchase of a customized wheelchair because they insist they will walk again.

Those with no disability (a temporary condition, it is said, for most people), recoil in horror at the thought of being "wheelchair-bound." In their minds, it is a mark of tragedy, of lost dreams, of pity, grueling effort, and regret. One becomes an object of charity—with some thanks to the fundraising symbol of the "poster child"—who needs care and lifelong medical management. It is an image fostered in the media in which films and television dramas emphasize either the tragedy or the heroism of people with disabilities rather than portraying the largely normal daily life that many chair riders experience. Newspapers typically use the phrase "confined to a wheelchair" and write about chair riders as human interest stories.

These beliefs are simply not true. The wheelchair is a tool that enhances quality of life. Wheelchair users are not always ill, not condemned to a life of no meaning or pleasure. Even for people with life-threatening illness, the right wheels facilitate their ability to be out in the world, continuing their life, partaking of the many realms of human experience.

The human spirit is remarkable in our capacity to adjust. We learn that our spirit can express itself even if we are unable to walk. We learn that we can survive and strive on wheels, just as well as we could on our feet. Thousands and thousands of people have proven this point, but the wider society has yet to take notice.

There is a huge gap between the way our culture views disability and the truth of the experience. More than 54 million Americans are thought to have a disability which significantly affects their lives. According to 1990 U.S. census data, there are nearly one and a half million regular wheelchair users in this country. All too many of these people are not living to their full potential because of obstacles placed in their way by society, or by their own beliefs—which were fostered by our culture in the first place. The census figures showed that only 18.4 percent of chair riders over the age of 21 were employed.

In the meantime, people with disabilities of ranging degrees of severity are getting on with having a life. Working, marrying, traveling, playing sports, being full members of their community. They have various limitations to deal with, but most will tell you that any difficulties they would ascribe to their disability are more about misguided cultural attitudes, and a political and architectural environment that places unnecessary obstacles in their way.

People with disabilities are not "broken"; neither are they heroes. Like everybody, people with disabilities are simply human.

What this book offers

This book offers an initial road map to the lifelong, complex, and fascinating road of the disability experience. This book is primarily a guidebook for those with a mobility disability, with practical information about how to adapt your home, choose a wheelchair, explore your sexuality, take care of your body. This book is designed to help people make their adjustments sooner and more completely by explaining how one adapts to disability, and by addressing misconceptions that only delay your ability to adapt. Throughout it I have tried to foster the principles of choice, of control, and of your right to pursue your interests and convictions.

Life on Wheels is also an effort to explain that inclusion is an innate right for everyone and that people with disabilities are excluded for reasons not based on a balanced or realistic understanding of what is possible. It's time our world caught up with the reality, closed that gap, and allowed millions of people with disabilities to play their full role in society.

There is a phenomenal amount of information concerning disabilities of all types. This book barely scratches the surface—it was extremely difficult to leave out so much interesting material. So its purpose is to be an orientation, to point you to some basic issues, and hopefully provide you with a strong start to continue your exploration of your own disability experience or that of someone you know and love.

There is an emphasis here on spinal cord injury (SCI). The fact is, I know more about SCI from personal experience, so feel better qualified to address it in depth. There is also a significantly greater amount of material available on spinal cord injury. At the same time, I have made a point to include other disabilities throughout the text. I regret not having the time or space to do them all justice.

However, the specific disability is irrelevant to the core issue of inclusion in society, and the process of managing one's health and discovering adaptive approaches which optimize the quality of one's life. To the degree that I focus on SCI, I hope I am shedding light on these core issues for people with all kinds of disabilities.

Why I wrote this book

I've been living the experience since I fell out of a tree and injured my spinal cord in 1973 at the age of 18. After thirteen weeks of hospitalization and rehabilitation I got a college education in architecture, have had an active professional life as a graphic artist, manager, and consultant, kept up my sidelines as a musician, juggler, and performer, traveled, moved to California, was married and divorced, pursued spiritual interests, developed enduring and deep friendships, gave and received support from my family…

Well, you get the idea. It's been a full life, marked by the whole range of experience that is the nature of being human—ups and downs, successes and failures. Not being able to walk has really been a pretty small part of it, in a way. In other ways, it essentially defines who I am.

This book comes from my desire to use my skills as a writer to express something about the truth of the disability experience, but it has also been a personal process of facing my own disability identity. I was a "mainstreamer." On a certain level I knew that I was not comfortable being seen in the world as having a disability. I wanted to appear as "normal" as possible, perhaps understandably because I had eighteen years of nondisabled identity still inside me. I pursued my personal interests and goals, and had little interaction with other chair riders.

But writing this book has deepened my sense of alliance with a disability community intent on gaining its entitled rights. I found out just how much I have in common with this large population of people with disabilities. We are not seen fully for who we are, but are excessively defined in the world's eyes by a mistaken conception of the meaning of our disabilities—rather than the deep and universal truth of our souls.

Who this book is for

This book is for anyone who is or will be using a wheelchair for a significant period of time who wants to make the most of every moment. This includes those with spinal cord injury, MS, amputations, and a host of other conditions and diseases. It includes those who are able to live independently, as well as chair users with more severe disabilities who direct the services of personal assistants and other staff.

This book is for people who are newly disabled and facing using a wheelchair, with background information on rehabilitation, wheelchair selection, emotional responses, and societal attitudes. However, it is also for those who are well past the shock of diagnosis or injury, who want to explore new options, take advantage of evolving technology, learn about the state of spinal cord research, reexamine accessibility in their homes, and optimize their lives.

While the voice of this book is directed to the wheelchair user, it is my hope that family, friends, medical workers, and people in public service or policy roles will read these pages. Perhaps the voice of the book will help you to place yourself in our "wheels" and help you better understand your own role in the lives of chair riders.

How this book is organized

This book first gives you background to understand your disability, then focuses on preparing for as active and independent a life as possible, and finally looks ahead to options for a full life.

- Chapter 1, *The Disabilities*, describes disabling conditions that might lead a person to use a wheelchair, giving most emphasis to conditions that have large numbers of people likely to be active with some degree of independence.

- Chapter 2, *Rehabilitation*, looks at the rehab process; facilities; the team of people who work with you during rehab; programs of physical therapy, occupational therapy, recreation therapy, respiratory therapy, and psychotherapy; and the transition to home and work.

- Chapter 3, *Medical Concerns*, looks briefly at medical concerns associated with various disabilities. Conditions common to many chair users—such as pain, pressure sores, and spasticity—are described at greater length.

- Chapter 4, *Staying Healthy*, addresses general health practices and topics for persons using a wheelchair, including exercise, diet, bladder and bowel programs, alternative therapies, aging, and personal care assistance.

- Chapter 5, *The Experience of Disability*, looks at some of the dynamics of what disability feels like from the inside, including identity issues and emotional responses to disability. It also looks at family responses, dependency, and public attitudes.

- Chapter 6, *Wheelchair Selection*, discusses funding, researching products, working with professionals who will advise you, and the many features and options of manual and power wheelchairs.

- Chapter 7, *Home Access*, looks at what you can do to make your home environment accessible and your daily life fuller and more convenient.

- Chapter 8, *Intimacy, Sex, and Babies*, looks at options for intimacy, finding partners, sexual activity, reproduction, and parenting.

- Chapter 9, *Spinal Cord Research*, gives a snapshot in time of the state of spinal cord research, as well as a discussion of using electrical stimulation to work with paralyzed muscles and some current research on behalf of other disabilities.

- Chapter 10, *Politics and Legislation*, looks at the disability movement and legislation. It also looks at the controversy of assisted suicide, access to transportation, enforcement of enacted laws, and remaining challenges.

- Chapter 11, *Getting Out There*, looks at getting around physically, using adaptive technology, education and employment, and the variety of sports and recreational activities you can consider.

Terminology

This book is addressed to wheelchair users, usually referred to as wheelchair users, wheelers, or chair riders. Yet, the term "people with disabilities" is also used freely throughout. This term I felt was the best solution to the ever-sensitive issue of words. It just gets too messy writing and reading "this person with spinal cord quadriplegia" or "persons with mobility limitations." I will trust the reader to know when the phrase "people with disabilities" refers to wheelers only and when it is a more inclusive usage.

The term "patient" has fallen out of favor. People with disabilities are trying to unbind themselves from a medical view of who they are. I have tried to avoid the use of "patient" in favor of the word "client." However, I did not change the quotes of medical workers who refer to patients, typically with regard to people who are residents in a hospital or rehabilitation center.

Throughout the book, I alternate in using he and she as third-person pronouns, so that no reader will feel excluded.

Acknowledgments

These pages come all the more to life thanks to the many personal stories and experiences included throughout. Some are in response to questions posted on my web site and others were drawn from online discussions, all used with kind permission for them to be quoted here. My sincere appreciation to the following people for sharing their heartfelt insights: Blane N. Beckwith, Blaze Henry Birinyi, Chris Bourne, George Buckner, Steven Edwards, Michelle Gallagher, Rebecca Gavin, Annette Hanna, Steve Hegg, Gary Hervey, Pauline Horvath, Paul and Jill Jacobs, Erika Jahneke, Jesse Kaysen, Dawn Kellman, Warren King, Douglas Kruse, Emmett S. Land, Constance Laymon, Linda Janine Lipe, Leeya Lowe, Kimber Mangiafico, Tracy L. Mankins, Francois Matte, Bob Mauro, Stan Melton, Carol Swedberg Meyer, Anet (AMARIS) Mconel, Lois Klesa Morrison, Tamar Magenta Raine, Dylan Ryall, Gary Schooley, Gale See, Gary Shakerdge, Marjie Smith, Viki Solomon, R.N., Michael Warner, Holly Waters, Chester M. Worwa, and those who wish to remain anonymous.

A number of very gracious souls took time from their busy schedules to lend support throughout the writing process. Special thanks to Ron Cohen, Barry Corbet, Carol Gill, Deborah Quilter, Stephen Rosenbaum, Mitch Tepper, and particular appreciation to Dr. Wise Young, for their ongoing and extremely generous help as the book evolved.

One of the most satisfying parts of the work was the process of interviewing people, including healthcare professionals at the forefront of their particular domain of the disability experience. For their openness and willingness to be quoted throughout these pages I thank Alex Barchuk, M.D., Cynthia Bishop, Michael Boninger, M.D., Mary Lou Breslin, Doe Cayting, Dennis Choi, M.D., Ph.D., Paul Church, Ron Cohen, M.D., Marcel Dijkers, Ph.D., Saunders Dorsey, Esq., Jeff Ewing, Ann Marie Fleming, M.F.C.C., Carol Gill, Ph.D., Sheldon Ginns, Jody Greenhalgh, O.T.R., Bob Hall, Deborah Kaplan, Esq., Naomi Kleitman, Ph.D., Sandra Loyer, M.S.W., Ron Mace, Providencia Morillo, Edward Nieshoff, M.D., Linda Noble, Ph.D., Margaret A. Nosek, Ph.D., Richard Patterson, Uli Salas, P.T., Marco Saroni, Michael Scott, M.D., Bonnie Sims, Denise Tate, Ph.D., Louis Tenenbaum, Mitch Tepper, M.P.H., Janie Whiteford, Karl Ylonen, and Wise Young, M.D, Ph.D..

Life on Wheels was reviewed prior to publication by a number of people who helped refine the contents. Thank you to Kim Beasley, Diane Conklin, Julia Dolphin Trahan, Richard Duncan, Martha Edwards, Richard Fessler, M.D., Carol Gill, Ph.D., Michelle Gittler, M.D., Pauline Horvath, Mark Johnson, Melinda Kelley, Ph.D., Dawn Kellman, Bill Lipscomb, Marca Sipski, M.D., and Ellen Winchell, Ph.D., for graciously taking time to read the draft manuscript, providing your honest and valued feedback.

I am, as always, deeply blessed by the enduring love and support of my family and friends: Marjorie and Morry Opperer, Carolynn, Stacey, Bruce, and Ken Karp, Mark Glasgow Johnson, David and Kate Downey, Bob and April Garrity, Dieter, Lynne, Sophie, and Lena Gloeckler, Jessica Jones, Alan and Elly Woontner, Frish Brandt, Richard Knight and Judith Lynch, Lawrence Elkus, Debra Waldman, Laurie Brown, the Malls, the Reveres, the Cassidys, Rob Robb, Lori Simon-Rosinowitz, Patricia Gleeson, Katherine Halsig, P.T., Sherrie Foster, O.T., and Oscar and Sarah Ichazo.

This book would not exist without the patience, experience, wisdom, and support of my editor, Linda Lamb. Thank you, Linda, for your belief in my work and my message, and for so skillfully guiding me through the mysterious straits and whirlwinds of first time authorship.

Thanks to editorial assistants Carol Wenmoth and Christee Styles for their dedication and skill in dealing with permissions, citations, file tagging, and much more that I'm sure I'm unaware of.

Despite the inspiration and contributions of so many, any errors, omissions, misstatements, or flaws in the book are my own.

Lastly, to people with disabilities everywhere, please accept this work with my prayers that it make a positive difference in your lives. I hope, at least, to have pointed the way to a few options you might not have known about, or given you cause to consider that your boundaries are a little farther out than you thought. It has certainly done so for my own life on wheels.

CHAPTER 1

The Disabilities

There are many reasons why a person might be a wheelchair user. Some, like spinal cord injury, result from accidental trauma or illness. Others, like muscular dystrophy, are genetic and might appear at almost any age. Some conditions are stable. Others are progressive, requiring a person to adapt over time. Each disability has physical features that require particular adaptations, such as the spasticity of cerebral palsy or the loss of grip associated with spinal cord quadriplegia. Despite the similar features of a given disability, each person's experience of it is different. The severity of disability can range widely. Your attitude and openness to adaptation also affect your experience, as do the resources available to you.

This chapter briefly describes disabling conditions that might lead a person to use a wheelchair. The disabilities described here illustrate how broad is the community of chair users—and how likely it is that any given person in this culture will eventually use a wheelchair, if only for a temporary disability. We list conditions in alphabetical order, giving more emphasis and space to conditions that have large numbers of people likely to be active with some degree of independence—the audience for this book.

Amputation

People lose parts of one or both legs from a variety of causes: vascular disease and infection, trauma, tumors, and congenital abnormalities that require limb amputation for better function or appearance.

Most people with single leg amputation ultimately walk with a prosthetic leg, often without even the use of a cane or crutch. They are capable of running and skiing. Losing a leg does not have to compromise mobility or require the use of a wheelchair. But in the early stages of the experience, those with single leg loss will use a wheelchair during rehabilitation and while being fitted for a prosthesis. They will wheel during the gradual process of adapting to the prosthesis or at a later time if sores or blisters form from prosthetic use.

People with bilateral amputation are more likely to primarily use a wheelchair, given the added difficulties of walking on two prosthetic legs.

Persons with amputation retain use of their posterior muscles and full sensation, and so are at reduced risk of pressure sores.

Amyotrophic lateral sclerosis (ALS)

Amyotrophic lateral sclerosis (ALS) is also known as Lou Gehrig's disease. ALS is a progressive condition. It attacks motor neuron cells, which control the movement of voluntary muscles. People with ALS gradually lose the ability to walk, speak, chew, swallow, and breathe. Bladder and bowel reflexes, vision, hearing, the sense of touch, and sexual function are unaffected. The intellect also remains completely intact, as demonstrated by the most famous example of someone living with ALS, physicist Stephen Hawking.

Most people with ALS eventually die from respiratory failure. The course of disease varies, depending on which area of the brain is affected first.

Only 10 percent of ALS cases have been found to have a hereditary, genetic cause. In some people with ALS, scientists have found high levels of glutamates, or excitatory neurotransmitters, in the spinal fluid. With high levels of glutamates, nerve cells are over-stimulated and damaged. Current treatments—none of which is a cure for ALS—are designed to partially block glutamates. Riluzole, marketed as Rilutek, is the first drug approved for ALS patients by the FDA. It has been found to slow the evolution of the disease. Gabapentin, marketed as Neurontin, is still in the process of human trials as of 1998.

ALS research is pursuing ways of providing nourishment to nerve cells to protect them. Antioxidants counteract the kind of oxidation that typifies the destructive process; vitamins C and E might have something to offer. General advancements in gene therapy might also contribute to management of ALS.

Cerebral palsy (CP)

Cerebral palsy (CP) is a permanent injury to the brain which affects its ability to send motor impulses to the rest of the body. CP is usually thought of as a defect at birth, but can also result from childhood injury or illness. It is characterized by muscle spasticity, paralysis leading to awkward movement and balance or complete inability to walk, and delayed development. A diagnosis of CP covers a very wide range of severity, from being virtually unnoticeable to complete paralysis and inability to speak.

The effects of CP are not limited to motor deficits. A person with CP can also experience difficulties with vision, speech, hearing, seizures, or mental retardation. The degree of muscle spasticity or paralysis is not determinative of other difficulties: a completely paralyzed child can have a high IQ. Although there is no cure for CP, early treatment and therapy can reduce some developmental disabilities and provide for better adjustment.

Physical barriers can be significant, but people also face some challenging social concerns, as noted by this man with CP:

> I think people in general have a harder time dealing with a person with CP than they do with people with other disabilities. It may be because of a number of things like the spastic movements, the drooling, or the lack of communication. I don't think the world as a whole views people with CP as very pretty people, but that's because they don't see beyond the outside. Once you get to know somebody then it changes, but getting past that barrier is very hard.

Many of the 500,000 Americans with CP function at a high level of independence and activity. Most people with CP-related mobility limitations have some ability to walk. They can adapt and move about independently with tools such as braces, a walker, or a scooter, and use a wheelchair at the times when it is appropriate:

> I am twenty-three years old with athetoid CP. I can walk around my house with help of the wall. I use a walker for short distance walks and a wheelchair for long distance. I wear a shoe insert on my left leg and an AFO on my right, along with a hand brace to straighten out the fingers on my right hand. My speech is affected, but if I talk slowly enough people can understand me.

Convulsive seizures and drooling can sometimes be managed with medication. The general approach is to make the most of braces, wheelchairs, and other adaptive methods along with counseling to optimize independence and reduce any psychological barriers to a productive life.

Friedreich's ataxia (FA)

Friedreich's ataxia (FA) is a genetic disease, marked by degeneration of nerve tissue in the spinal cord. FA appears between the ages of five and fifteen, first affecting the upper limbs, head, and neck. Within eight to ten years, the nerve damage of FA impairs the ability to walk. One loses balance and coordination, often exhibiting a "drunken" walk:

> With FA, you continually lose your coordination and balance (particularly in the legs). A wheelchair is definitely a benefit, because it's safer. I've also found that a wheelchair seems more dignified than attempting to hobble around on a cane. Also, by being in a wheelchair, I don't get accused of being intoxicated anymore—I've almost been arrested for public drunkenness because of that damn cane!

Multiple sclerosis (MS)

Multiple sclerosis (MS) is a condition in which the myelin coating around nerves in the brain and spinal cord is attacked and destroyed by the body, for reasons researchers have yet to confidently identify. Lesions occur in many locations, leaving behind scar or sclerosed tissue: thus the name multiple sclerosis. The majority of initial lesions occur in the brain.

Messages which normally travel at 225 miles per hour are slowed, causing loss of coordination and strength, though intermittently and incompletely. Other symptoms include loss of balance, emotional disorders, vision problems, bowel and bladder dysfunction, impaired sexuality, paralysis, or pain. Both the sensory and motor systems can be affected by MS. The emotional center of the brain can also be a target of MS, leading to unexplainable depression or even uncontrollable laughter or crying.

Jimmie Heuga was an Olympic skier in 1964 at the age of fifteen. Eight years later he was diagnosed with MS, as he relates in an interview in *New Mobility Magazine*:

> The neurologist who diagnosed me seemed to feel a little sorry for me, but I was in good shape and I thought I was indestructible. The morning before I had run five miles in under twenty-five minutes.

> I had vision problems, spasticity. My reactions were off and I knew it. In the spring of 1967, I was twenty-three. I'd never been twenty-three before, and I thought these things just happen at that age.[1]

The majority of people with MS have the relapse-remitting form of the disease, where symptoms appear or are accentuated during a period known as an exacerbation and then recede again. There is a less common type of benign MS, in which a person may experience only minor difficulties throughout his or her lifetime. At the other extreme is the chronic-progressive form of MS, marked by a continual decline. Fortunately, only 2 percent of cases take this form. A conservative estimate of 350,000 people in the United States have some form of MS. Most of them continue to function at a high level.

Exacerbations

MS symptoms are typically intermittent, with symptoms present or accentuated during periods of exacerbation. When the myelin sheathing around nerves is damaged, the body responds with an inflammatory process as part of its attempt to heal the area. The swelling further blocks nerve conduction. Once the inflammatory process is over, symptoms can recede or disappear. Still, damage has been done and scar tissue formed. A significant amount of myelin needs to be destroyed before symptoms become permanent, so it is common for people with multiple sclerosis to have breaks from the condition, essentially symptom-free, especially in the early stages. About 70 percent experience complete remission in the early stages of the condition.

Subtle symptoms of an exacerbation are early fatigue and general muscle weakness. More extreme indications include speech disorders, tingling sensations, frequent urinary infections, double vision, or sharp pains, among others. Difficulty in walking is the most common symptom. One or both legs can become weak. Walking at home might still be manageable. However, during significant exacerbations the person needs to avoid fatigue; fatigue can aggravate an exacerbation and other symptoms. Between exacerbations, therapy and exercise can help minimize effects and improve walking capacity.

A number of drugs have helped limit frequency and severity of exacerbations. Beta interferon drugs have been given a lot of attention, including Avonex, which gained FDA approval in the U.S. Diet also has great impact. MS is more prevalent in societies that eat more fatty foods, such as dairy products. Myelin is largely made up of polyunsaturated fats, so it makes sense that diet can have some impact on the disease.

While the cause remains a mystery, certain conditions are understood to increase the likelihood of an exacerbation. In *Living with Multiple Sclerosis, a Wellness Approach*, George Kraft, M.D., and Marci Catanzaro, R.N., write:

> *Emotional stress, immunizations, infections and other illnesses, changes in the weather, and trauma have all been credited with causing multiple sclerosis exacerbations.*[2]

MS seems to be particularly sensitive to elevated body temperature. Swimming has proven to be a good form of exercise for people with MS, since it keeps body temperature down during exercise.

Physical limitations

Multiple sclerosis does not necessarily lead to being a full-time wheelchair user. Some people with MS only use wheels during significant exacerbations, while others with chronic progressive MS or in later stages of the relapse-remitting form will find themselves using wheels much of the time. A scooter is popular for occasional use outside the home.

Walking can be affected by foot drop, which might be compensated for with a brace. MS can cause spasticity or muscle tightness, which can interfere with gait. Medications can help with this problem. Loss of balance or ataxia can be severe enough to require use of an assistive device. Sensory ataxia can cause numbness in the feet of such severity that the floor cannot be felt.

Multiple sclerosis can be an invisible disability, since many people walk and appear normal, except during exacerbations or the significant onset of chronic-progressive MS. During times of remission, it can be a challenge to maintain the health and social habits needed to limit relapses; there is the natural desire to enjoy a period of relapse as a chance to take a break from the disease. People do learn to manage their relapses, make adaptations, and continue to have active lives.

Muscular dystrophy (MD)

Muscular dystrophy (MD) is a group of nine genetic diseases that affect muscle proteins. They are progressive, degenerative disorders which are sometimes fatal. Effects are usually limited to skeletal muscles that control voluntary movement. Some forms of MD can also impact involuntary muscles such as the heart.

While many muscular dystrophies occur in childhood, others occur as late as sixty years of age. MDs which could result in being an adult wheelchair user include the following:

- Myotonic dystrophy is the most common form of MD. It generally appears between the ages of twenty and forty, and its progress is slow, spanning as much as sixty years. This form of dystropy exhibits myotonia, the delayed relaxation of a muscle after contraction. One of its most troublesome symptoms can be the inability to release the grip of a hand. The first symptoms tend to appear in the face, neck, hands, forearms, and feet, although weakness is eventually experienced in all muscle groups. Myotonic dystrophy can affect other body systems.

- Becker dystrophy generally has its onset between two and sixteen years of age. Survival into middle age is common. Becker dystrophy is similar to Duchenne dystrophy, but milder. Symptoms appear first in upper arms and legs, and pelvis.

- Duchenne dystrophy is among the better known dystrophies, perhaps because it strikes children between the age of two and six. Some people with Duchenne dystrophy have survived into their twenties.

- Limb-girdle dystrophy begins in the shoulder or pelvic girdles and strikes at any time from late childhood to middle age. It progresses slowly and is ultimately fatal, usually as a result of complications with the heart. However, some people have a normal life span.

- Distal dystrophy occurs later in life, between the ages of forty and sixty. It primarily affects the hands, forearms, and lower legs. It advances gradually and rarely reaches the stage of complete disability. It is the rarest form of MD.

Myasthenia gravis (MG)

Myasthenia gravis (MG) is a neuromuscular disorder. It is a chronic muscle disease that results in weakness and quick fatigue.

Nerve impulses are transmitted to muscles by means of the chemical acetylcholine, for which muscles have receptors to receive the messages. Medical evidence exists that the body's immune system attacks these receptors in people with MG. The thymus gland is linked to the production of acetylcholine receptor antibodies, which would have a destructive effect on the receptors. Many adults with MG have abnormalities in their thymus glands which normally shrink after infancy to a level of having little function in the body. The relationship of the thymus to MG is not yet well understood, but there is enough suspicion to justify further research.

Onset of myasthenia gravis may be sudden and severe, but early symptoms are usually more subtle, making MG difficult to diagnose. The first symptoms tend to appear in the eye muscles, leading to blurred or double vision. People might experience intermittent fatigue for a lengthy period before gaining a proper diagnosis. Weakness in the muscles caused by MG is variable, often worse at the end of the day and exacerbated by exercise. Rest usually helps alleviate extreme fatigue. Difficulty in swallowing or breathing generally precede difficulties with mobility.

MG is managed with drugs or surgery. Drugs known as anticholinesterase agents can extend the effect of the body's acetylcholine, although the drugs do not repair damaged receptors. At a later stage, the thymus might be surgically removed. After removal of the thymus, more than half of the people treated show remission or substantial improvement.

Polio and post-polio syndrome

Polio—or poliomyelitis or infantile paralysis—is a virus which at its most severe causes paralysis and even death. Children are the most vulnerable targets, although symptoms can develop in adulthood as well. The two types of polio—paralytic and non-paralytic—have a wide range of possible effects. Some people have a mild case and mistake it for the common flu, while others are completely paralyzed, dependent on assistive breathing devices such as an iron lung or a ventilator.

The polio virus kills neurons in the brain and spinal cord. If the cranial nerves are attacked, the disease is fatal. Attack of the spinal cord can also cause death, but paralysis is more often the result. A polio attack only lasts as long as a common cold, so is not a progressive disease. Neural damage in the spinal cord is random, and healthy nerves are able to resume work when the virus passes. Damaged nerves also send out sprouts in an attempt to reestablish contact, some of which hit their mark and allow for some functional return. Once the polio virus has done its initial damage, a person can begin a process of recovery and sometimes walk out of the hospital, even after having been in an iron lung.

Polio is considered eradicated in the U.S., with the last known, active case of polio in 1979. However, the virus continues to appear in other parts of the world.

In the '70s, people in the U.S. who had polio in the epidemics of the '30s, '40s, and '50s began to experience a return or increase in symptoms. This return of symptoms is now termed post-poliomyelitis syndrome (post-polio syndrome or PPS). One theory holds that people made a degree of recovery when nerves branched out and found new connections. Muscles also found ways to do more work with less than all of their fibers fully able to contract. The result was that fewer nerve and muscle tissues were doing more work than they were meant for. After years of use, the tissues began to give out from sheer wear and tear.

People with PPS have been surprised to find themselves becoming weak again, many years after the initial onset of and recovery from polio. In a National Institutes of Health study, 42 percent of people with non-paralytic polio have experienced PPS. Over 75 percent of polio survivors record new muscle weakness and pain. More than 90 percent reported both physical and mental fatigue.

Some people with PPS have reacted to the change in their health by beginning a vigilant program of exercise. They believe they can build supplemental muscle strength to make up for the late-appearing weakness. This, it turns out, is the wrong approach. Overtaxed nerves and muscles are simply pushed harder, accelerating the PPS process.

All evidence points to the need to pace one's activities as the best way to reduce weakness, fatigue, and pain from PPS. In a study performed at the Kessler Institute in New Jersey, polio survivors who got regular therapy demonstrated 22 percent less weakness and fatigue than those who did not continue their therapy program. Survivors in the therapy group conserved their energy, took two fifteen-minute rest breaks each day, and appropriately used assistive devices such as canes, braces, wheelchairs, or scooters.[3]

There are efforts toward a pharmaceutical solution. Mestinon, a drug that prevents the breakdown of ACTH in the muscle, might reduce fatigue in some polio survivors. Parlodel, used with some persons with Parkinson's disease, has helped increase attention and wakefulness. There could be a danger, though, in covering up symptoms. Continuing to overuse the body could lead to more severe symptoms later. The more conservative, common-sense approach emphasizes good health and appropriate levels of activity.

Rheumatoid arthritis (RA)

Rheumatoid arthritis (RA) is an autoimmune disease in which the body essentially attacks its bone and the cartilage of joints—for reasons that science has yet to determine. Our joints are lined with a lubricating layer called the synovium. In people with RA, the synovium becomes inflamed and then releases enzymes that literally digest bone and cartilage. RA eventually affects the joints of the entire body, although statistically it tends to attack some parts earlier than others. The hands and feet are common early targets of the disease.

Once damage is done to bone and cartilage, it is irreversible. Treatment and therapy is focused on slowing the progress of the disease and reducing symptoms, which include pain, swelling, limited range of motion, and deformity of joints. Research increasingly shows that early treatment can make a difference in long-term prognosis. Once enough damage has occurred, joint replacement surgery is the only remaining option.

Eighty percent of people with RA experience remission, although not for long periods. As RA progresses, walking aids such as canes, ankle braces, and crutches are used while it is still possible to walk. At some point, the knees and ankles become deformed, inflexible, painful, and increasingly unable to support the weight of the body. A scooter might be used during a period when moderate walking is still possible around the home. Once walking is inadvisable or impossible, a power wheelchair is the likely solution, since the arms usually experience frailty at the same time as the legs. It is important to continue to stand and walk to the degree possible:

> I am supposed to use my chair when I am tired, have swollen ankles,
> or need to carry files at work. It is very important for me to walk and
> weight-bear, for bone strength and protection, at appropriate intervals.

Most drugs used to control rheumatoid arthritis—even widely used non-steroidal anti-inflammatory drugs—can produce significant or unacceptable side effects. Pharmaceuticals like methotrexate can, in many cases, prevent deformities and the progression of the disease.

In a 1991 study, it was found that diet can have an impact on a range of RA symptoms. The study group—compared to a control group which ate a normal diet—fasted for seven to ten days and then ate a non-dairy, vegetarian diet, adding dairy foods later on. Not only did they experience reduced pain and swelling and an increase in strength, the effects lasted longer than in the control group, which received traditional drug, physical, and occupational therapies.[4]

Spina bifida (SB)

Spina bifida (SB) is a neural tube defect which involves the incomplete development of the brain or spinal cord in the womb. The spine fails to close properly during the first month of pregnancy. Spina bifida is the most common birth defect, involving one of every 1,000 newborns in the United States. It is now very common for children to survive into adulthood, thanks to modern surgical and rehabilitation developments. Some children are able to walk with crutches, or have sufficient upper body strength to use a manual wheelchair.

Many children born with spina bifida also have hydrocephalus, an accumulation of fluid in the brain. The excess fluid can usually be relieved by the surgical placement of a shunt system. Many children with SB develop latex allergy. Tendinitis, depression, gastrointestinal disorders, learning disabilities, and obesity are sometimes associated with SB.

A low level of folic acid in the mother increases risk of spina bifida. The Spina Bifida Foundation says that if women were to consume a sufficient daily amount of folic acid prior to pregnancy and during the first trimester, 75 percent of folic acid-preventable SB could be prevented.

Spinal cord injury (SCI)

Spinal cord injury (SCI) can result from trauma (automobile crashes, acts of violence, falls, sports injuries, and so on) or from other causes, such as aortic aneurysms, tumors, radiation, and infections. An estimated 250,000 people live with spinal cord injury; about 10,000 join the ranks each year.

The spinal cord is the conduit from the brain to the rest of the body and its muscles and sensations. All impulses sent out to tell the muscles to contract and all sensory messages the body returns to the brain travel through the spinal cord. Injury to the cord cuts off communication to some portion of the body, depending where on the cord the injury occurs.

The higher the physical level of injury, the more function and sensation is lost. Level is defined according to the vertebrae of the spine. Survivors of cervical spinal cord injury have all four limbs affected and are known as quadriplegics. Those with injuries at or below the first thoracic vertebrae, or T1, retain full use of the hands and arms and are known as paraplegic.

Following is a discussion of the impact of spinal cord injuries at various levels of the cord. More than half of spinal cord injuries are considered incomplete with some nerve function intact, so these descriptions are not absolute.

Injury to the lumbar spinal cord

When the injury is above the fourth lumbar level, the ability to stabilize the pelvis is lost and thus the capacity for independent walking. Below this level, although the ability to push off with the foot is compromised, short leg braces and crutches can allow mobility without a wheelchair.

Injury to the thoracic spinal cord

At T12, the brain is essentially out of contact with the legs, including the muscles of the buttocks which are used to brace the body at the hips. Muscles of the trunk and abdomen remain intact so that the person retains relatively good upper body balance, helpful for wheelchair skills. At this level, there is the greatest loss of sexual function, since the reflexes of orgasm and ejaculation take place at this point.

Below T5, all of the chest muscles remain active, including those involved in breathing. Abdominal and lower back muscles begin to be affected as this level is approached, affecting upper body balance and posture.

Injuries at the top four thoracic levels begin to affect the chest and trunk, although the hands and arms remain fully functioning. Upper thoracic injuries have less impact on sexual function, since some of these functions travel between the genitals and the spinal cord without involving the brain.

Injury to the cervical spinal cord

At the seventh cervical level the hands become affected, beginning with the fingers, costing the ability to grip. Now categorized as quadriplegic, the person can still use a manual wheelchair because arm and shoulder strength are unaffected.

At C6, there is still total shoulder control, but movements of the hand and forearm are limited to certain directions as specific muscle groups lose their link to the brain. With grip completely gone, there is a greater dependence on adaptive devices. The trunk is very weak, so balance is a challenge, sometimes suggesting the need for a reclining wheelchair back or the use of belts.

A C5 trauma begins to limit full shoulder movement and the ability to straighten the arm, although lifting the arms with the biceps remains unimpaired.

In C3-4 injuries, considerable head and neck control is retained, the ability to shrug the shoulders, and—in most cases— control of the diaphragm. Some quadriplegics at these levels will have difficulty breathing for lack of abdominal and trunk muscles, so may rely to some degree on a ventilator. Use of the arms is very limited, making the use of chin controls or puff-and-sip controls the options of choice.

It is rare for a person to survive a spinal cord trauma above C-3.

Spinal muscular atrophy (SMA)

Spinal muscular atrophy (SMA) is a genetic disorder that affects the anterior horn cells of the spinal cord. Its impact is on voluntary muscles, usually those closest to the trunk of the body. The legs tend to be affected more than the arms. Sensations are not affected. People with SMA have normal intelligence.

SMA is often listed with the muscular dystrophies. SMA types that could result in being an adult wheelchair user include the following:

- Type II Chronic SMA can result in early death, but people with this type of SMA can also survive into adulthood. Children can develop the ability to stand, often with use of bracing.

- Type III—also known as Kugelberg-Welander or juvenile SMA—is a mild form in which many people are able to walk but become weaker later in life. Survival into adulthood is common. Scoliosis can become a problem over time, and might require spinal fusion to prevent the restriction of breathing that accompanies severe spinal curvature.

- Type IV is an adult-onset form in which the symptoms typically appear after the age of thirty-five. This type of SMA is characterized by very slow progression.

- A variation of adult onset SMA is the X-linked form which occurs only in males. It is also known as Kennedy's syndrome or Bulbo-spinal muscular atrophy. It tends to progress slowly, but is sometimes stable.

As SMA progresses, use of a wheelchair usually becomes necessary. Ultimately a power chair will be needed, although a manual chair can be appropriate at earlier stages.

Stroke

The most common form of stroke is the result of a sudden disruption in the flow of blood to parts of the brain. The oxygen supply is cut off and brain cells die. Sometimes, blood vessels burst (hemorrhage) and blood spreads into nearby brain areas. Either way, brain functions are affected, causing unconsciousness and/or partial paralysis. Paralysis on one side of the body—hemiplegia—is common.

The number of strokes in the U.S. annually is estimated at between 400,000 and 730,000. Stroke does not only affect the elderly. Although two thirds of strokes happen to people over sixty-five, young people can and do suffer stroke, sometimes at the peak of their working lives. With good medical care, survivability of strokes has improved markedly.

Traumatic brain injury (TBI)

Traumatic brain injury (TBI) is a result of an impact to the head that affects brain tissue. Any tissue in the body swells when it is injured. When the brain becomes inflamed, danger is increased because the brain is contained inside the skull without much extra space to accommodate swelling. Leaking blood vessels cannot drain easily, further increasing swelling. Controlling swelling and maintaining oxygen levels are key strategies during the acute period after brain injury.

Doctors have found that there is continuing, secondary damage during the first twenty-four hours after injury, similar to the secondary damage that occurs with spinal cord trauma. Among other biochemical events which take place, free radicals are formed which destroy fatty acids of cell membranes, in a process known as lipid peroxidation. Reducing the impact of this progression is a focus of research in emergency treatments.

Most long-term, chronic effects of TBI are the result of secondary damage. Long-term effects include cognitive problems such as memory loss, difficulty concentrating, or trouble communicating. Physical problems might include headaches, loss of smell or taste, speech impairment, fatigue, muscle spasms, or seizures. Temporary paralysis can affect the ability to use a foot or leg. Some people must relearn how to walk, so might be temporary chair riders. Others will sustain permanent paralysis from brain cell death.

Each year, 373,000 Americans are hospitalized with TBI, 99,000 of whom experience lifelong disabling conditions. Often, multiple injuries are associated with TBI. Spinal cord injury and TBI are an all-too-common combination.

Many people who experience a brain trauma will spend time in a coma. Being in a prolonged coma does not necessarily mean a poor prognosis. While in a coma, a person requires specialized care to minimize the risk of conditions that can be disabling after the coma. He must be moved often to prevent pressure sores, to support respiratory functions (some people require a ventilator), and to prevent contractures—the shortening of muscles and tissues. Left alone, a person in coma would curl up into a fetal position. This constant, curled position would affect his ability to walk after he returned to consciousness.

Temporary and age-related disabilities

Statistically, including temporary and age-related, disabilities make the population of people who will use a wheelchair at some point in their lives very large indeed.

People break legs. They have surgeries. People have extended illnesses that weaken them enough that they can only walk limited distances. Temporary injuries requiring wheelchair use are growing, particularly because of the popularity of riskier sports like in-line skating, skateboarding, and rock climbing.

Older people face risks to their mobility. Many older people break arms, legs, or hips when they fall and might find themselves using a wheelchair—even if temporarily. Joints, such as the knees and hips, are common sites of age-related wear—or of arthritis and rheumatism, which are statistically more present in the elderly—and can affect the ability to walk.

A wheelchair is a powerful symbolic image of aging. Many people try to avoid using a wheelchair as long as possible. As with any disability, if people can view the wheelchair as a tool—possibly one that they only need to use temporarily or occasionally—often they will find a higher quality of life available. Wheelchair use does not have to be an all-or-nothing proposition. A rider could use a wheelchair for trips outside the home, while walking at home to maintain as much capacity as possible in an environment without as much risk of a fall or overstrain of the body.

CHAPTER 2

Rehabilitation

As a wheelchair user, optimizing your physical capacity and learning new skills are the key to being as independent as your body and medical condition allow. A rehabilitation hospital or clinic is the place where you develop these abilities. It is a place of hard work, unique relationships, and challenges and opportunities at every level of your life—emotionally, physically, intellectually, socially, and for some, financially.

The rehabilitation process is designed to reduce the negative effects of disability so you can enjoy life again and adapt to physical changes. Do your best to make the most of it. Your time there is brief, and you may not get another chance to work with a group of highly trained professionals assembled to help you adapt to your disability.

This chapter looks at issues encountered in rehab. We first look at the process itself: the goals of rehab and how rehab is changing. We then look at facilities—the range of centers, rehab accreditation, insurance coverage, and the admission process. Next we discuss the team of people who will be working with you during rehab: your case manager or social worker, physician, and therapists, as well as family and peer support. We look at programs of physical therapy, occupational therapy, recreation therapy, respiratory therapy, and psychotherapy in the rehab setting. We end with a brief look at the transition to home and work.

Hope and adjustment

Rehab is a place of safety, where you have the benefit of a controlled environment in which to do the work of returning to your life on the outside. Being in rehab is also a challenging process of considerable adjustment and emotion.

This woman with an L1 spinal cord injury expresses the dichotomy:

> *The whole experience was valuable. I could never have progressed to being so independent without it. However, I found it unpleasant, because living in the rehab unit for four months was like being in prison. The schedule of therapies was stringent. No freedom whatsoever.*

Rehab is a chance to explore possibilities. You might walk out with braces and crutches or using a walker. Or you might wheel out. You and your medical team should question what is physically possible and set your goals accordingly—preferably with a little room left for that occasional miracle.

Dr. Michael Scott of the Rancho Los Amigos Center in southern California tries to be realistic when people with brain or spinal cord trauma ask him the "cure" question:

> *I think we're on the road to a cure. But I tell people that cure doesn't necessarily mean that you're going to be up and running around again. A cure probably means we're going to find a way for you to be a little better and able to do more. I think it's going to be a combination of rehabilitation and whatever the cure is.*

Dr. Wise Young, Director of the Neuroscience Center at Rutgers, State University of New Jersey, is concerned that some rehab centers are too pessimistic when it comes to recovery from spinal cord injury:

> *I certainly agree that rehab is a place of safety, but many places are still discouraging the hopes of people who are interested in recovery. Most rehabilitation centers, in my opinion, are unnecessarily pessimistic. They emphasize that the goal of therapy is to make the most of what they have, and many people are told that they should not expect much recovery. This is applicable only to a minority of severely injured patients. The vast majority of patients with spinal cord injury recover substantially.*

Use the rehab experience to keep yourself in optimal condition. By waiting for recovery rather than working with what you have, you risk robbing yourself of motivation to gain skills that might contribute to your degree of independence. Do the work available to you, adapting as much as possible to your condition while working to foster your recovery. Learn skills being taught, even if you don't expect to be using them for long:

> *Believing I would walk really didn't affect my participation in rehab. I guess it goes back to my being an overachiever or something. I've always*

been the best at whatever I've done in many ways, so I set the hospital record for getting out with my level of injury.

How rehab has changed

The rehab experience has changed much in the past twenty or so years. Rehab has gotten shorter. You no longer have the luxury of many months of adjustment and training. There are fewer resources available for many patients.

There are plenty of things about rehab that are better than twenty years ago, including:

- The evolution of wheelchair design has advanced so far that rehab professionals are now able to fit a person to the ideal chair and extend their independence in ways that had not previously been possible.

- Bedding and cushion technology have significantly reduced the risk of decubitus ulcers which have often interfered with the rehabilitation process.

- Assistive technology has evolved recently that gives people with limited arm use much more control over their environment. Rehab centers increasingly have dedicated staff who identify such solutions and provide training during the rehab stay.

- Psychological, sexual, family, financial, and political dynamics of disability are addressed in ways that they were not in the past.

Shorter stays

Stays of several months were once common. Longer stays might have allowed people more opportunity to develop strength, gain skills, and make psychological adjustments. People were nonetheless caught in an environment that imposed a lot of control over their lives, according to this quadriplegic woman injured in the '70s:

I spent nine months in rehab. I really got a flavor of what institutionalization is like, and how the needs of the institution eventually prevail over the needs of the individual because the institution has a schedule and needs to function. And the needs of one individual don't really compare in scope.

Stays of several months are now very rare, given current insurance coverage. A person's claim must prove that he is continuing to make gains in order to be allowed to stay. However, much rehab work is slow and small gains are the natural pace. The pressure to show progress can cause great stress.

Rehab starts early, during the acute stage. Most people with traumatic injury are up and out of bed as soon as reasonable after their injury has stabilized. Some people still will need to spend significant time on bed rest. For example, some high quadriplegics require more time for their body to adapt before they can be physically active.

The common practice now with spinal cord injuries is to mechanically stabilize the spine (for example, with a halo or back brace) and get you up. There are advances occurring in these technologies. As Dr. Wise Young describes:

> Many of the more advanced centers no longer use halos. Instead,
> neurosurgeons are stabilizing the cervical spinal cord with either anterior
> or posterior plates which are screwed into the bone. People with such
> plates do not need halos and can be mobilized earlier after injury.

For some injuries that require stabilization, surgeons install rods in the spine, which make it possible to sit someone up within days of injury and begin the rehab process. It is open to question whether installation of rods to stabilize the spine in order to begin rehab is wise. This device restricts the movement of several vertebrae; newer designs are better able to accommodate normal contours of the spine. Your posture is forced into a more upright position, and greater forces are exerted on neighboring vertebrae because of the loss of flexibility imposed by the rods. There is some potential for future problems due to the strain on the spine.

It can be beneficial to initiate the rehab process sooner so you can begin to develop strength and skills. The goal of early rehab is to make the healing process more efficient—which saves costs and also speeds your return to independence. This early rehab approach can also head off the risks of extended bed rest, including progressive weakening, medical problems such as pressure sores, contracted muscles, infection, and falling into a depressive or angry state, which can interfere with your commitment to the rehab process.

A downside of shorter stays is that many people are not ready to commit emotionally to the rehab process, much less accept that they should learn how to use a wheelchair. The initial, acute period of medical recovery can be an important phase in making the emotional adjustment to disability and in finding out more about what the level of impairment will actually be. Some people do regain function, after all.

A person with a traumatic injury needs more than medical stabilization. The psychological shock and its social implications are massive, but the short rehab periods that are now typical barely allow people to begin these adjustments. Dr. Marcel Dijkers, Director of Research at Detroit's Rehabilitation Institute of Michigan, observes:

> *The compression of length of stay forces us to treat people as "patients" rather than being a socio-emotional development center where people can take time and think about what has happened to them. In Europe they still have lengths of stay of four and five months with a very low-key treatment program. It might look like they are just hanging around, but they talk and interact and have the opportunity to adjust. Here, we essentially kick them out just as they are starting the mental change process.*

Short stays also put the squeeze on patient services staff who are trying to organize equipment, modifications, support resources, and financial coverage you will need when you leave. Bonnie Sims directs the Patient Services Group at Denver's Craig Hospital. She says:

> *Resources may be out there, but the challenge is to call them into play within the time allotted.*

High quadriplegics have a number of unique issues to deal with. They might use a ventilator to breathe, and rely more on others to get dressed and get in and out of their chair. They are unable to do their own pressure relief lifts and have more extensive muscle atrophy, so are at greater risk of developing pressure sores. Sores limit the ability to participate in therapy and might make a longer stay necessary.

At some centers, it has become common practice to send a quadriplegic home with a halo on and discontinue therapy until it is time for it to come off. Rich Patterson is a C5 quadriplegic who directs the peer support program at the Santa Clara Valley Medical Center in California. He says:

> *They will send people home with a halo on because they feel that their therapy has stopped. Once equipment can come off, they come back*

for therapy. People have to use their own equipment or rentals and loan-
ers. Most of those people come back with pressure sores or are very
dejected, confused, and frustrated.

That does not have to be the case. A quadriplegic man in his twenties states:

I was happy to be sent home until my halo could come off. I got to be
with my family and spend time with my friends. They would take me to
restaurants, and we had a great time. I was in a much better mood by the
time I went back into rehab.

The pressure from insurance has motivated providers to tighten up their systems, as well as to pursue more detailed research into what really works. Dr.
Scott of Rancho Los Amigos states:

I don't know that shorter stays are all bad. I think we've learned to
become more efficient, working at how to be more critical about what we
do, about what works and what doesn't work. There's a lot more atten-
tion being paid to functional outcome.

Rehab practitioners must squeeze in much more treatment into much less
time. Many mourn the fact that they know they are unable to accomplish as
much as they want, that people are not being given the time they need to
adapt to what has happened. Since rehab now begins so soon after injury,
the focus is placed more on medical stabilization. Says Dr. Alex Barchuk,
physiatrist at the Kentfield Rehabilitation Hospital in northern California:

Basically all rehab is doing is providing a good environment for the
body to heal. There are so many things that can go wrong—blood clots,
pressure ulcers, things like that— which really can affect the long-term
rehab of an individual.

Sandra Loyer, clinical social worker at the University of Michigan Rehabilitation Unit, sees that rather than being able to complete rehab, staff must
teach people to do it for themselves after they leave:

All we can do is get them medically stable, teach them basic skills like
bowel and bladder management, help them attain what strength they can
in that time, and then they're gone. We have to help them be able to advo-
cate for themselves, because we just can't follow through for them.

Despite shorter stays, rehab can become comfortable, especially compared to
the outside world which can seem quite scary to someone who is returning

for the first time to that world on wheels. Rehab staff is very aware of the danger of allowing people to get too settled into rehab, where they are taken care of, don't need to discipline themselves thanks to a built-in schedule of activities, and are generally surrounded by people who understand their disability. At some point, it is time to move on.

Adaptive technology

Technology has made a tremendous contribution to the range of options for people with disabilities, especially more severe disabilities such as high quadriplegia. Computers contribute in four areas:

- **Control of mobility.** Power wheelchairs have evolved in quality and flexibility. Speed and acceleration can be finely controlled. Voice-controlled wheelchairs are not far off. Digital controls for vans are also making driving an option for more quadriplegics.

- **Control of the environment.** Commercial products allow remote control of doors, lights, telephones, or almost any electrical device from the wheelchair. The remote controller might be a keypad similar to the television remote control or a puff-and-sip device for people with limited arm use.

- **Communication.** The Internet connects people to the world. It has discussion groups and is a powerful resource and research tool. For those with limited ability to get out of the home—however temporary—the Internet can become a place of community and support. It can extend the rehab process by helping people discover possibilities they didn't know existed.

- **Vocational possibilities.** Research has shown that computer skills erase the pay gap that people with disabilities otherwise experience in the job market. Adaptive keyboards and voice control systems provide full computer access and thus access to jobs that have nothing to do with physical labor. Many rehab centers with fully equipped computer labs include computer training during the inpatient rehab experience.

Finding the right center

Rehab services are offered in a range of settings: acute care hospitals, nursing facilities, local rehab clinics, or large regional facilities associated with major, urban medical centers. Each must be evaluated for their ability to offer what you need in order to achieve the greatest degree of independence.

During the acute stage of injury, you might find yourself in a local hospital which may or may not have rehab staff. Resources might be very limited. Perhaps a physical therapist will visit your room to guide you in simple exercises or perform range-of-motion exercises. After you stabilize medically, you will probably need to go someplace else for rehab. If you were first taken to a medical center with extensive resources, you might stay in the same complex from initial traumatic treatment and simply move between units—from medical care to rehab, for example—until released.

Where you get injured can make a difference in your recovery and rehab. This quadriplegic woman explains:

> When I got to the hospital, the neurosurgeon had a lot of experience. I was injured in Santa Cruz, which is a resort area. They get a fair number of spinal cord injuries moving through the hospital there.

Specialized facilities

A person with a disability is likely to need a very focused rehab program, delivered by people experienced with that disability. Spinal cord injuries, tumors, infections, localized or diffuse brain injury, the onset of MS, ALS, and certain MDs all have specific features which need the support of staff specifically experienced in these areas. Dr. Alex Barchuk of Kentfield observes:

> There are specialists who say that they specialize in spinal cord injury or head injury or another disability, and they really don't. You need to have a team of people who work with people in your situation on a day-to-day basis.

The eighteen rehab centers which comprise the Model System offer specialized care. They are multi-disciplinary facilities with comprehensive departments in each form of rehab therapy and service. Their facilities tend to be substantial—computer labs, recreational options, larger grounds—and are often related to a large, urban medical center or university hospital system. Centers include Craig Hospital near Denver, Shepherd Center in Atlanta, the Rehabilitation Institute of Chicago, the Kessler Institute in New Jersey (where Christopher Reeve did his rehab), and Detroit's Rehabilitation Institute of Michigan. These rehab centers share data that is gathered by the

National Institute of Disability and Rehabilitation Research, which provides them with grant monies.

The makeup of the Model System lineup changes as grants are reconsidered after the five-year life of each funding cycle. If a center is dropped from the Model System, this does not mean that the center has been found lacking. The center might have simply chosen not to devote its resources to the research which the Model System status demands of its members. Model centers are not necessarily the best of what's available, but they might offer you a chance to participate in a study or therapy still in the research stage.

The Veterans Administration operates a significant network of rehab facilities. Some facilities are engaged in research or the development of new technologies for use by people with disabilities. If you are a veteran, the government will cover all of your costs.

Other centers

Rehab used to be the province only of specialized centers. In recent years, rehab has begun to show up in many places. It is big business, so general hospitals and nursing facilities are attracted to the idea of establishing rehab services. They can keep clients in their facilities and attract the insurance funds. By providing complete care in one location, the facility can also avoid making someone endure a transfer.

As hospitals start to dabble in rehab services, they begin to learn what it really takes to deliver services well and cost-effectively. Bonnie Sims of Craig Hospital describes what happened when local HMOs tried spinal cord rehabilitation:

> There were some attempts to develop specialty care in acute settings, only to find that it was no less expensive. Spinal cord and brain injury rehabilitation was not their expertise. And so HMOs began to refer patients to centers that specialize in treating and rehabilitating persons with catastrophic injury.

The question is whether the scale of rehab services provided by these non-specialized services is appropriate for a given situation. Ask about the program you will be on as an inpatient. Even a ventilator-dependent quadriplegic should be scheduled for therapy several hours per day, five days a week. A rehab center that does not schedule an aggressive program might not be offering you all you deserve.

Geographical differences

Different rehab hospitals specialize in certain conditions. Urban facilities are likely to be better equipped to address victims of violence, understanding both the details of entry wounds from gunshots or stabs and also the psychological dynamics of a disability as a result of personal attack. Rural hospitals will have more exposure to farm-related accidents, which often result in amputation. Both settings see their share of the great number of automobile accidents that result in disability.

Rehab centers become experienced with the particular populations in their immediate vicinity. The large regional centers will have a much more mixed array of people, while others will have a more specialized experience. Dr. Michael Scott directs the acute spinal cord unit at Rancho Los Amigos near Los Angeles:

> As with all other regional spinal cord injury centers, we have seen an increase in violence-related injuries. This presents a whole new set of challenges for the rehabilitation team. However, we have the experience and have developed programs to meet the needs of patient population.

Rehab staff members do their best to accommodate you and to help you reconsider attitudes which might interfere with getting the most out of rehab.

Transfer from acute care to rehab

You need rehab provided by a Physical Medicine and Rehabilitation (PM&R) specialist—a physiatrist. If you are receiving acute care in a hospital or have been sent immediately to a nursing facility, you should have a referral with a PM&R doctor who can evaluate your needs and help you identify where you should go for rehab services. Director of Occupational Therapy for Stanford Rehabilitation Services, Jody Greenhalgh states:

> Not all hospitals have PM&R in-house. If the doctor is a primary care physician, they might refer someone to an orthopedist, a neurologist, a cardiologist, or a plastic surgeon. What the person really needs is to deal with the disability.

Janie Whiteford is a chair user and peer support coordinator at the Santa Clara Valley Medical Center. She has seen hospitals keep people in their facilities when it was not appropriate:

> Spinal cord injury is a big cash item for hospitals that aren't well prepared to deal with them. They might not refer someone to a spinal cord center. You'll get a hospital that might only have one SCI case a year, but they'll keep the person. They'll come out with pressure sores, contractures—just a mess.

It falls to the rehab staff at the acute care location to urge transfer to an appropriate program. Says Greenhalgh:

> I have actually recommended other hospitals. If they truly have a specialty need that we don't serve all the time, where the patient needs the support of other people who are going through the same thing, and there's a center a reasonable distance away, we need to work together to use those resources. We should not be competing with them. Sometimes, even high quadriplegics might not get referred by a facility to a specialized rehab center.

Rehab accreditation

Accreditation is the approval of an organization that reviews programs and sites. Hospitals and rehab facilities are motivated to pursue accreditation to attract patients, convince referring doctors of the quality of programs, and get paid by insurers.

You should ask about accreditation if you are shopping for a rehab center, whether you are presently in an acute care hospital or have moved to another city and need to establish a working relationship for continuing rehab support. Accreditation is an indication that the center is concerned with refining and improving its services. Accreditation is not a guarantee of perfection.

Accreditation not only tells the public the facility has met a stringent set of standards, the accreditation process is also a means of achieving high-quality care. Accrediting organizations conduct training conferences, publish educational materials for professionals, and develop systems for measuring the outcome of programs to determine the effectiveness of their work, including consumer satisfaction. Certification also saves government agencies, the insurance industry, and rehab administration from the cost of conducting their own standards development and evaluation from scratch. The following are some common certification credentials:

- CALS is an overall hospital certification group which reviews all types of facilities, including rehab.

- The Joint Commission on Accreditation is another widely sought credential by facilities of all types.

- CARF, the Commission on Accreditation of Rehabilitation Facilities, certifies programs within a given facility, not the entire rehab center. In medical rehabilitation, certified programs could include inpatient or outpatient programs, spinal cord rehabilitation, pain management, brain injury, or pediatric programs, for instance. It is a not-for-profit, nongovernmental organization. To date, 3,000 organizations in the United States, Canada, and Sweden have earned CARF accreditation.

Other entities, such as state-sponsored organizations, concern themselves with the quality of services delivered in hospitals and clinics.

Most insurers will not approve coverage in a facility without accreditation. The specific accreditation a facility pursues will be driven very much by what the insurers want to see. Rehab hospitals might pursue Joint Commission status, since most insurers accept that, while being less concerned with CARF. However, according to Uli Salas, P.T., Spinal Cord Program Director at HealthSouth Rehabilitation in Albuquerque, New Mexico:

> CARF has marketing value for us as a rehab facility. It means something to the physicians and hospitals who refer patients to us. We also value the process of evaluation that it requires us to go through.

The accreditation process begins by having the facility evaluate itself in preparation for application. Self-evaluation lets facility staff identify issues for improvement and increases prospects for approval in the accreditation process. Next, a survey team of experienced professionals comes to the center for a comprehensive site visit. The team files a report to the organization. Based on this report, various levels of accreditation will be offered. For example, CARF offers either a three-year, one-year, or provisional accreditation. A one-year or provisional accreditation indicates some deficiencies, but also that CARF believes the organization is capable of correcting them. A facility can be refused accreditation altogether.

Nontraumatic disabilities

Someone in an accident who acquires a spinal cord or brain injury will find him- or herself in a medical facility and will generally be transferred to a rehabilitation services program. But what of people with a condition from birth such as muscular dystrophy or spina bifida, or with a progressive condition that appears later such as multiple sclerosis or ALS? How are they helped to adapt to a disability, particularly when the progressive nature of a condition demands continuing attention and adjustment?

Organizations dedicated to specific disabilities sponsor services at major medical centers or sometimes finance their own facilities. The National Multiple Sclerosis Society is very active in making support available nationwide, as are the Muscular Dystrophy Association, American Syringomyelia Alliance Project, United Cerebral Palsy, and the Spina Bifida Association, among others. If you are facing a late-onset progressive disability, your doctor should have referred you to such sources. However, doctors are not always well-informed about what options are available for you. If you haven't been referred to a program, do the research to find out what programs exist. These groups and services may be able to help you adapt to the condition in ways which your present doctor might not be aware of, and possibly even reduce its progression or impact by informing you of recent advances in research.

For example, Shepherd Center in Atlanta has established an MS Center— one of thirty-two in the U.S.—which provides both inpatient and outpatient services. Shepherd Center is a medical unit capable of diagnosis and treatment, and participates in research and clinical drug trials, at the option of the client. A study published in *Archives of Physical Medicine and Rehabilitation* found clear benefits to a period of inpatient rehabilitation for people with MS. People in the group with intensive treatment learned greater degrees of adaptive skill and came out with better attitudes about their ability to function with MS than the group who came as outpatients.[1]

Rehab practitioners are sensitive to issues with which physicians in general practice might not be familiar. People with MS or ALS typically establish a working relationship with a neurologist. However, if the neurologist is attending to many people with other conditions, he might not gain the same detailed experience as someone working in rehab who spends all her time with people with a given condition. Cynthia Bishop of Shepherd's MS Center notes:

> Neurologists may have a very small percentage of patients with MS. The doctor is not able to be completely current in the many developments happening in MS and its treatments. We might see a patient and notice that they're starting to experience foot drop, and will refer them to our brace clinic and help them with their gait in therapy. A neurologist might not notice that. A person with MS commonly has problems with bladder or bowels. A neurologist is not an expert in that type of thing. You really need someone who knows rehab to address those problems. The patient might be getting good medical treatment from her neurologist, but still have a lot of symptoms or mobility difficulties—day-to-day life issues—that aren't being addressed.

It is the role of the neurologist to refer someone to rehab and to be informed about the existence of resources such as the MS clinics and centers or aquatic programs sponsored by the MS Society. If you have never had access to rehab services, explore options that might be available to you on either an outpatient or inpatient basis. You will need to evaluate how well-informed your doctor is about resources. If it is a good working relationship, work together to do research.

Transition from childhood disability

The rehab system discussed in this chapter is largely targeted to adults, many of whom already work or are educated. Many disabilities are work-related; conditions such as MS typically occur in adulthood. Children with disabilities such as cerebral palsy, spina bifida, or muscular dystrophy are serviced under a different system.

With the passage of the Individuals with Disabilities Education Act in 1975, children began to be integrated into public schools and those systems were required to provide services to those children. In effect, rehab for children got delivered through the school system. Physical therapists would work with disabled children at the schools. Equipment and medical services continued to be supplied by charitable organizations.

The difficulty with this delivery system is what happens when children become adults. For some, the transition is not smooth. This man with muscular dystrophy is angry about what happened once he became an adult:

Throughout my childhood and adolescence, the Muscular Dystrophy Association (MDA) and Easter Seals were very good about providing various things I needed such as wheelchairs, orthopedic shoes, braces, clinics, etc. Unfortunately, when I became an adult, the MDA forgot I existed. I no longer fit their marketable, "dying child" image.

MDA has refused to help me with anything on several occasions over the years. Even when I first became ventilator-dependent in 1982, they refused to even consider helping me buy a ventilator even though Medi-Cal was also balking at this major expenditure. They refused to help purchase replacement ventilators in 1988 also. I also requested their help, to no avail, to get a badly needed automatic page turner so I could read. They only offered me a donated manual page turner even though I couldn't use it. I now hold the MDA in complete contempt.

Once children with disabilities leave the school system where they were receiving medical and therapeutic services, they need to establish a relationship with physicians and facilities qualified and equipped to address their needs. New issues also appear in adulthood, such as weight gain, sexual activity, living independently, driving, or alcohol use. People in such transition need a specialized set of services, and the family doctor is not in a position to provide them. As Jody Greenhalgh describes the transition:

When they turn eighteen, where do they go? Hopefully the children's services doctors refer them to a rehab doctor, but it doesn't always happen. If they get a job and go on an HMO program, they get assigned a primary physician who may not know much about their disability. The physician may not know their equipment needs or that they need ongoing therapy.

The primary physicians don't know what questions to ask, and the people don't know how to advocate. People need to know the services they can ask for. They need to say, "My wheelchair's falling apart because I'm sixty pounds heavier. I'm an adult and I'm still on this pediatric cushion."

Dealing with insurance

Many medical professionals believe that insurance companies have gained excessive control of medical treatment. Spending limits tie the hands of physicians, whether limits are set by an HMO, private insurance, or government programs like Medicare. Medical professionals chafe at decision-making control being out of their hands. Insurers complain of cost pressures—rising prices, shrinking profits, and a healthcare system too expensive for many people to afford. The issue is too complex to simply demonize insurers.

Alex Barchuk of the Kentfield Rehabilitation Hospital in northern California states:

> All these new products coming out are great, but no one can afford to buy them. Insurance doesn't pay for them. In the past five years, we've all transitioned into managed care. We get reimbursed at a per diem rate. No matter what we do in the hospital, the insurance company doesn't care—they pay us a certain amount. Somebody can cost us $2,400 a day, and the insurer pays $750 a day. In that situation you have to go with cheaper medications that have good efficacy. You can't compromise somebody, but…
>
> We look sideways at all these new drugs, because they're not affordable. Unless the drugs really show something very special or unique, they don't get used. A lot of the new wheelchairs—the ones that stand or recline—the insurance companies don't want to go with. We have to really fight for those.

Cynthia Bishop of the MS Center at Atlanta's Shepherd Center knows that inpatient stays are very effective in certain situations for people with MS:

> We have all the research articles about the value of inpatient stays for people with MS, because the difficulty we have is getting insurers to pay. Since MS is a progressive disease, the insurer's position is, "What's the point? You can rehab them now, but they'll only be worse later." It seems ridiculous, but that's what they say. The insurance people can see that if you have a spinal cord injury, there's a major life change and you need rehab. It's one time, and then they're done with it. But with MS, a person might need rehab five different times. It's a hard sell.

The new insurance environment has affected a critical piece of equipment for Bob Mauro, a writer and disability activist with severe post-polio syndrome. His Medicare coverage—now administered by a private HMO—has begun to deny coverage for a second ventilator, which allows him flexible mobility by being able to use one by his bed and the other on his power wheelchair. More importantly, the second ventilator is a backup in case the primary ventilator breaks down—which they inevitably do.

I cannot express the terror these routine denial letters give me. I only have two ventilators, and both are vital. I must have two ventilators to stay alive! I am permanently disabled, will not get better, and will probably get worse as I age. I must be on a ventilator twenty-four hours a day and cannot be off it for more than five minutes!

By the book

The services and coverage you get are increasingly defined by manuals and policies developed at hospitals and insurance offices. Managed care can lead to cookie-cutter classifications and treatments, with some danger of not seeing the case or person as a whole. According to Jody Greenhalgh:

> *Insurance has disability ratings, and people get plugged in. "This is how many days you're going to be seen, this is where you should go." But not everyone fits the mold of the way insurers see these cases. There might be other conditions along with the one they've rated, and it makes a big difference in what someone really needs. There's a lot of education [needed] to get insurance to look at the bigger picture.*

There can be advantages to these automated, modular approaches to care. Once you have been given a disability rating, any member of your health-care team might recognize a certain condition. By reporting it, they will initiate a trigger which automatically leads to a pathway of treatment. When these triggers and pathways are clearly defined, the doctor is spared having to diagnose and prescribe every last detail of treatment. It makes his job more efficient, and can get you into the treatment process sooner, keep you from losing strength, and get you back to your life sooner. In the process, the insurer saves money, which is not in itself a bad thing.

One of the great challenges of managed care is to improve the efficiency of a medical system with immense demands, while being certain that care is appropriate for the individual. Your medical care cannot be entirely automated. Attention needs to be paid throughout the process and there needs to be flexibility to adjust to changes.

Not always a battle

It is easy to elicit stories of frustration—from clients and providers—at the hands of insurance. Stories of people coming up against insurers' limits are increasingly common: shorter stays, restrictions on medical testing and procedures, limited funding for mobility or medical equipment.

But frustrations are not always the case. Viki Solomon is a nurse case manager who works with traumatic brain injury cases. When the coverage is from Workers' Compensation, she finds:

> Once the injury is determined to be compensable, most things are authorized when it comes to rehabilitation and related needs. In my experience, there have been homes and vans purchased by the funding source.

A man with spinal cord injury and private insurance states:

> I recently had severe shoulder pain from overuse. I was able to see my physiatrist, have an MRI, and get physical therapy at my rehab hospital. My private insurance paid with no complaint. I'm confident that I can get what I need. Yet I know there are limits to what they'll approve.

The Veterans Administration often does well by injured soldiers and veterans. Although far from perfect, the VA is a system involved in extensive rehabilitation research. It is the largest buyer of wheelchairs in the United States and provides services with very little out-of-pocket costs to the veteran.

While some people are fortunate to have good coverage, the insurer is going to limit reimbursement. Bonnie Sims finds that insurers want to get people on government rolls, so they can reduce their exposure.

> On catastrophic claims, health insurance companies and HMOs rely on the state and federal system to provide long-term care and to supplement gaps in coverage. When persons become eligible for Medicare, companies are settling Workers' Compensation claims with the idea that Medicare will provide primary coverage for future medical needs.

That situation makes for a bad bind. The only way to get Medicaid is to have little income and assets. In order to qualify—particularly when insurance coverage simply does not exist—people find themselves having to sell property and use up savings until they reach the requisite financial level.

Ironically, facilities in low-income areas sometimes struggle less with funding issues. As Dr. Michael Scott of the Rancho Los Amigos rehabilitation hospital near Los Angeles explains:

We're not under the same pressures as private institutions. We're a county facility and many of our patients have MediCal (California's Medicaid program). We do get reviewed by MediCal in terms of justifying patient stays for rehabilitation, but I think the private sector experiences that more.

The admission process

Your primary physician will refer you to a rehab center, according to an evaluation of your needs, ability, and appropriate timing. Even if you are in a major medical center which includes a rehab facility, it is not guaranteed that you will gain access to its full range of services. Some people are never inpatients, but access rehab services on an outpatient basis. The rehab facility will have an admission specialist who will oversee the complex process of admission to the program.

High-risk admissions

The process of admission relies on an estimate of what you would be capable of in terms of independence. Sadly, the determination will depend on finances more than anything else. A high quadriplegic might require expensive mobility and ventilation equipment, significant personal assistance, major adaptation or purchase of a new home, and transportation between facilities—sometimes by private jet. In these extreme cases, the rehab center or the insurance company being asked to pay might decide it is not cost-effective to provide you rehab services.

In their paper "Preadmission Screening and Secondary Transport," Suzanne Nyre and Virginia McKay of Craig Hospital in Englewood, Colorado, state:

> *It is the height of cruelty to introduce the patient and family to these options and freedoms in the rehabilitation program, to provide that temporary lifestyle of increased mobility and independence, only to take it away when lack of resources demands a discharge back to an acute hospital setting or to an institution that cannot allow patients out of bed, their rooms, or the facility.*[2]

If you do not go through rehab, there are two options. One is to be in a restrictive facility where you will probably spend more time in bed without access to productive activities. The other is to be supported in the community.

The cost of care in a nursing home—including the higher incidence of medical episodes like infections and sores that are likely to occur with an inactive, institutionalized life—is probably more expensive than the cost of having people in the community. Bonnie Sims notes:

> While it is not our philosophy to institutionalize people with catastrophic injuries, it is usually not an option anyway. Long-term nursing facilities are not eager to take persons who are quadriplegic, since the costs often exceed the reimbursement.

This parent of a child with a traumatic brain injury comments:

> The system does not provide financial assistance to people so that they can have equipment and in-home care and make modifications to their homes. They conclude that there is no point in giving patients a taste of what they can't have. This is typical bureaucratic thinking. Clear-headed people would start with the premise that every life has value and should be lived to the fullest, so what has to be done to make this possible?

A decision to deny admission to rehab—which you should know is far more the exception than the rule—would be the result of a comprehensive review of your medical status, an evaluation of your home, and a great deal of research into your family's financial resources—including the possibility of selling land, redeeming life insurance, or borrowing money, as well as charitable funding sources or community fundraising options. In the course of this process, your family and a social worker on the team should leave no stone unturned to identify the resources which would demonstrate your ability to function outside of a nursing facility—or else you might find it your only option.

During the admission process, consider seriously the kind of attitude you demonstrate about your future. It will be taken into account in the decision as well. All other things being equal, someone who does not appear committed to doing the work of rehab might be considered less "deserving" of admission.

Persons who are more severely disabled will be made to prove their capacity to benefit from rehab in ways that a lower level spinal cord injured person might not. Such persons will need significantly greater financial support to be out in the world. It is equally true that plenty of high quadriplegics using ventilation are living full lives. There is plenty of precedent to demonstrate that rehab makes a substantive difference in the life of someone with a severe disability, and that it can be well worth the investment.

Despite the possibility of being denied admission, it is rare that someone is not admitted, even if on a reduced program more focused on medical stability and basic self-care skills. Some rehab hospitals have transfer agreements with acute care facilities which may not allow them to deny admission.

In rare cases, when there is no coverage, a major rehabilitation center will take someone on and absorb the charges. For obvious reasons, they are only able to do this for a very few people. This might happen in an emergency situation, where someone nearby had to be admitted before all the details could be worked out. Once the person is there, the hospital might agree to continue providing services.

The admission process as planning

The physicians and other team members design a treatment program for you in advance. Staff want to have a fair idea of how long you will be there, what departments will be involved, and what kinds of resources will be committed to your rehab. The pre-admission process is used to estimate costs for your funding source. The program is designed around the conditions you will be released into when you leave. The admissions coordinator should be doing his best to demonstrate to the insurer that your rehab program will lead to lower costs in a noninstitutional setting after discharge.

What you want out of the treatment plan is to be offered a range of services which will allow you the chance to accomplish the greatest level of health and function with your disability. Whether you are considered high risk or not, the team should involve you and your family intimately in the planning process. According to Nyre and McKay:

> [The coordinator should identify the family's] areas of concern and provide some counseling and guidance that will help them prepare for the rehabilitation program. It is not necessary for families to make decisions in the area of discharge options, community resources, and finances at this time, but [these] should be brought up and discussed as options they can begin to consider. Up until this time, they have been fighting for survival and have had little time to look into the future. When they have, they have been frightened of the unknown and unable to identify any realistic goals for future independence.[3]

No one should get an unfair advantage over someone else who might otherwise have gained a place, but a family will understandably want to do everything possible for a loved one who needs rehab and pull strings when possible. A quadriplegic woman relates:

> My father was head of Clinical Social Work at Stanford Medical Center. He got me into Santa Clara Valley Medical Center, because he heard that was the best at dealing with spinal cord injuries in northern California. He later started a one-day program for Stanford medical students on disability where students spent a half day at the disabled students program in Berkeley and a half day at Santa Clara Valley Medical Center. At that point, nothing was being taught about disabilities.

Is it time to be admitted?

The insurer is usually anxious to see someone transferred to a rehab program as soon as possible. Most insurance policies limit the number of days you can stay in rehab. Such a limit might not exist for time you spend in acute care at a general hospital, so insurers want to admit you to rehab to start the clock running and limit their costs.

Because you are getting pressure from the insurer to transfer does not mean it is the right time for you to do so. It might make more sense to stay in an acute care hospital longer, and then be in a better position to benefit from a specialized rehab facility. As Bonnie Sims explains:

> The system depends on establishing and maintaining good relationships with insurers. Therefore, it is difficult for case managers and physicians to resist pressure to transfer or receive patients into rehabilitation. Often patients still require acute treatment and are not ready for rehabilitation activities. Because they are now in a rehabilitation facility they are using rehab days which are often limited by coverage. Since we are licensed as a hospital, we can sometimes negotiate for medical days during these down times, saving the rehabilitation days for active therapy.

The rehab team

You have arrived. You have access to rehab services, which means that a group of dedicated and highly trained professionals are at your service—the rehab team. The team consists of a case manager and others in patient services, a physician, and a range of therapists, depending on your needs. The team is committed to helping you reach the highest possible level of function with your disability.

Dr. Gary Yarkony of the Rehabilitation Institute of Chicago observes:

> *The foundation of a comprehensive rehabilitation program is an interdisciplinary team. The staff must be willing to work together while breaking down the boundaries of individual disciplines for the betterment of those they serve.*[4]

Jody Greenhalgh notes that the role of team members is important:

> *Regardless of what discipline you are from, when you go into assess rehab needs, you find yourself advocating for the patient's needs. Although I'm an occupational therapist, I'll point out a physical therapy need, when I see it.*

You, your family, and peer support persons will also function as part of the rehab team.

Patient and family services

Patient services—often referred to as the social work department—will deal with finding resources, determining insurance coverage, and making sure you get all the benefits you are entitled to. Even before you arrive, your case manager is looking into insurance policies and participating in the admissions process. Case managers deal with insurance adjusters, bureaucrats at federal, state, and local levels, charitable agencies, and the team at the facility who will serve you.

The people who do this work might have a social work degree or not. Bonnie Sims explains:

> *We have counselors with varied degrees in our department, but all have a masters degree in their field. We hire with an eye to experience as well as a degree, which gives us differing viewpoints.*

Your case manager or social worker is a key member of the team with whom you might develop a close relationship. Sandra Loyer, clinical social worker at the University of Michigan Medical Center in Ann Arbor states:

> *I am often one of the first people to make contact with the patient and the family. That is a chance to develop a close relationship from the*

start. I try to make them comfortable enough to ask me whatever ques-
tions are on their mind, and then I get the chance to find out more about
their needs. I often discover important details that I pass on to the rest of
the rehab team.

It is a challenge for a case manager or rehabilitation counselor to spend as much time as they'd like on each person's case. With the pressure to contain costs and the complexity of the job, there is only so much time available to be a good listener. Many times case managers feel they can do their best for you by getting back on the phone to explore services and benefits to meet your needs. Sims observes:

The counseling relationship can be very supportive to some people.
However, the opportunity to create this relationship has become limited.
Counselors spend so much time on the financial and discharge issues that
it becomes difficult to spend quality time with patients.

You might be unaware of some of the benefits you have. For example, you might have credit card insurance or a policy for your mortgage or auto loan that makes payments if you become disabled. A case manager should ask these questions and help you research all possible ways to ease your financial burden.

Unfortunately, much of the case manager's time is spent trying to make up for coverage you don't have. Sims notes:

When people buy insurance, they assume they have coverage for all
their needs, including healthcare. This is usually not the case, and so
much of their care ends up falling to the family.

Often people must take extreme measures to qualify for state Medic-
aid to fill the gaps left in home care or equipment. They are required to
spend their savings and assets before they qualify for assistance. Basi-
cally, they become paupers to get the care they need.

Medicare is a federal program related to Social Security. People who collect Social Security disability benefits for two years become eligible for Medicare, which covers some equipment, physicians, therapy, and/or hospitalization. The case manager will explain these programs and help you understand the application process and your eligibility.

There is a huge array of details involved in government programs like Medicare, Medicaid, Workers' Compensation, or Vocational Rehabilitation, in the particulars of any given policy from any of hundreds of insurers, in the offerings of charitable groups like Easter Seals or the local Rotary Club, programs offered by Independent Living Centers, and so on. Sims says:

> *We have to spend almost as much time researching as we do working on the actual cases. I spend an inordinate amount of time just keeping up with changes and what programs are out there, trying to keep current and keep my staff current. I don't have time as a supervisor to actually take cases. We've got so many resource listings, packets, and handouts—it can be overwhelming just keeping up.*

There is also work to prepare for the day you leave rehab and go back to daily life in the outside world, a process that begins even before you arrive. Patient services arranges transportation, sets up the relationship with a home healthcare agency, or assists you with finding personal assistance services, as necessary. Sims finds that discharge is often difficult:

> *The transition out to the community is always chaotic. We never know why everything breaks down at the last minute. You get the whole thing set up, you get the home health agency ready to come in, then the patient gets sick and you have to cancel everything. Or when you implement discharge, you forget something, so the transportation goes awry, and so forth. Some chaos is typical.*

Take good advantage of the patient services staff. Get to know them early and learn all you can. Plan for departure as much as possible, and you have a better chance of making a smooth transition from rehab.

The physician

The physician, most often a physiatrist, is the leader of the team. The physiatrist coordinates the members of the team, is responsible for maintaining clear records that everyone on the team will share and contribute to, and oversees the common strategy. The physiatrist relies on input from other team members who are spending time with you. Dr. Scott explains:

> *The physician is the team leader, but the leadership shifts depending on the topic on hand. For instance, if a psychological issue is at hand, then the psychologist takes the lead.*

The doctor's goal is to help you be in the best possible health so you can get the most out of rehab. There is a tremendous amount of research and information for a doctor to keep up with, to bring the latest resources to bear in supporting your rehab effort. The quality of your relationship with the doctor has tremendous impact. In the past, doctors were likely to play a very strong leadership role, taking little stock of the personal experience of their clients, making unilateral decisions, or at least making it difficult for someone to disagree. To this day, many people find themselves intimidated by their physicians, afraid to speak up, hesitant to challenge them. But this attitude is changing, both on the part of people who now prefer to be "clients" or "consumers" rather than "patients" and on the part of some doctors exploring a more holistic point of view.

With restricted budgets and pressure for hospitals to work efficiently and profitably, doctors' schedules are very tight. As much as they might want to be good listeners, or take time to learn more about your life and experience, they are hard-pressed to be able to devote the kind of time you might prefer. You can help by being prepared with questions and being informed. Take advantage of therapists, nurses, other rehab consumers, and a rehab center library, if one exists.

Doctors are human. They aren't perfect. The nature of your relationship with them is not one of absolute trust, but one of respectful cooperation. If you suspect someone is not competent or fully committed to your needs, pursue your right to ask for someone else. If you are not getting what you need, or if you can tell that something is not right, speak up. Statistically, mistakes are far more the exception than the rule, but they do happen.

> *When my halo was removed, I was told it would not hurt. There were originally two people removing my halo, but one got called away in the process. He had only unscrewed half of the screw on the front left side before he left, and the other doctor pulled on it thinking it was completely unscrewed.*

Rehabilitation nurses

Perhaps more than any other team members, your central relationship will be with the nursing staff. Nurses are part of your daily life and always on duty on the floor where your room is located.

Rehabilitation nursing is a certified specialty, supported by organizations such as the Association for Rehabilitation Nursing and the American Association of Spinal Cord Injury Nurses. The associations provide continued education required for certification. Rehab nurses are trained in being able to recognize and attend to the unique needs of people with disabilities. Nurses in a general hospital might not ever see autonomic dysreflexia, deal with pressure sore management, or understand the respiratory needs of someone with post-polio syndrome, for instance.

Rehab nurses play many roles. They treat. They advise the client, the family, and the physician. They teach. They interact with and support the rehab team. They are crucial to the rehab process, since they have regular contact with you and because they are generalists, able to recognize any of many different needs you might have. They also direct the nursing aides who do much of the hands-on daily work, such as assisting you with bladder and bowel care, washing, or dressing.

Rehab nurses tend to think in terms of increasing independence and helping people move from the role of being sick to the role of being well. Many have a holistic view of health and could bring healing modes such as visualization or massage into your treatment.

The family dynamics and emotional experience of early disability are best supported by people experienced with the complex set of adjustments you are called upon to make in rehab. Nurses can be a source of tremendous emotional support:

> I was in rehab to have a large sore closed surgically. After weeks of not sitting while it healed, I was at last allowed to start to sit for brief periods in preparation for going home. It turned out that the sore had not healed properly beneath the skin, and it broke down again, leaving another large, open wound. In that moment when I realized that I was about to spend another several weeks there, having the rehab nurse just sit with me after showing me the sore and explaining what had happened was a great comfort. She knew she didn't have to say anything. I could tell she understood how upset I was. It meant so much to me that she would commit her time to me and not leave me alone.

Therapists

Therapists who specialize in rehabilitation must strike a balance between hard work and keeping an upbeat and friendly atmosphere. Their work is to encourage and support you in applying yourself to the process of rehabilitation.

There will always be some people who don't connect or a therapist who is difficult to work with, as this paraplegic woman found:

> The only trouble I had was with one of my physical therapists. I ended up firing her because we had no rapport at all. She was patronizing and mean.

But the following view is probably more typical:

> My therapists made a huge difference in the process of getting back to my life after my injury, and I think I have been more successful because of it. I bless them for their contributions to my life.

Your therapy will be customized to your needs and the issues of your disability. Someone with multiple sclerosis will have a very different program from someone with a spinal cord injury, as explained by Cynthia Bishop:

> With MS, the problem is not inability to walk, it's a combination of gait difficulties and severe fatigue. MS causes very, very severe fatigue. Physical therapy for MS has to take this into account, along with the problem of overheating. Even a core temperature increase of .5 degree in an MS patient can affect his or her ability to function. It's not anything like spinal cord injury where you just work, work, work, work, work 'til you drop!

The ranks of specialized therapists include physical therapy, occupational therapy, respiratory therapy, recreational therapy, and speech therapy. These people are experts who have worked with other people in your situation, and have seen them master the skills they will be teaching you.

Whether you were injured, are feeling the first effects of a progressive condition, or have spent your life with a disability, you might feel weak, fragile, uncoordinated, or insecure about testing your physical limits. When you first come into rehab, some goals might seem unattainable—whether lifting yourself easily in and out of a wheelchair or becoming accustomed to breathing with a ventilator. These doubts are a common and normal reaction, particularly to sudden trauma, with its dramatic change in physical capacity.

Your rehab program will be based on goals developed by the team along with your input. Members of the team are unlikely to suggest a course of rehab work unless they think that your medical status allows for it. They will have seen others in situations similar to yours, and know from past experience what is possible. They might know that you can go beyond limits that seem unreachable to you. They will ask you to put a certain amount of faith in them—and yourself.

Therapists must set reasonable goals for you, day by day, and let you know what to expect. You might make very gradual progress that seems too slow to you, but is expected for a person in your situation. The better you understand the expected pace of your rehabilitation, the more you will be able to celebrate your advances, instead of pressuring yourself and feeling that you are failing because things are going too slowly. As you give your therapist honest feedback about your experience, you can work together to adjust your program as you go.

Physiatrist Michael Scott says that the process of setting goals has become easier thanks to a growing body of outcome studies:

> We have more information these days in terms of predicting neurologic recovery. Instead of saying, "Time will tell"—which we still say!— we have a better idea what the realistic expectations are. Our director, Dr. Waters, has done work looking at where patients are one month after injury and where you can expect them to be a year down the line in terms of what muscles are moving, how strong they are. We can give the patient more information about what to expect.

Your roles

A successful rehab experience makes a tremendous difference, but rehab only gets part of the credit. Its contribution is of no use unless you choose to make the most of the experience, use the tools and skills offered, and continue your own process of growth and evolution after you leave. This woman with C6/7 quadriplegia observes:

> The public approaches me with the attitude I was "taught" independence in "therapy." Nothing could be further from the truth. It took years of personal exploration and peer examples to get where I am.

Many rehab centers will include you in team reviews of your case. How much you participate is up to you, but it is your right to ask questions and have your say. Of all the members, you are the most important person on the team.

Your main role is the hard work you will do, which offers you the chance to believe in new possibilities and to gain capacity. Novelist Reynolds Price, after being paralyzed by cancer, describes his rehab experience in his book, *A Whole New Life*:

> *Few sessions passed without my learning at least one skill, and soon I felt surprising new strength in my arms and chest—more upper-body strength than in my past life. Throughout that summer my chest size went from forty-two inches to forty-six, and my arms and wrists thickened proportionally. Best of all, the new skills produced in most of us a heady sense of control and choice. Those physical choices are obviously more limited than the almost limitless array that's offered to the able-bodied. But in time I was skilled enough in the homely detours and reinventions to put myself through almost all the motions I needed for the necessary work of my life.[5]*

You will also need to advocate for yourself to make your hospital/rehab stay as humane as possible. If you find yourself faced with a staff member who won't or can't take the time to listen, choose an ally who has time to campaign for your needs. It can be helpful to talk to patient advocates, social workers, peer support volunteers, psychologists, or simply someone who has taken a personal interest.

The role of the family

Your family also plays an important role in your rehab experience and impacts your attitude. It is of inestimable value for you to have regular visits, to know that family members are seeing to personal business outside of the facility, and that they are sharing the emotional adjustments of the rehab process. Rehab staff knows the importance of family involvement. Rich Patterson of Santa Clara Valley Medical Center notes:

> *It's important for us to get to the family as soon as possible, to help them make sense out of the situation, explaining how rehab is going to help, what physical and occupational therapy are about. In general they know what those people do, but they don't know how it's going to apply to their family member. We have to go into a lot more depth.*

Family members also need to learn the line between reasonable expectations and hope. This is a delicate line, says Patterson:

> It is more common than not that people think they're going to walk out. You have to tread lightly on that one because you can easily upset the family and the person by saying they won't walk out. Their denial is a coping mechanism.

A disability experience is a potent test of the quality of family relationships. It reveals the depth of commitment and ability to adapt to a crisis. Family response can express itself in extremes. Christopher Reeve's wife, Dana, is entirely involved in his support and has said she will stay with him for the rest of his life. On the other hand, according to Margaret Nosek who researches women with disabilities at Baylor University:

> It could be a very minor injury and the spouse is out the door. This is not related to the level of severity. It has more to do with the quality of the marriage before the disability.

Peer support

While in rehab you are likely to get a visit from someone who had an experience similar to the one you are going through, or be invited to attend peer support meetings. While everyone's experience is different, the chance to talk with someone who has a similar condition can be very powerful. Janie Whiteford, peer support coordinator in Santa Clara, California, explains:

> Though doctors and therapists talk about these things, sometimes it is more validating to hear it from a peer. Sometimes there are things going on in the hospital that the client needs to talk about, such as relationships with staff.

Not everyone is ready to meet someone who has made the adjustment to disability. It is very common to operate on a belief in recovery during the acute stage after an injury, or to feel committed to resisting a progressive disease. This quadriplegic man describes his first visit from a peer supporter:

> I remember somebody coming to visit me, and he was in a chair. He was talking to me about life in a chair and what had happened to him, and I just refused to accept that I was anyone like him. I kind of resented him being there, although I realized it was a nice gesture on his part and he was trying to help.

After rehab, some people participate in outreach programs sponsored by the rehab hospital. At Rancho Los Amigos they have a program called Teens on Target. Says Dr. Michael Scott:

> *Teens on Target is a violence prevention program for adolescents. They meet on a regular basis and go out to talk to kids in schools. It is an effort to do proactive outreach to prevent injuries. It has a rehabilitative effect for the people going out to speak, too.*

Peer support doesn't have to happen in a formal, organized manner. People build relationships as they encounter each other in rehab, whether inpatient or outpatient. Cynthia Bishop has seen people create close bonds:

> *We have formal support groups, but I think a lot of the best peer support is the informal stuff that happens at the aquatic classes, or in PT, or in our waiting room! It gets to be a social thing, too. People make their appointments together so they can hang out with their friends while they do it.*

One benefit of a specialized rehab center is the chance to share the experience with others who are facing the same challenges and process. This bonding is encouraged by rehab staff, who are often surprised by the deep friendships that develop.

Friendships are also a source of some fun in rehab, particularly during an inpatient stay. This quadriplegic man was injured at the age of fourteen in 1977:

> *I made some great friends. Most days after training classes, we would get together and party a little. Just off the corner of the rehab property was a place we called "The White House" where we would party in the front yard. A few times, in the fall when it started getting cold, we would build a small fire. During the cold months, we would sneak in some orange juice and rum and party in a friend's dorm room.*

Not all rehab centers allow people freedom to come and go from the property, but people have a way of finding places to meet. Bonnie Sims notes that Craig Hospital has a Friendship House where families, friends, and patients meet, away from the hospital atmosphere.

Physical therapy

Your strength and mobility are the main concerns of physical therapists. The physical therapist will work with you in areas such as:

- Exercising specific muscles and muscle groups
- Stretching and range-of-motion exercises
- Developing balance
- Wheelchair skills
- Transfer training
- Bed mobility
- Aquatics
- Standing programs
- For some people, gait training

When you first arrive in rehab, or are at a point where your condition is medically stable and you can participate in therapy, physical therapists will work with you on issues as basic as sitting up or turning in bed.

As a wheelchair user, you will need a certain level of strength for many activities. For paraplegics and many quadriplegics with sufficient upper body function, your arms will take on much of the work that you used to do with your legs. Not only will you push a wheelchair, but you will also carry your body into and out of the wheelchair, lifting your body weight without the aid of your legs. Your legs are more weight to carry, instead of supporting your body.

The strength you have will determine how much you can do on your own, without having to be assisted. A sufficient level of strength will allow you to function with less fatigue, handling your body and the wheelchair with less exertion and strain. The physical therapist will help you gain the ability to perform daily functions without unnecessary exertion.

Muscles and stretching

Physical therapists know your anatomy and what muscles allow you to move or balance. Based on the nature of your disability and an evaluation, the therapist will know exactly what muscles you have control of, and will design exercises and use equipment to make the most of what you have.

Physical therapy is a precise process. To exercise a certain muscle in your arm you need to apply resistance to that muscle in a particular direction in order to make it work and become stronger.

Each person and each condition involves some special need. Many wheelchair users will need to develop strength for pushing wheels and for pressure relief push-ups in their chair. A quadriplegic might have control of only some muscles in the upper arm that need to be strengthened enough to lift the forearm at the elbow. Someone with a traumatic brain injury and resultant cognitive difficulties needs to have a simply designed program that he can remember. Someone with a lower limb amputation will need a program for the residual limb, so that the muscles do not contract or get weak. (The muscles in the limb are not getting used for walking during the acute and rehab stages; if a prosthetic leg is to be fitted, it cannot happen until later so that healing of the socket can take place and swelling can be reduced.)

In rehab, you will probably need to do some serious stretching. Your muscles, tendons, and ligaments have a natural tendency to shorten when they are not used. The initial period after a traumatic injury is marked by very limited physical activity during which your tissues tighten up and become weak. You might not have been in great shape before the injury. The physical therapist will do stretching work with you, to soften up these tissues and increase the range of movement of your joints. Stretching is also part of the strength program. Elastic muscles that can travel a greater distance during a contraction are stronger.

Balance

Being immobilized for a period of recovery compromises your sense of balance. The physical therapist will help you recover and increase your sense of balance, strengthening the muscles which will help you achieve greater upper body stability. An activity as simple as playing catch with balls of various sizes is a common PT technique for improving balance.

> *I remember how surprising it was to sit up in that bed for the first time in six weeks and find that I had to hold on to something to keep from falling over. My upper body was just dead weight. Sitting up was now foreign to my body. My center of balance was entirely different given the loss of weight from muscle atrophy below the waist, and from the fact that I no longer had the use of my legs to stabilize my upper body.*

After an injury, the map of your body changes. Your new center of gravity depends on the level and type of injury. Lower-level spinal disabilities leave more trunk muscles in contact with the brain. Use of the hips and abdominal muscles make a big difference in your ability to maintain balance and stability while sitting and while engaged in any physical activity. With the loss of control of trunk muscles, more support is required from the wheelchair, and you will rely even more on arm strength to move your upper body. Strengthening can make the difference between independence and reliance on support.

Without the use of your legs or the gluteus maximus muscles of your buttocks, your ability to keep from falling forward is seriously changed. Those with lower-level spinal injury begin to rely more on the back muscles. It is not a good habit to force those lower back muscles to continually support you; they can become easily overworked. The typical adaptation is to steady yourself with your arms, for example, by reaching an arm around behind the wheelchair or grabbing onto a wheel to hold yourself as you lean or reach forward. If you don't hold on, you can fall on your face. Double lower limb amputees experience the change in their center of gravity to an even greater degree than those with SCI—legs that you cannot move still serve as a counterweight.

Wheelchair skills

In addition to building the muscles you will use when you propel your chair, you also need to gain experience using the chair. Your body learns from doing, and your nervous system and muscles adapt. At first, using the chair will feel awkward and foreign. You will have to think carefully as you wheel, whether by pushing on wheels, operating a joystick, or using breath control. It will not feel natural, because you are unaccustomed to it.

The physical therapist's goal is to help you develop expertise in your chair. There are some refined movements that you'll have to think about at first, but eventually it will become second nature. For instance, when you turn a manual chair, you might either pull back on one wheel or else hold one wheel in place as you push the other, depending on the turning radius you need to achieve. You will apply just the right pressure in the right direction on a joystick, letting go to allow the precise time the chair needs to decelerate. To help you develop these refined responses, the therapist will also take you on outings so you can experience cracks in the sidewalk, curbs, ramps, grass, and other terrain you are likely to encounter in daily life.

If you have sufficient strength and balance, you are likely to be taught to do a "wheelie," to negotiate curbs or single steps, going up and down. The technique is also helpful on uneven terrain. These skills extend independence and are worth learning to the degree you are able. Most physical therapists you meet can do a wheelie. It's part of their training.

Your therapist should prepare you for falling out of a wheelchair. If you play a sport like wheelchair basketball, hockey, or rugby, you can count on falling out. Even if you are careful and have excellent wheeling skills, like not wheeling too close to the edge of a curb, accidents can happen. The therapist will teach you how to fall, practicing it with you so you will not be afraid. You can develop a natural, habitual reaction which protects you by breaking your fall properly. The therapist will teach you techniques for getting back into the wheelchair. If you have the strength, you can get back into your chair directly from the floor, or by lifting yourself onto successively higher surfaces. Or you can learn to guide the people who will be helping you.

Is a wheelchair necessary?

It is not always clear that someone should be using a wheelchair or for how long. Someone with MS might need one during a severe exacerbation or in the later stages of progressive MS. A person with brain injury might need one early on, but later might reach a stage of needing wheels only for trips and when away from home. Viki Solomon is a rehab nurse who works with brain injury clients:

> My concerns are for the ones who have cognitive problems and who make strides in physical rehabilitation. I find they are often kept in the chair as a primary mode of transportation because it is a way to restrain a person who has poor cognitive abilities. In other words, the wheelchair is used for staff convenience. What happens next is the person "learns" that he is wheelchair-bound and so do the therapists and other professionals who treat the person.

The process of rehab should be about determining your proper relationship to a wheelchair, not to make you dependent on it when it might serve you best as a part-time tool. Therapy in that case would be to develop skills for using wheels while at the same time working to optimize your walking abilities.

This woman in her forties is a spinal cord quadriplegic, but she has limited ability to stand and walk. For her, the wheelchair proved to be the better solution, despite the beliefs of rehab staff:

> *I'm an incomplete quad. It's a funny disability because it doesn't fit any of the categories. When I got out of rehab, I started off walking with a cane, which I still use in the house to some extent. This was back in the early '70s when the goal was to get you up on your feet if at all possible. My balance was very poor. I was just tottering around. The rehab staff thought it was great, but it was really dangerous. Eventually, I changed to using a chair. That was liberating because then I could cross streets by myself.*

Gait training

There are many benefits to being in a standing position, although not all physiatrists agree on the extent of these benefits. No one argues the range of motion benefits. When we stand, our muscles and ligaments are kept from developing contracture—shortening chronically in a flexed position. Standing can be a psychological boost. You can be at eye level with others and make practical use of your legs. Proponents of standing say that having weight on your legs also helps bones remain strong, improves circulation, and aids bladder and bowel functions which are constrained by the sitting position and limited movement. Standing frames are discussed in Chapter 4, *Staying Healthy*.

Another way to get the benefits of standing is to walk with braces and crutches. Based on the rehab team's assessment of your abilities and prospects to gain strength and balance, you might be considered a candidate for gait training. People are attracted to this option more often in the early stages of disability when the desire to stand is very strong. People also find that gait training allows them to reach high surfaces or get into bathrooms which are difficult to adapt. Walking with braces allows some people to return to their previous work. Being able to return to a job makes the cost of braces more acceptable to insurers, who might otherwise resist paying thousands of dollars for equipment and therapy just so you can reach a kitchen shelf.

The work it takes to develop the strength and skills to use braces is intensive. It is not for everyone. Dr. Michael Scott of Rancho Los Amigos describes how he approaches the option of gait training:

> We definitely motivate people with incomplete injuries who have gait potential, to maximize their locomotor ability. We evaluate complete paraplegics on an individual basis. We explain what it would be like walking with long leg braces with locked knees and crutches, and how it's not like walking before. We show them videotapes of what that would look like, talk about the tremendous energy expenditure, and how it's not really practical. They would still end up using a wheelchair as their primary means of locomotion. Some patients understand all that, but they'll say, "I want to get up, I want to exercise, I like the idea of standing, or on certain occasions be able to look people in the eye." For those who are motivated and have enough upper body strength, we proceed.

Uli Salas states:

> Standing is very motivating for some people. The chance to get on their feet helps involve them more in the rehab process. Then there are people who find very quickly that it is more effort than they care to make and are satisfied with using a wheelchair.

Gait training involves being fitted for braces to keep knees from buckling and feet from dropping as you propel yourself using crutches or a walker. Some braces provide support for the hip as well. Most are made of metal or plastic. Braces in general have become lighter over the years, and some can be worn discreetly underneath clothing.

One approach, known as the RGO (reciprocal gait orthosis) uses cables to assist the movement of each leg. Roy Douglas of the PEERS program in Southern California patented a version of RGO with few pieces, including only one metal support for a leg, rather than one support for each side of a leg. The unit cost approximately $10,000 in 1998, not including the training period.

If you have little strength in the buttocks and upper leg muscles (which lock the knees), walking in this way is done almost entirely with the arms and shoulders. Some people walk with a "swing-through" gait, in which both legs are swung forward through the two crutches. The other option is an alternating gait, in which one leg and crutch are moved at a time. The option selected is a matter of strength, upper body balance, and personal preference. People with higher level spinal injuries are less likely candidates for gait training because of limited control of trunk muscles. Generally, people with injuries above T12 are not considered candidates. Even then, gait training is not for everyone.

> I found gait training very painful. I could not tolerate it for very long.
> It made me tilt my pelvis, and even when I was totally stretched, I
> couldn't handle it for more than three minutes. I was afraid of falling, and
> it never seemed practical.

You might be a candidate for FES (functional electrical stimulation) walking, in which electrical impulses make your muscles contract to reproduce the movements of walking. This technology is still primitive, but some people are using it in their daily lives. It can be used by some people with injuries higher than T12, although it still involves intensive training and sufficient strength. FES is discussed in Chapter 9, *Spinal Cord Research*.

Since walking with braces is tantamount to being on stilts, there is a risk of falling, breaking a bone, or developing a sore if you accidentally bump yourself or are forced to sit on a hard surface in order to rest. If you have atrophied buttock muscles, you will have trouble finding properly cushioned surfaces when you eventually need a break from standing. Carrying a bag while walking with braces is awkward and you do not want to add more weight to your body when your arms already have to do so much work. Most people find that using a wheelchair is easiest and safest for their daily activities, but some like to be able to stand and walk, perhaps maintaining the skill to be used in certain situations—such as walking down the aisle at their own wedding.

There are a number of programs that offer intensive walking therapy employing braces, of which the PEERS programs is one example. They typically involve months of work, and are not associated with a formal rehab center or hospital. Take care not to be drawn in by someone who promises what you feel you are not being provided by formal rehab. These extracurricular walking clinics might not be as well equipped or have sufficiently trained staff. Check out walking clinics carefully and talk to others who have gone through the program. People give mixed reactions to these programs. Some say they were drawn in by a desire to stand based on elaborate promises which did not come to pass. Others say they were urged to have reasonable expectations from the start and gained functional abilities beyond what they were able to achieve in rehab.

Gait training and amputation

Gait training is central to someone with a single lower limb loss. Not all persons choose to use a prosthetic leg. Some find they are afraid of falling or that walking with crutches seems easier.

There is a lot of work involved in getting the prosthesis properly fitted and in learning the skills to use it. Your PT will help you learn how to walk on ramps, up steps, and on uneven terrain, to sit down and stand up. The residual limb is usually very sensitive at first, and is unaccustomed to supporting weight and being used in this way. These adjustments are challenging, but the physical therapist is there to help you understand how your residual limb becomes desensitized over time, and how to use the prosthesis with the least amount of fatigue.

If you are a person with an amputation, wheelchair skills are still important for times when you might not be able to use the prosthesis, while it is being repaired, or when you must allow a blister to heal.

Occupational therapy

The occupational therapist is primarily concerned with the practical activities of your life. The OT will condition and train you to optimize self-care and your ability to work and perform typical daily tasks. The therapist's expertise is in techniques and tools to increase your independence. Occupational therapists will teach you methods for making transfers and for performing bowel and bladder management. The occupational therapist is usually the person involved in wheelchair selection, often in cooperation with the wheelchair vendor (see Chapter 6, *Wheelchair Selection*).

Jody Greenhalgh compares occupational and physical therapy:

> *OT adapts people to their disability to be functionally independent or to optimize their function. PT is more purely about physical capacities. OT is physically oriented, but we focus on functional skills so people can perform daily activities. There is definitely overlap.*

In occupational therapy, you might find yourself making cookies or doing a craft project like stringing beads. Some people make the mistake of thinking they're being trained to perform a menial job. Such tasks are used therapeutically as a way to improve your dexterity, your ability to recover cognitive skills (especially in the case of brain injury), and to retrain muscles that might have become weak or lost coordination. Making cookies might help you pursue a career as a medical technician. Don't judge the task. Consider the goal.

Sometimes the occupational activity is also exercise, as a man with SCI recounts:

> *I worked on a special loom designed by an occupational therapist. As I made a rug, I was also lifting weights.*

OTs are very involved with orthotic devices. They might fabricate splints or braces, working with an array of materials they can shape to your body. OTs might make a functional brace that gives you greater leverage for a task or keeps your hand and fingers from curling with muscle contracture.

Perhaps the greatest portion of the OT's work is in activities of daily living, or ADL. Every rehab facility has a kitchen, a bathroom, and often a bedroom or other areas of a home where they can simulate conditions, helping you learn to function in these spaces. ADL addresses such activities as:

- Grooming
- Bathing
- Dressing
- Feeding
- Housekeeping
- Using of automated environmental controls
- Driving (this might also fall to the PT or a specialist)

In the bathroom, you might have sufficient control to transfer from the wheelchair to the toilet for bladder and bowel activities. Transferring from the chair involves body strength, dexterity, and balance. Some people will always empty their bladder from a catheter or leg bag. Your bowel program might be more easily performed in bed with a bed pan. You may never need to transfer to the toilet. If your abilities and program make transferring appropriate for you, the therapist will have you try the transfer from a variety of positions, since in public you will encounter restrooms with limited space near the toilet.

You will explore the best method for getting dressed, which might be done lying down, using assistive devices. There are extended shoehorns, button pullers, and grabbers to help pull up your pants. Getting into and out of your clothes is another task that some people will need to perform in the bathroom, a task which is very doable with sufficient arm strength. You might have no need to undress in a public restroom, reserving your bowel program for home or using a leg drainage bag for your bladder.

More adaptive methods and devices come into play in the kitchen than perhaps anywhere else in the home. You can use a grabbing device to extend your reach to high shelves. There are utensils for quadriplegics which require no grip strength to use. There are lap tables for cutting and other tasks that are awkward at typical counter heights. The OT will teach you to be extra cautious of handling hot items, since you cannot move away from a sudden spill as easily. If you lack sensation, you are at greater risk for burns.

John Hockenberry, a journalist and spinal cord paraplegic, tells of making stuffing for a Thanksgiving turkey in his book *Moving Violations*. The turkey was in a dish that had been refrigerated after cooking on the stove. The handles of the dish were cool, so he set it on his lap to work with. After a time he noticed unusual spasms. It took a while to realize he had set a hot pan on his lap. But then, he writes:

> *Removing my trousers revealed the place where the hot dish had sat for perhaps two full minutes. The skin was gathered into a leathery, shrunken depression on the top of my thigh. The hairs had all been cooked into a blistered white wound.*[6]

Occupational therapists are concerned with more than techniques and tools. Their task is also to train you to change your habits and views. Hopefully you will not have to suffer burns, falls, or urinary slips before you build an awareness of these risks into daily life. Your therapist will tell you that new habits will seem unnatural at first. But if you make a point of doing them, they gradually become transparent, part of your daily routine and lifestyle.

Recreation therapy

While in rehab, you are removed from your daily life in the outside world. You face considerable psychological adjustments, do hard physical work in the therapy gyms, and possibly live with pain. A little fun is an important element of successful rehab. And, like other forms of therapy, recreational therapy helps you develop and optimize your strength and skills.

A recreation therapist is a trained professional. Recreation therapists understand the physiology and psychology of your disability and what physical and cognitive capacities are necessary for a given sport or activity. By bringing that information together, recreation therapists help determine athletic options and are aware of adaptations which make a sport available to you, such as the mono-ski or sip-and-puff controls for target shooting. They will work with the OT and PT to design supplemental activities that give you the chance to use the strength and skill you will develop in the therapy gym.

There is a remarkable and expanding set of sports and recreation options that are increasingly open to wheelchair users. Choices include wheelchair basketball, quad rugby, snow skiing, kayaking, water-skiing, archery, billiards, Ping-Pong, tennis, shooting, and many other sports accessible to chair users, often by means of adaptive devices. Many sports are available to people with limited arm strength, including swimming, archery, bowling, camping, sailing, and even throwing a Frisbee, thanks to the Quad-Bee designed by Foster Anderson, a quadriplegic in northern California.

The recreation therapist will discuss what interests you, what you did before your disability, and then point you to organizations that sponsor events where you can observe activities that interest you. You might even get to try some of these things out during your rehab stay.

Rancho Los Amigos uses sports as a way of finding out what interests people have. The center offers hockey and wheelchair basketball games, as described by Dr. Michael Scott:

> We have a very active recreation program. We introduce people to various sports to make them aware of options. We have developed a highly competitive sports program. The recreation therapist also takes them on outings in the community.

Many rehab centers take you on field trips, organized and overseen by the recreation therapist. Therapists know the value of contact with the outside world, to help you through those early moments of feeling conspicuous as a wheelchair user and to give you a taste of an accessible recreational activity. The outing might just be a stroll around the block or going to a movie, but recreation therapists do their best to get a little fun into the experience.

HealthSouth Rehabilitation Hospital's Uli Salas takes people to local wheel-chair basketball games:

> People might just sit and watch, or join in depending on their ability.
> It is a good way for us to get them out and thinking in terms of still being
> athletic.

Outings show the recreation therapist your reactions to disability and help you learn how the world will react when you begin to appear in the world as a chair user. Dr. Scott explains:

> Based on how they do when they go out, we give them counseling
> about how to handle certain situations. The first time they go out they
> might come back and say, "People were staring at me!" or "People were
> much nicer to me!" It really depends. Everyone has a little different expe-
> rience.

How much exposure you'll get to various options depends on the facility, and the space and resources it is able to devote to recreation. Some smaller rehab hospitals will not have a space devoted to recreation. Your room might become the principle gathering place. Visitors will have to come to your room—usually shared with one to three others—and you might feel like there is nothing much more to do than be in bed. Recreation therapists in such settings will try hard not to let that happen, being as creative as they can by renting videos and setting up an evening "theater" in the therapy gym or throwing parties around a holiday. Their goal is to keep you active and, to the degree they can, give you a taste of available athletic options.

Respiratory therapy

Oxygen is essential to all metabolic processes and to life. Breathing is partic-ularly an issue for people with post-polio syndrome, or high level spinal cord conditions. The muscles that cause the lungs to expand and contract are often weakened by these conditions, limiting the amount of air you can draw in. Higher level paraplegics can also face breathing difficulties from limited use of trunk and abdominal muscles, and a reduced ability to cough and clear mucus.

The respiratory therapist's job is to ensure that you are getting sufficient oxy-gen into your lungs. Respiratory therapists determine the efficiency of your breathing by measuring "vital capacity," based on body size and age.

Therapists can measure oxygen saturation in the capillaries of the ear or finger. They listen to your lungs with a stethoscope to judge air movement and the presence of secretions. If you fall below a certain percentage, the therapist will take measures to improve your breathing.

Doubts about your ability to breathe are often a source of deep fears and insecurities. Respiratory therapists are acutely aware of the anxiety associated with breath; part of their job is to reassure you. If you have respiratory issues, the RT is one of the first people you meet and one of the first to spend significant time with you.

RTs will work with occupational and physical therapists to select activities that help strengthen muscles in the chest and diaphragm used in breathing. RTs interact with other rehab team members, advising them how your respiratory status needs to be considered in the work they are doing on your behalf, instructing them about respiratory issues, and in some cases teaching basic methods such as use of a resuscitation bag.

If your vital capacity is low, RTs might recommend a stretch program. A ventilator machine literally inflates your lungs to stretch them out—hyperexpanding them—to increase their capacity. Pressure is increased gradually, taking your comfort level into account. This is usually done for ten to fifteen minutes, four times per day.

In some cases, breathing needs to be assisted with a ventilator. Not all centers are equipped to work with ventilator-dependent quadriplegics; this requires special skills and facilities.

Volume ventilation

One of the strongest images associated with the polio epidemic of the '40s and '50s was the iron lung. It was the assistive breathing device of the day, using negative pressure to create a vacuum which would cause the lungs to draw air. Now the most common approach is positive-pressure ventilation, in which a machine delivers a measured volume of gas into the lungs. The machinery has become very advanced. There are a number of portable products that can be installed on a wheelchair. They are equipped with alarm systems that indicate either volume or pressure drops; the sensitivity can be adjusted. Machines even have the ability to simulate a sigh, to recreate the normal pattern of breathing as much as possible. Settings control respiratory rate, humidity, and pressure.

Assisted breathing settles into a routine part of life for those who rely on it, as this ventilator user notes:

> I have had my trach and vent for a couple of years now, and it just seems like it has been part of me for a long time. But I do remember when they took me off of the hospital vent and put me on my personal one that I coughed and choked a lot until they got the vent settings adjusted correctly. When you get used to it, using the vent is no more traumatic than brushing your teeth!

Successful use of a ventilator depends on good training provided by a respiratory therapist, not only for yourself, but for people who will be assisting you:

> When I first got the permanent trach and vent over four years ago, the respiratory therapist and doctors were excellent in training my partner, me, and my personal assistants in trach cleaning, suctioning, vent settings, etc. I was not allowed to go home until both my partner and my PA were taught CPR. I must say that the training was excellent.

The tracheal tube

With a ventilator, breathing occurs through a tube inserted through the neck, nose, or mouth. An inflatable cuff tracheostomy tube is often used in the neck to maintain pressure into the opening and prevent respiratory gases from escaping around the outside. The cuff precludes the user from being able to speak, although it can be deflated for periods to allow speech.

After the acute stage, some people pursue the goal of using a Jackson tracheal tube, which allows speech. The tracheal opening requires greater care to prevent infection and drainage of secretions than when the inflatable cuff is used.

The acute period in rehab when a cuffed ventilator user is unable to speak is very frustrating for the user and family. Communication options are reduced to smacking the lips or clicking the tongue to get attention. Lip reading, eye blinks, or a spelling board are sometimes tried. You might be afraid of not being heard over the sound of the machine. Experienced rehab nurses are very aware of these issues and will teach various options. They will do their best to be readily available, responsive, and to encourage the presence of family to help reduce everyone's level of anxiety.

The tracheal tube needs to be changed, depending on the sensitivity of the opening to infection and the amount of secretions. Some people change the tube every two to three weeks, but each person finds a pattern, as does this quadriplegic woman with post-polio syndrome:

> Trach changes depend on what both patient and doctor agree on. I have gone as long as six months without a change. I was checked by myself, doctor, and partner for signs of infection. If cleaning the trach area occurs daily, the tube can be kept in for months. My doctor doesn't like me to change a lot, due to irritation of the tracheal wall which could cause bleeding.

Ventilator users are generally unable to cough up secretions on their own. The respiratory therapist or rehab nurse might use a technique of assisted coughing, in which pressure is placed in an upward motion at the base of the rib cage to release mucus from the deep sacs of the lungs. Suctioning secretions is part of the ventilator experience and is done as often as every eight hours for some people. It is important not to do suctioning more than necessary, since it irritates the trachea and can increase secretions, as well as the risk of infection. A suction machine is usually kept near the bedside, and portable models are also available. Family and assistants can be trained in suctioning.

> At first suctioning is a scary thing—having the air sucked out of you to try to get mucus up. But as time goes by, it is just a way of life.

Weaning

Some people will always need to use a ventilator twenty-four hours a day. Others wean from ventilation and are able to breathe on their own. Whether you are expected to breathe on your own or not, the respiratory therapist will develop a weaning program for you.

Using a ventilator at all times allows respiratory muscles to atrophy. Even five minutes of breathing on your own several times a day helps maintain some tone. A typical goal is to achieve the ability to breathe unassisted for ten to fifteen minutes. In the case of a mechanical disruption, the ability to breathe without the ventilator for a brief time until assistance arrives obviously means the difference between life and death.

Since depression is a very common feature of the acute stage of high quadriplegia, the rehab team will typically suggest that you wait until you are more stable psychologically. It takes a certain degree of motivation to participate in the weaning process, which can be frightening. A respiratory therapist will always be present during any weaning session, and all staff are trained in the use of a manual resuscitation bag, which should be kept with you at all times.

Psychotherapy

The goal of the psychologist is to work with you as an ally to help change mental patterns which can limit you. In the past, you would only have been referred to a therapist if you were considered a "problem patient" or in such deep despair that staff was concerned for your safety. Present day rehab therapy takes a different view. Powerful feelings, confusion, or rebellion are widely recognized as understandable reactions to sudden disability. Rather than stigmatize people who experience extreme emotion, now psychologists work with everyone to help them deal with their feelings.

There are many possible emotional responses to a disability. Many factors come into play, including age, degree of injury and impairment, financial and class status, cultural expectations, and so on. How the disability occurred is also crucial, as peer support coordinator Rich Patterson explains:

> Whether it was an accident, someone else's fault, or gang-related—
> this makes a big difference in how everyone responds. It's hard enough to
> feel that you made a stupid mistake, but when someone does something to
> you and puts you in a chair, that tends to be pretty hard to swallow.

Depression and suicidal feelings are common during acute rehab—although not everyone experiences them. The staff is trained to recognize behavioral signs of these feelings. Depression and suicidal feelings are treatable and generally temporary.

The overall work of rehabilitation depends on commitment—an attitude that promotes full participation and cooperation with the process. The psychologist helps you sort out what drives your behavior in ways that limit you, cause you unhappiness, or compromise the potential you can reach in the rehab process. Types of behavior that could interfere with your ability to gain from rehab include:

• Passive-aggressive behavior, in which one is indifferent to the value of what is being offered and places responsibility on others' shoulders

- Extreme dependency, in which one fails to participate proactively, and loses the chance to feel personal accomplishment
- Severe anti-social behavior, in which one possibly represents a danger to self or others

Rehab doctors and therapists know they must adapt their approach to each person according to how that person is coping. Says Dr. Michael Scott:

> Everyone copes in a different way. Some people are more energetic, gung-ho and motivated. Some are depressed. Everyone does their best, and we try to motivate them and get them going. Some are able to do a little more early on, and we try to adjust for that. If someone isn't up for a vigorous weight lifting class or tires out we try to space things out to accommodate what they can and can't do.

The fact that someone is depressed or angry while in rehab does not mean they will fail to adapt to disability. Saunders Dorsey was a young attorney in Detroit when an angry client attacked the office with a rifle. Saunders jumped out of the third-story window and became a spinal cord paraplegic:

> I was extraordinarily dependent. I needed twenty-four-hour attention. I wouldn't do anything. I was virtually helpless. It was obviously more emotional than physical. I was so angry, I laid there for two years and wouldn't do a thing.

Dorsey has since returned to a thriving law practice, established a successful accessible transportation company after seeing the flaws in the services he was receiving, and is living in a comfortable home with his wife and children. He just needed time before he was ready to move forward with his life.

Working with a psychotherapist

The rehabilitation period is recognized as an important time for psychological support. Psychotherapists are typically included in the rehab team. Many rehab clients have the opportunity to spend time with a therapist as part of their daily schedule, where they are free to ask questions and discuss their feelings confidentially.

Many people who find themselves in rehab will never have met with a therapist before. Those persons might feel as if therapy is being forced on them and is an invasion of privacy. Psychologists expect that some people will be unwilling to participate at first and will have negative ideas about the psychotherapeutic process.

Meeting with a psychologist means revealing intimate facts and exploring deep and often troubling emotions. Although the process can seem threatening at first, the therapist's job is to be an ally—not a friend, because this is not a personal relationship—who listens openly and explains what he or she has to offer. Psychotherapists can affirm the validity of what you are going through and help you begin adapting.

Jeri Morris, Ph.D., of the Department of Rehabilitation at Northwestern University Medical School in Chicago, writes:

> The immediate goal of the psychologist is to encourage a willingness by clients to think about the long-term effects of their injury. The psychologist must get on the side of clients rather than make himself or herself their adversary.[7]

Thinking about long-term effects can be especially hard for people with progressive conditions, such as MS or ALS. People with MS fight hard to maintain their health. One of the most difficult moments is when it is time to begin using a wheelchair, as explained by Cynthia Bishop:

> A lot of people see using the wheelchair as giving up, as giving in to their disease. We hear that over and over, "I'm not giving in to it, I'm not using a wheelchair." We have to do a lot of talking. "How does it affect your day-to-day life function? If using a wheelchair would make it possible to go to your child's Little League game—would you rather go or would you rather stay home? How about using the wheelchair at work so you still have the energy to stay up with your family when you get home, as opposed to walking at work and becoming so tired that you just come home and collapse in a heap?"
>
> Generally speaking, it's not something that people receive warmly. We have to continue the process over several visits. We have to gently bring them to the point where they say, "Okay, I'd like to do that, I think it might be a good idea."

Most rehab centers emphasize education, offering programs on an array of topics to enhance your sense of control and sense of self. Dr. Michael Scott describes the offerings at Rancho Los Amigos:

We have a program that all patients go through called Starting Out class. Every day of the week there's a different topic. One is called Take Control, basically an assertiveness training class. It's given by one of our former tetraplegic patients, who does a great job with it. Other topics are Attendant Management, Funding and Resources, and Learning Your Rights, which is an introduction to the ADA. We let them know what the resources are and how to stick up for themselves.

Sexuality

The presence of a psychologist on the team helps foster more openness in discussing this crucial topic. You might be hesitant to bring up questions as personal as what kind of sex life you might be able to look forward to. Dr. Michael Scott describes his approach to helping people ask about sex:

Most patients are reluctant to bring up sexuality initially. They're definitely thinking about it. We use the approach of giving them permission to talk about it. I'll say, "You've had a spinal cord injury, things are different for you now, you probably have some questions, and one thing people usually want to know about is sexuality and sexual function. If you have questions about it, then please let me know." Usually they'll say, "Oh yeah, I've been wondering about that, doc."

The priority of sexuality to the person depends on many factors, including the type of disability, age, and sexual experience. Dr. Ed Nieshoff, Rehabilitation Institute of Michigan, talks about younger men with a spinal cord disability:

They're still in the grip of their raging hormones like any teenage guy, and all that energy is hard to redirect. It is very hard—and often angering—for them to have to redefine their sexuality. It adds to the pain. People think that walking again is the most important, but I'd say for most people it's about number five on the list. For a quad, first of all you want your hands back, second you want to be able to urinate, third you want to control your bowels, and then your sex life, and last of all walking. When you're nineteen, you'll take the sex before the walking!

Much of the information offered in rehab is about male sexuality. Since women with disabilities are generally not prevented from having children, the emphasis often falls on male fertility. And since maintaining erection is an issue only for men, this also tends to weigh the discussion in their direction. There is a lot of information about penile implants or injections, and harvesting sperm is now possible.

Yet women also face questions regarding vaginal lubrication, positions, bladder control, and how to attract men in a culture that doesn't encourage women to be the pursuer. Women need to hear about birth control, pregnancy, and gynecological care. Margaret Nosek has been researching sexuality in women with disabilities, and says:

> I've heard from women who said they were put in groups with men and were very uncomfortable with that. They felt it was introduced at a time when they didn't feel ready to deal with it. It's just that rehab centers have people for such a short period of time now that they try to cram all this stuff in. Women need more time to adjust.

Women might have underlying issues of abuse. Their disability might even be the result of spousal abuse, which is sadly responsible for a share of brain injury and spinal cord injury from gunshot, for instance. A past history of sexual abuse will certainly be aggravated by becoming a woman with a disability. Women become more attractive targets for abuse by being in an increased position of vulnerability.

It is common for women's menstrual cycles to be interrupted for up to six months to a year after a spinal cord injury. Says Nosek:

> Something seems to happen to a woman's hormone cycle. Some women have observed a relationship between how long they have been without periods after a disabling injury and problems they have later in life.

This raises psychological issues about the desire to have children—the loss of a feature which is a matter of feminine identity for some women—and anxiety about whether the cycle will return, despite what rehab staff says.

A skilled psychologist can help women begin to address these and other issues in order to achieve success in their sexuality. Nosek again:

> The key is self-esteem. Our studies have shown that when women feel good about themselves, disability has no effect on the quality of their relationships. But there is so much more to study. We want to find out more about what makes women have high self-esteem.

Psychology for the family

The rehab psychologist is there to support the family, too. When you are in rehab with a traumatic disability, other family members have to deal with a lot of difficult emotions. They might doubt whether you can have a high quality of life, particularly if they have no models of people with disabilities who made the kinds of adaptations you are facing.

Initially it may be even more difficult for your family. You have something to do. You will be involved in hospitalization and rehab, getting the attention of medical staff, being visited and called, doing the work of recovery and gaining independence. Family members are often left wanting to do more, wishing they could help, and having too much time to think about what has happened to you. Your family is caught in a storm of emotional experience immediately after your trauma. Joan Anderson writes that:

> Families understandably display anxiety and stress. They are confronted with a medical emergency, questions of life and death. Few people are prepared to respond to such an overwhelming catastrophic event. Patient and family are rarely able to comprehend the implications of the injury.[8]

They are wanting answers to a flood of questions: "Will my family member survive? What has happened to her? What is being done to her? How do I help?" Your family might feel quite helpless. Psychologist Ann Marie Fleming says:

> The family is so petrified by the near-death experience that it reels them in to take care of their family member. If they are parents, then they go back into the over-protective, hyper-vigilant mode they were in when their child was small. This is a natural reaction of anyone to trauma. I think that reversion is important. It makes them really celebrate each achievement, whether it is taking a step or going to the bathroom without a catheter. It needs to happen.

Family members also need to avoid smothering or allowing their lives outside the hospital to disintegrate, causing further stress and trauma. Psychologist Joan Anderson writes:

> Families feel torn between their need to be at the hospital and their need to care for other children at home or to attend to a job. They bear

*the burden of the emotional crisis plus all the mechanics of reorganizing
their lives to accommodate the injured family member.*[9]

When family members are able to reach out to other families they encounter at the hospital, they can benefit from their experience and learn coping skills by example. Other families can pass down what they have learned during stages of the rehab process that you and your family might not have reached. Being able to help others keeps families from becoming too engrossed in their own trauma.

When you observe other families adapt, you can envision a new future for yourself.

Vocational rehab

A primary goal of rehab is for you to be able to work, if at all possible. Rehab staff want to foster your opportunity to return to your previous or some other kind of job. The anticipation of returning to a productive role in the world can increase your motivation to participate in rehab.

You will work with a vocational counselor—sometimes known as vocational rehabilitationist—who might be employed by the rehab center, assigned by the insurer, or hired as a contractor by your State Vocational Rehabilitation agency. Vocational Rehabilitation (Voc Rehab) is a government program that exists at both state and federal levels. Legislation dating as far back as 1917 has authorized money to help injured workers get back to work. Your insurer might also have vocational rehab services and funds to offer you. If you get back to work, they figure you will not require as much expensive continuing healthcare or long-term disability benefits.

Counselors you work with will have varying loyalties, depending on who employs them. Those loyalties can limit their effectiveness, as attorney, quadriplegic, and disability activist Deborah Kaplan of the World Institute on Disability notes:

> *The Voc Rehab system is sometimes helpful, often not. And very frustrating, very bureaucratic, very rigid. These days, they don't want to spend much money per client. You have to be a fairly sophisticated user of government entitlement services to get anywhere with rehab, unless you happen to luck into a good counselor who is genuinely trying to facilitate life. Counselors usually want to put you into a community college, get you*

a trade and say that they rehabilitated you. If you get a job, they have succeeded, whether you keep it or not.

The hard truth is that your State Voc Rehab agency will generally work with you only when they consider you employable. How that gets defined might be up to the particular case worker you encounter. This man with advanced muscular dystrophy reports:

> *I went to their office, did the entire intake process, interviewed with a case worker, but nothing ever came of it. They said they would call me, but never did. I talked to other disabled people more familiar with the workings of the California rehab system, who told me the reason they probably didn't follow up is because they considered a person with MD in his late thirties a "bad risk." That is, I would probably die before I would work enough to make the money spent on me worth it. As cold as this may sound, I believe it to be true. I've heard about this type of thing many times before.*

State Vocational Rehabilitation services are getting tighter these days. There has been greater demand on these programs, in part due to the increasing number of repetitive strain injuries resulting from computer use in offices. In some states, legislation limits the money that can be spent for a given case—this limited amount can be small if you need an education and adaptive tools such as a computer or a modified vehicle.

You always have the chance to advocate for yourself. For instance, you don't have to accept the first counselor who is assigned to you. If there is someone in the rehab facility to organize your vocational rehab, she might work harder on your behalf because she has no association with the funding source. When a counselor is doing her job well, she does the following:

- Takes a history of your past job experience and skills
- Learns about your medical status and prognosis
- Considers how your disability affects your ability to return to previous work
- Evaluates new career possibilities and make suggestions to see what interests you, if your previous work is not possible
- Surveys the job market to help identify realistic options
- Explores sources and means of funding, if you require training or education

- Coaches you on job seeking and interview skills
- Advises you and your employer on possible modifications and accommodations that make it possible for you to perform the job

Vocational counselors want to make the most of your physical and psychological rehabilitation, accomplished with hard work by you and the rehab team. They want to make a smooth transition to work or to education, and take best advantages of your accomplishments in rehab.

Beyond rehab

There is not always time for you to make full adjustments before leaving rehab. States Dr. Michael Scott of Rancho Los Amigos:

> In the past when there were longer stays, people had the support of staff to go through some of the psychological adjustment issues. Now they're going through them in the community. It's probably more difficult.

Once you are out of rehab, how can you find out how much more progress is possible in gaining strength and skills? How do you make that progress on your own? This is the challenge of shorter stays.

Rich Patterson of the Santa Clara Valley spinal cord unit notes:

> It is very tough to see people who don't get the chance to make adjustments while they're in rehab, though it depends a lot on where they were at socially, their communication skills, and level of education. If they don't have these skills, then they run into some serious difficulties dealing with all facets of life, from family and neighbors to doctors and equipment suppliers. They need to learn how to develop these skills. We try to help that by matching them to a peer supporter, but we run into the problem of people who, when they are released after three months, don't want to talk to anybody. They're still very insecure about their disability. They don't think that other people have the same problems they do. They're still in the denial stage.

Your rehab experience might be unpleasant for you. You might resent the controlled environment or feel you just want a break from all the hard work. But the resources there exist for you, and it is a mistake not to take advantage of them. Don't wait until you find out how limited you are by having stopped short of gaining your optimal strength and skills. Even people who hated rehab reconsider. Bonnie Sims says:

> I am sometimes surprised when people who seemed so dissatisfied during their rehabilitation return for treatment. I guess it's true that we look a whole lot better looking back!

It is much harder to achieve your optimal level of function without the support and regulated schedule of a rehab facility. Nonetheless, take advantage of outpatient services your rehab center offers, find similar services nearby if you live too far from your inpatient center, or at the very least be sure that you have a home program designed for you when you leave rehab and do your best to stick with it. There is always more you can achieve. Once you are home, don't let the rehab process stop.

The transition to home

The question of what you will go home to comes up quickly once you arrive in rehab. There is a lot to do to get ready, so the process should begin as soon as possible.

The first question families have is usually about the adaptation of their home. As discussed in Chapter 7, *Home Access*, this may not be a simple matter of adding a ramp or putting in grab bars. Contractors may need to get involved, doors might need to be widened, lifts installed, or full additions built onto the house. Some people find they must sell their homes and find another more accessible place to live. These things take time—and money.

Equipment is another key to the discharge process, but the task of identifying a wheelchair is difficult to accomplish early in the rehab process. As Bonnie Sims explains:

> In the first weeks of rehab, most people plan on walking out. The last thing they want to do is order a chair when they believe there will be no need for it. Power chairs can be especially complex. There isn't sufficient time to prescribe, fund, order, and fit the chair prior to discharge. We do have a loaner system that makes timely discharge possible in most cases.

Many major rehab centers have special apartments designed as transitional living locations, but most insurers will not pay for a stay at such a facility.

Building a support system

You want to create an environment for yourself that helps you continue coping. The choice of people you interact with makes a big difference.

Your relationships will change with some people. A disability has a way of flushing out relationships, of showing who is really committed to you as a friend or even a family member, and who is unwilling or unable to accept you on new terms. There is both heartbreak and joy in this. You will find a deeper connection with some people in your life, and you will be disappointed in others, facing the loss of their presence because they are unable—perhaps only for now—to face their fears raised by your disability.

> *I found out years later that some of my closest friends felt my life was over once I had become paraplegic. A couple of them did not see me for years, and when we reunited later they said that, at the time, it was just too painful for them.*

You will also meet new people and develop friendships in ways you might not expect.

You have control of who you interact with and in what ways. You have new priorities for maintaining your health and redefining an active, satisfying, and meaningful life. You have to choose how you need and want to live, give people you've known the chance to understand your new terms, and try to have enough people in your life who inspire you and support you.

Relationships take work. Expressing emotions to each other is part of the process of deepening your connection. Even if others grieve about your disability or tire of the caregiver role, keep communication open. The relationship can grow, so long as people are expressing themselves.

In her book, *Coping with Limb Loss*, Ellen Winchell, Ph.D., describes aspects of a successful support system:[10]

- Our lives are enriched by emotionally nourishing relationships.
- We are innately social beings who turn to each other in times of need.
- Knowing people love and care about you reduces your sense of isolation and the burden of the experience.
- One "best friend" is not a complete support system, but is an overwhelming responsibility for that person.

- You are not a burden to people who care enough to want to contribute and will find meaning for themselves by doing so.

- Accepting support is not a matter of shame—everyone needs support in some way at some time in their lives.

Family caregivers

By speeding the date of discharge, insurers have placed more responsibility for care on families. Coverage for home nursing and personal assistance is also limited, so families end up carrying much of the load. In the case of a ventilator-dependent quadriplegic who must have someone nearby at all times, this is a large task indeed.

According to a June 1998 article in the *San Francisco Examiner*:

> *Managed-care companies and hospitals conscious of the bottom line have weighed in, pushing to get clients home faster and, many critics contend, sicker. The result has been an explosion in family caregiving. A poll by the National Alliance for Caregiving found that the number of people providing free care to a family member grew to 21 million, up from 7 million in 1987.*[11]

Some families have a great deal of trouble with the caregiver role. It is, at the least, a financial strain. Often at least one family member must leave a paying job to perform a caregiver role which produces no income. Caregivers take on medical responsibilities, such as assistance with a bowel program or suctioning secretions for a ventilator user, but might not have received sufficient training. They might have an emotionally difficult time performing such intimate and invasive tasks.

Many people who use personal assistance say that they would not recommend a family member playing the role of primary caregiver, especially a spouse. It alters—sometimes seriously strains—family relationships. When a parent assists an adult child, the quality of the relationship can revert to when the adult child was young, as the protective instincts of the parent resurface. Even when a parent-as-caregiver relationship succeeds, parents will have increasing difficulty with the physical tasks as they age.

Some families succeed by sharing the caregiver tasks among parents and siblings. No one person is overwhelmed, they learn to perform tasks and procedures effectively, and everyone knows the first priority is preserving the disabled family member's rights of decision-making and control. People can discover that tasks which they considered unpleasant—like providing bowel assistance—become more accepted with experience.

> *I know a family with a son who has severe cerebral palsy. He is unable to walk or speak. He has deformities in his spine and arms, and is spastic, yet with the support of his large family he has graduated with high grades from high school, uses computer technology by means of a mouth switch, and travels often with the family in a specially outfitted recreational vehicle. They even developed a special system of communication in which he clicks with his mouth in response to a system of prompts. The father says that he wouldn't change a thing, that the experience has been a remarkable gift for his family.*

When the caregiver role falls to a family, there are choices about how to approach it and what to make of it. With appropriate training and support, a family can settle into a routine which is not burdensome and makes a full life possible for their loved one. Chapter 4 has information about personal assistance services.

Use outside resources

Rehab is only the start of the process: there is more to accomplish. You might not be a resident at a rehab hospital anymore, but your insurance might cover continuing therapy on an outpatient basis. Even if you live in a different city from the major rehab hospital where you stayed, there are an increasing number of small rehab hospitals or therapy groups which can work with you closer to home.

There is likely to be a Center for Independent Living in your area. While not a rehab hospital, a CIL can help in many ways. If you are struggling with your insurer about coverage for continued therapy, the CIL might be able to offer you advocacy training and support to gain funding for your needs, possibly even for home adaptation. Many CILs conduct support group meetings that give you the chance to meet others who share your circumstances. You get to learn from the pros, who will gladly share their "tricks of the trade." Of course, each CIL has its own programs. Offerings vary widely. At the end of Chapter 10, *Politics and Legislation*, there are descriptions of some of the range of programs found at CILs.

Just because the insurance industry calls the shots on how long you get to stay in rehab does not mean that you are denied the chance to be as strong and active as you can be. It just means you have to do more of it on your own.

Janie Whiteford of Santa Clara Valley Medical Center notes:

> *When you're discharged, you are definitely not what you're going to be a year from now. We really push people not to think in terms of where they are now. Consider where you might be a year from now, because it will be a totally different picture.*

Rehab is inevitably a sheltered environment where you can begin adjustments. Once you get out, there will be new stresses, even for the person who has good coping skills. Kentfield Rehabilitation Hospital's Dr. Alex Barchuk comments:

> *Psychological adjustment is very, very, very, very individual. People who don't have a history of depression and usually have felt okay about things will go through a period in the beginning of not knowing what the heck's going on. Then, they realize, "Oh boy, this is a whole new life!" But it isn't until they get out of the hospital that it really hits them hard.*

Ongoing healthcare

Your disability will need continuing medical management. Maintain a relationship with your physiatrist. If you traveled to a regional rehab center, identify a place that can offer ongoing physical medicine services. Ask your rehab doctor for a referral.

You are also going to have general medical needs. You'll get the flu, sustain a deep cut, deal with allergies, and so on. Don't neglect your standard healthcare. Get checkups and have a relationship with a family practitioner.

You'll have to educate these doctors about your disability. There is much they will not understand, since they do not deal with disability on a daily basis. You will have to ask whether their office has an accessible bathroom, for instance. Believe it or not, the office itself might not have room for the passage of your wheels.

Even if you have been living with your disability for many years—whether you had a formal inpatient rehab experience or not—the rehab community still has something to offer you. Says Margaret Nosek, researcher at Baylor University in Houston:

> There are a lot of people in this world who got their rehab a long, long time ago, and have never made contact again, so they don't get the benefit of current knowledge. Despite all of the setbacks due to managed care, rehab has improved and learned a great deal over the years.

CHAPTER 3

Medical Concerns

Your disability might entail a risk of certain medical complications. You'll need to be aware of those that affect you, so that you can take preventive actions, know warning signs, react promptly, and participate in treatment decisions.

This chapter looks briefly at some medical concerns commonly associated with various disabilities. There is far too wide a range of conditions to fully cover all medical concerns that might apply to you in this chapter. For your particular medical profile, do your own research and cultivate an open and cooperative relationship with your physician. After a quick look at overall concerns, conditions are presented in alphabetical order:

- Autonomic dysreflexia
- Bladder cancer
- Deep vein thrombosis
- Heterotopic ossification
- Pain
- Pressure sores
- Scoliosis
- Spasticity
- Stress
- Urinary tract infections

Conditions common to many chair users—such as pain, pressure sores, and spasticity—are described at greater length.

General concerns

As a person with a disability who uses a wheelchair, you have additional health risks and must work harder to maintain your health. If you lack sensation, you must be alert for other signals from your body. Primary care doctors might not understand specialized needs you have; specialists in a particular condition or body system might not understand how your disability changes how they would normally treat a condition.

The 1998 National Organization on Disability (NOD)/Harris Survey of Americans with Disabilities notes that those with disabilities are less likely to be able to afford healthcare, get insurance, or have special needs covered by insurance:

> One out of five (21%) adults with a disability did not get medical care that they needed on at least one occasion during the past year, compared to one in ten (11%) adults without a disability....

> One in four (28%) adults with disabilities postponed getting healthcare they thought they needed in the past year because they couldn't afford it.

> Although nine out of ten (90%) adults with disabilities are covered by health insurance (a marginal increase over 1994, when 86% were covered), adults with disabilities are more likely than other adults (23% vs. 13%) to say that they are dissatisfied with the healthcare services they and their family have used in the last few years.

> Among those with disabilities who are insured, one in three (32%) say they have special needs because of their disability (such as particular therapies, equipment, or medicine) that are not covered by their health insurance.

> Among adults with disabilities who are not covered by health insurance, one in five (18%) were not able to get insurance because of a disability or pre-existing health condition.[1]

It is wise to find out what you can about healthcare and advocating for yourself before an emergency or serious health threat arises. General precautions you might want to take to prepare for potentially serious medical situations are:

- Educate yourself about insurance options and your coverage.

- Know your medical history.

- Know your medications. Know what types of medications you are taking and which ones you're allergic to. Before you accept a prescription from your doctor, let him know what medications you are presently taking, and ask him to check his *Physician's Desk Reference* (PDR) for any possible conflicts.

- **Establish a good relationship with your physician.** Be comfortable talking with your doctor and jointly solving problems. Nancy Keene, in her book *Working with Your Doctor*, suggests the following strategies:[2]

  — You and your physician should compare definitions of the problem, goals of treatment, and preferred methods of treatment.

  — Ask the doctor why she thinks the recommended treatment is best and if there are any guidelines for treating your illness or condition.

  — Explain as clearly as you can your life circumstances that make one treatment more appropriate than another. If, for instance, you have three preschool children at home, you might not want to take an anti-seizure medication that would cause you to sleep most of the day.

  — Repeat back instructions and explanations to make sure you understand. One way to do this is to say, "Let me see if I fully understand. You think the problem is _____, caused by _____. You want me to take _____ medication and call you back in a week if things improve and sooner if they get worse."

  — If you find yourself getting overwhelmed by information during an appointment, say so and ask to come back another time to complete your discussion.

- **Tell others about particular health risks.** Inform those closest to you and most likely to be present should an emergency arise about particular health risks. For example, if autonomic dysreflexia is a possible complication for you, give close family and friends enough information so they know how to recognize it and how to respond.

- **Become a MedicAlert member.** Consider getting a MedicAlert bracelet or necklace to help alert emergency medical services personnel and others in case of an emergency, particularly if you have difficulty communicating or have a non-obvious medical condition. The initial membership fee for MedicAlert is a minimum of $35, depending on the style, metal, and size of the bracelet or necklace you order. After that, the annual renewal fee is $15. Your fee provides one-year membership, including:

— Setting up and maintaining your computerized medical file with personal ID number, and unlimited free record updates.

— Custom engraved emblem with chain.

— Twenty-four-hour Emergency Response Center (ERC), which is staffed around the clock to receive calls from people who call with information from your bracelet in case of an emergency. Information that can be accessed includes: your ID information, emergency contacts, doctors' contact information, health coverage information and emergency approval phone number, medications and the dosages you are taking.

— Membership card to carry in your wallet or purse; member publications.

• **Execute Durable Power of Attorney document.** A Durable Power of Attorney for Health Care (DPAHC) is a legal document that must be signed by a competent adult. It allows you to transfer medical decision-making authority from yourself to a person you designate as your *agent*. Obviously, the person you select to be the agent of your DPAHC should be someone you know and trust, and someone you feel is capable of making decisions based on your wishes. The DPAHC guarantees that your healthcare choices will be carried out according to your wishes, values, and beliefs. Once signed and witnessed by either a lawyer or a notary public, the DPAHC can only be executed if you are unable to make the decisions yourself, for example, if you are unconscious, comatose, or cannot speak for yourself.

Autonomic dysreflexia (AD)

Autonomic dysreflexia (AD) is also called autonomic hyperreflexia or paroxysmal hypertension (among other names). Autonomic dysreflexia is particular to people with spinal cord lesions at or above the sixth thoracic vertebra, although it has been reported with injuries as low as T8. It is marked by an increase in blood pressure and should be taken very seriously. AD can cause stroke or seizures, and can be life-threatening.

The nervous system tries to send a message to the brain when it perceives an irritant to the body, such as a full bladder or a wound. Since the message can't get past the spinal cord lesion to the brain, and since the brain can't respond by sending inhibitory agents down the cord past the injury, a "hyper reflex" occurs. The body keeps trying to send the messages, and blood vessels tighten below the injury level. Above the injury level, vessels open, which causes the typical red, blotchy skin seen with AD.

Stimulations that can produce this response include:

- Urinary tract infections
- Impacted bowel
- A full bladder
- Pressure sores
- Bladder, kidney, or gall stones
- Hemorrhoids
- Deep vein thrombosis
- Burns to skin, including sunburn
- Open wounds
- Ingrown toenails
- Sexual arousal
- Fractures
- Labor and childbirth
- Some surgical or diagnostic procedures
- Tight-fitting or wrinkled clothing

As you can see from the list, you have control over most causes. Bladder distention is the most common cause of autonomic dysreflexia. Users of indwelling urinary catheters need to manage the catheters well to make sure they do not become clogged or bent into a kink which blocks the flow. Fecal impaction is the second most common cause. A well-managed bowel and bladder program is very important, not only to decrease the chance of an occurrence of AD, but to prevent secondary conditions like infections and stones which can also cause an event.

When blood pressure rises, any of the following symptoms might occur:

- Pounding headache
- Red, blotchy skin above the lesion level
- Profuse sweating above the lesion level

- Cool, clammy skin below the lesion level

- Nausea

- Blurred or spotty vision

- Nasal congestion

- Goosebumps

- Slow pulse

- Anxiety

Many people learn to recognize the signs of high blood pressure early, and find they can manage episodes of AD. However, if signs persist, it is very important to get immediate medical attention. There might be a fracture you are unable to feel or a urinary infection you are unaware of.

If symptoms appear, the first thing to do—after removing the offending stimulation, if possible—is to sit up. Elevating the body helps reduce blood pressure by encouraging pooling of blood in the lower extremities. Check if your leg or bedside urinary drainage bag is full. This could indicate a distended bladder which is backed up and causing the event. Empty your bladder if you can, but no more than 500cc at a time, since this can cause spasms which would aggravate the situation.

If you need to go for medical attention, the first thing a physician should do is check your catheter or take measures to empty your bladder. You might need to be catheterized. The act of catheterization itself could increase stimulation to the nervous system. The treater might use an anesthetic jelly such as lidocaine to minimize sensory input and relax the urinary sphincter muscle to avoid aggravating the problem. A physician should also check for fecal impaction. A physician might gently clear some stool at the opening of the rectum. Again, an anesthetic agent might be used. In some cases the physician might give you an antihypertensive drug to quickly bring your blood pressure under control while he continues to work to identify the cause.

If you are being treated in a general emergency department or by your family physician, it might be necessary for you to educate them about AD, since they will probably not have treated AD very often.

During medical treatment, your blood pressure will be monitored closely, since it can change quite quickly during an episode of AD—as quickly as every two minutes. You might be watched for as long as two hours to ensure the episode does not recur. It is necessary to be certain that the cause is removed, rather than simply improved by short-term treatment. If the episode of AD is serious enough, you might be admitted to the hospital for closer observation.

A medical alert card for autonomic dysreflexia is available from the Paralyzed Veterans of America. The card includes instructions for how to help if someone needs to assist you in an emergency. Information on how to contact the Paralyzed Veterans of America is given in the Appendix.

To prevent AD:

- Wear loose, comfortable clothing
- Maintain a regular bladder program to prevent infection
- Keep catheters clean and flowing
- Keep stool soft and follow a regular bowel program
- Check your skin for signs of pressure sores or circulation problems
- Protect your skin from burns, bruises, and wounds

Bladder cancer

Bladder cancer is not widely seen in the general population, but its incidence is slightly higher among people who rely on catheterization for bladder management. In a study of 2,660 records at Craig Hospital in Denver of people with spinal cord injuries, only thirteen cases of bladder cancer were found, or less than 1 percent. Still, it is worth knowing what measures you can take to reduce the chances further.

Bladder cancer is more likely when there is repeated irritation to the bladder. Tumors have been seen inside the bladder at the point where a catheter makes regular contact. Indwelling catheters and suprapubic catheters are thought to be the greatest potential risk. People who use intermittent catheterization are less vulnerable. Infections are also an irritant—whether you are a catheter user or not—as are the presence of stones. Smoking is also thought to contribute—carcinogens from smoke can be carried in urine.

Some physicians feel the risks of bladder cancer are already lowered by the development of modern antibiotics, and safer nonrubber materials now used for catheters. Anticholinergic drugs such as Ditropan, Propanthline, or Daricon are bladder relaxants which are sometimes prescribed to aid a bladder program, and which can secondarily reduce bladder irritation.

The most common symptom of bladder cancer is blood in the urine. Blood in the urine does not mean that cancer is necessarily present. Blood can also be present with urinary tract infections or other causes. But take the symptom seriously and get examined by a urologist.

The urologist might suggest a cystoscopy, a diagnostic procedure in which an instrument is inserted into the bladder. The physician can then visually search for tumors. If a biopsy seems justified during the examination, he will take a small amount of tissue for testing.

Some cystoscopic biopsy reports come back with a diagnosis of "squamous metaplasia," a form of cellular change often seen in the bladder. Physicians do not widely agree that this is an indicator of cancer—many people, disabled and nondisabled, have squamous metaplasia but never develop cancer. Yet some doctors feel this change sometimes is a precursor to bladder cancer.

The strategy for preventing bladder cancer is to limit irritation to the bladder. Prevention measures include:

- Control infections and stones by drinking enough fluids. See the discussion of bladder management in Chapter 4, *Staying Healthy*.

- If you have a suprapubic catheter, keep the area around its insertion in the abdomen clean and shaved.

- Clean drainage bags and tubing with chlorine bleach and water.

- Reduce or quit smoking.

- Switch sides with your leg and/or bedside drainage bags. This changes where the catheter contacts the bladder, rather than having it always contact the same spot.

- Use catheters that are less irritating. For example, hydrophilic catheters are softer than other catheters and are lubricated.

- Take antioxidant vitamins such as E, C, and B6, thought to reduce the effects of carcinogens on cells.

- Have regular cystoscopic exams, as frequently as every two years if you are a longtime indwelling catheter user.

Deep vein thrombosis (DVT)

When we do not walk, circulation through the legs is reduced. Contractions of the leg muscles are part of the circulatory system—an important mechanism for how blood is pumped through the body. For people with paralysis in the legs, blood may be pooling in the lower extremities.

The danger is that blood could begin to clot in a vein, coagulating into a more solid state, known as deep vein thrombosis (DVT). DVT limits circulation further, at the least. At worst, the clot could dislodge and travel through the body into the lungs or brain, causing a stroke or death. This is called a pulmonary embolism. A 1979 study found 35 percent of people with DVT who were untreated died of an embolism.[3] A clot in the thigh is the greatest concern, since this location gives a more direct route to the lungs.

DVT is a greater concern at the acute stage of a spinal cord injury, when someone is inactive for an extended period of time. DVT has been observed as soon as seventy-two hours after injury. Researchers suspect that 80 percent of acute spinal cord DVT occurs within two weeks of injury. Studies of people at this stage have found incidence rates from 15 to 47 percent. Studies have also found slightly higher rates of DVT for those with complete spinal cord injuries compared to incomplete injuries.[4]

During periods of extended inactivity and bed rest, pneumatic compression stockings or wrapping with elastic bandages is often recommended. The drug Heparin is sometimes used to reduce blood viscosity, improving flow. Electrical stimulation of calf muscles has also been explored.

Heterotopic ossification (HO)

Heterotopic ossification (HO) is a condition in which bone develops outside of the normal system, potentially clogging joints, limiting or freezing movement. It occurs in acute spinal cord injury, brain injury and other neurological traumas, and takes a year or more to develop, making it hard to diagnose early. Remaining active and keeping up regular range-of-motion exercises play an important preventive role.

Heterotopic ossification only occurs below the level of injury, commonly at the hips. It can lead to scoliosis problems as the nonneutral position of the pelvis puts curvature pressure on the spine. The condition can ultimately require surgical intervention. Some doctors use anti-inflammatory drugs to manage HO. Although studies have reported from 16 to 53 percent of occurrence of HO in people with spinal cord injuries, adequate acute management substantially reduces the need for surgery to free joints or correct scoliosis due to HO.

Pain

There are many reasons why a chair user might experience pain—far too many to detail here. The causes may or may not relate to your disability.

Pain is usually thought of as a message telling us something is wrong in our body. The International Association for the Study of Pain defines pain as:

> An unpleasant sensory and emotional experience associated with actual or potential tissue damage.[5]

But a disability might involve conditions in which pain is a continuing feature. When the nervous system is affected by injury or an autoimmune event like multiple sclerosis or ALS, nerve messages get mixed up. Impulses fly through the body and can be experienced as pain. In these cases, you manage and adapt to pain, rather than always thinking of it as an indicator of something to be fixed.

> I had a lot of pain the first couple of years after my spinal cord injury. I don't know exactly what it was. No one could tell me. It was in my back. I think it was because the bones were fusing. One day a friend said to me, "You haven't complained about your back hurting for days." It was just gone all of a sudden. I thought I would always be in pain because of my injury.

Pain is a very personal experience. What is unbearable to one person might be no big deal to another. Many people with disabilities experience sensations that stem from their disability, but define those sensations as discomfort rather than pain. Other people experience pain more disabling than their physical condition.

It is your task to identify your boundaries and manage activities to minimize pain. Some people find that sitting or lying for extended periods exacerbates pain, while others experience greater pain when active. Extremes of either will probably increase pain. The body requires variety of movement, but has limits to how much it can endure. Even sitting still involves muscular exertion and can become fatiguing. Your attitude affects your experience of pain and your ability to respond. Being overrun by fear of pain will increase it. The ability to stop and breathe can abate pain.

Stronger measures might be required to interrupt the pain if it interferes with your ability to function. This woman with SCI finds her pain from spasticity disabling:

> More than spasticity, the pain has limited me socially. I had to quit a part-time job because I cannot sit for eight hours a day (the pain is usually worse in the buttocks, aggravated by sitting). I have often said that the pain is the real disability, not so much the paralysis.

As time progresses after an injury or disability, people tend to report less pain. Studies have shown large differences between what people report while in the hospital and what they report later in follow-up meetings with their doctor. In a 1985 study, 60 percent reported pain while in the hospital compared to 17 percent as outpatients.[6] This difference is partly explained by the lesser response of the nervous system as we age, but probably more so by our capacity to adapt. What was once frightening and uncomfortable simply becomes an accustomed sensation we don't even notice unless we put our attention to it. This paraplegic man, twenty-five years after his spinal cord injury, reports:

> I have a strong tingling in my legs and feet that feels like I have been shot with a lot of Novocain, like the dentist uses. But I'm not even aware of it unless I think of it. I know that anybody else feeling what I do in my legs would be very upset and scared by it. To me it's just normal.

To the degree that someone experiences greater pain over time, it is often a result of poor health maintenance which allows urinary, gastrointestinal, skin breakdown, or other health problems to occur.

Of people with spinal cord injuries, estimates of people who experience pain range from 33 to 95 percent. A very small number of these people describe their pain as severe. Dr. Elliot Roth of the Rehabilitation Institute of Chicago estimates that:

> Between one third to one half of all people with SCI have pain and about 10 percent to 20 percent of all patients have severe, disabling pain. Only about 5 percent of them or less undergo surgery for pain.[7]

Most spinal cord pain develops within the first year. In a 1979 study, two thirds of people with spinal cord injury reported onset within six months. It has been observed that those people injured by gunshot are more likely to experience chronic pain.

If pain appears significantly later after a spinal cord injury, your physician can explore the possibility of syringomyelia, the presence of fluid-filled sacs in the spinal cord. This is found in a minority of cases of late onset pain and in only 5 percent of all spinal cord cases overall. For quadriplegics of level C4 and higher, syringomyelia needs to be caught early if it occurs. At that level of injury, breathing is a critical matter, possibly already assisted with a ventilator. Syringomyelia can effectively raise the injury level and further threaten respiratory function.

Syringomyelia often appears early. After an injury, testing with MRI can be complicated if a halo-vest is still being worn to stabilize the neck; however, there are halos made of metals that do not interfere with the imaging process.

There has been a correlation made between pain and intelligence—among other factors—as Dr. Roth notes in his study, "Pain in Spinal Cord Injury":

> Interference with daily activities by the pain tended to occur in patients who were older, of higher intelligence, more depressed, experiencing greater levels of distress, and involved with more negative psychosocial environments.[8]

Difficult to judge

Pain is hard to diagnose. Doctors do their best, but there are so many possibilities that the task is daunting. Descriptions of pain are subjective, not exact. People variously describe pain as being burning, tingling, stabbing, achy, pins and needles, numb, shooting, throbbing, cramping, freezing, stinging, or crushing. X-rays do not show soft tissue, often the source of pain. MRI or CAT scan tests are expensive and sometimes uncomfortable.

The difficulty of diagnosis forces doctors to use a process of elimination. They make an informed guess of the cause and treat accordingly. If the treatment doesn't work, they move on to the next possible theory. They will do this process conservatively, beginning with the least invasive approach. Some doctors might suggest beginning with biofeedback or self-hypnosis. Most doctors will save surgery for the last resort.

Symptoms can overlap or be misdiagnosed. Pain is sometimes referred—experienced in a different part of the body. With tissue pain, trigger points can be activated in the muscles, but the pain is usually experienced in another location. This is known as myofascial trigger point theory, and not all doctors subscribe to its concepts. Yet most doctors do understand that a disorder in one part of the body can express itself elsewhere. For example, gall bladder pain can sometimes appear as pain in the shoulder.

Doctors might not take your pain seriously. If examination and tests reveal nothing physical, they might say it's "all in your head" and leave it for you to deal with. This was the experience of a woman with post-poliomyelitis syndrome. After feeling stable for many years, she began to experience pain:

> I have been reluctant to talk to my doctor about my muscle pains, because every time I go, she insists that it is merely a muscle pull or tendinitis. I have gone to her so much about these "muscle pains" she thinks I am a hypochondriac and refuses to believe that post-polio even exists!

Tissue pain

Musculoskeletal or mechanical pain involves muscles, tendons, ligaments, or bony abnormalities. It can result from overuse. This type of pain is increasingly typical of longtime chair riders.

Muscles are generally able to recover with rest, stretching, and appropriate exercise. When tendons or bursae—fluid-filled sacs which help lubricate and cushion movement in joints—are involved, recovery can be more difficult, and chronic recurrence is more likely. There is less blood flowing to these tissues, so the body has more difficulty repairing strained cells.

Shoulder tendinitis is the most common tissue pain in longtime chair users. Chair users, particularly manual chair users, use their arms to replace the work of legs and place an increased workload on shoulders. For quadriplegics, shoulder, arm, and neck pain are also common because those muscles are the only ones available to do the work once shared by muscles in the trunk. In spinal cord injury populations, studies have found rates of shoulder tendinitis as high as 31 percent. Another study equated shoulder pain to years of disability; it found 52 percent reporting pain after five years, 62 percent at ten years, 72 percent at fifteen years, and 100 percent at twenty years.[9]

Learn optimal transfer techniques to minimize tissue strain which can produce pain. Transferring to and from your chair from different heights, over a distance, or without brakes (which requires you to grip with more force or throw yourself into the chair) are more likely to cause pain or injury.

Carpal tunnel syndrome is common for manual wheelers. When wheeling, the wrist is in a position of extension (bent backwards at the wrist) while applying pressure on the palm. This strains the median nerve which travels through a narrow opening in the wrist called the carpal tunnel. Symptoms usually include tingling in the fingertips, thumb, or palm. Nerve injuries such as this—including ulnar nerve entrapment at the elbow and wrist, or thoracic outlet syndrome in which nerves are compressed in the neck and shoulder—are serious and can become permanent if allowed to be become advanced.

When muscles are weakened or unusable, and if a joint is limited or bone fused—as in a spinal fusion of neighboring vertebrae—more stress is placed on nearby tissues and joints. If a muscle is not doing its share, other muscles must pitch in to make up the difference, and so the risk of overuse is increased. In the same way, if a vertebra cannot move, more force is transferred to the next vertebrae. Spinal fusions are common in spinal cord injury, as are the installation of metal rods to either manage scoliosis or reduce the time of acute hospitalization prior to rehab. The resulting overuse of neighboring tissues and structure becomes a source of musculoskeletal pain.

These measures will help you minimize mechanical pain:

- Be active. Keep your body flexible and strong.
- Move patiently and with awareness, avoiding unnecessary force, exertion, and strain.
- Design exercises that do not stress tissues.
- Reduce stress in your environment—the spring tension in doors, the weight of objects, an incorrect or poorly maintained wheelchair, etc.
- Adjust the wheelchair for optimal propulsion, keep tires inflated, etc.

Visceral or abdominal pain

Visceral (deep) pain is equated with abdominal pain. It can be caused by bladder and kidney infections, bowel constipation and impaction, peptic ulcers, gall bladder or kidney stones. Sweating, changes in blood pressure, or increased spasticity are often associated with visceral pain and pressure sores.

When control of the abdominal muscles is lost, internal organs have a weakened support structure. The lack of support can stress kidneys, bladder, stomach, etc. Initial sensations, such as spasticity, nausea, or fever, might not be perceived or could be mistaken for something else, such as a urinary infection. Dr. Roth writes that, "acute abdominal catastrophes were responsible for up to 10 percent of deaths in patients with SCI" (in two reviewed studies).[10]

Spasticity in abdominal wall muscles can be very painful, and possibly mistaken for problems in internal organs. As with spasticity in general, movement or sensory stimulation might evoke the spasm. Spasms localized to the abdomen could indicate a deeper, systemic problem. Your physician should first attempt to rule out spasticity as the cause of pain before settling on a diagnosis of a deeper organ disorder.

Most visceral pain involves constipation and impaction, which can be experienced as a feeling of fullness or bloatedness. Keeping a regular bowel program helps your doctor diagnose pain. Your doctor can more easily rule out the bowels and determine the source of your pain sooner, avoiding the chance of a problem escalating into a life-threatening emergency.

Neuropathic pain

Many disabilities affect the nervous system. Pathways that generate and carry messages of pain are functionally impaired; pain signals can result from sensory confusion in the body. Spasticity is an example of how the nervous system gets caught in a loop, with muscle impulses bouncing around in muscles because the brain can't turn them off. Sensory signals are thought to be capable of behaving in a similar way. "Phantom" pain, experienced by people with amputation, is a case in point. The limb is no longer there, but the sensory system still thinks it is and continues to generate sensations which seem to come from the missing limb. Pain from brain and spinal cord conditions seem to share some of the mechanisms related to phantom pain.

Pain can signal that something is going on in the body that merits attention, just as muscle spasms can signal infection, a full bladder, or other conditions:

I don't experience spasmodic muscle contractions, but when I have an infection, or a sore, or even the flu or a cold, there is a spot on my right thigh that will spasm with pain. Sometimes it is just like someone plunging a knife into my leg. The spasms only last for seconds at a time, but if I am really sick, it can happen many times an hour and is really exhausting. I have learned to pay attention very early if I feel the smaller shocks that usually appear at first. Sometimes it just means I've been sitting too long.

The same therapies used to manage muscle spasticity often help with pain, although doctors can't always explain why. The drug 4-Aminopyridine is presently in tests as a method of increasing function for people with spinal cord injury and multiple sclerosis. It helps by amplifying nerve impulses past areas of myelin damage, the material which insulates nerves. Researchers were surprised to find that a drug that increases nerve impulses also helped to temper muscle and sensory spasticity in some people.

Pain management

Pain management demands a good working relationship with your physician to develop the best strategy. Physicians can't magically identify the exact cause and make it go away. Dr. Roth, writing for other spinal cord physicians, states:

Successful treatment of pain relies heavily on the patience, cooperation, collaboration, and ingenuity of the patient and the professional alike. This means that active listening and taking complaints seriously are keys to successful diagnosis and management.[11]

The least invasive approach to manage pain is always preferred. Start with an active lifestyle—even if it is only performing regular range-of-motion exercises with an assistant, or alternating time in and out of your wheels as you're able—and maintain a healthy diet. Avoid factors that cause pain, such as infections, sores, or bladder and bowel disorders. Don't abuse alcohol, drugs, or tobacco. These things might seem like a source of relief from your pain, but in the long term they only aggravate it.

People are increasingly exploring what are called alternative (or complementary or holistic) measures to manage pain.

Emotions have a great impact on pain and don't have to be treated with drugs. Dr. Roth writes:

> Emotional well-being appears to exert a great positive effect on pain relief. Psychological stress, hostility, anxiety, or depression may precipitate or exacerbate pain.[12]

Fostering friendships, having satisfying activities, getting out into the world, or watching a funny movie can play important roles in your health. They help keep you out of pain. They help you remain focused on the external rather than dwelling on the internal.

Biofeedback is a method in which electrodes are placed on your head to read brain waves. A readout of brain activity appears on a meter or a computer screen. By relaxing and noticing the effects of your thoughts and breathing on brain-wave activity, you can learn to control stress and muscular tension. Biofeedback training allows you to take these skills into your daily life, using what you learned while using the machine.

In the film *Mask*, a young man has a disfiguring disease which sometimes puts great pressure on his brain and spine, causing great pain. His solution is to visualize a beautiful place and describe it in detail, closing his eyes and breathing deeply. Although this example is fictional, visualization is a valid pain management technique.

This woman found benefits in acupressure, a form of massage therapy that uses some of the same theories as Chinese acupuncture:

> I never believed in acupressure. My fiancé took a course in it before I met him. He did the acupressure and it worked. For the first time in fifteen years I was pain-free. I can't tell you how much massage and getting the blood to flow makes a difference. I can't move at times. I lay down and he does his thing and I am pain-free the rest of the day. My problem has been insurance and doctors not believing me.

There has been much interest in electrical stimulation as a means of pain management. TENS—transcutaneous electrical nerve stimulation—stimulates peripheral nerves and has the effect of diminishing pain. A TENS unit can be used at home without skilled assistance, after it has been set up by a therapist or trained professional and explained to you. It is a small unit—the size of a transistor radio—with electrodes which are applied to the surface of the skin. Its effect is temporary, but a 1977 study of seven quadriplegics and thirty-two paraplegics showed that half of them found complete or nearly complete relief with TENS. Another 41 percent had moderate relief. TENS was more effective with musculoskeletal pain. Pain rooted closer to the spinal cord or brain did not respond as well.[13]

Strong pain elicits strong emotions, and at some point you need a break. If you are disabled by pain, if it interrupts your sleep cycle, prevents you from being able to maintain your health with exercise and activity, then it might make sense to cautiously and carefully employ drugs to manage your pain.

Many drugs are used to manage pain. Some of them have significant side effects, such as reducing your sexual impulses. Many pain drugs are also sedatives which will affect your clarity, cause constipation, affect your appetite, and so on. A pain medication could interact badly with a drug you are taking for another reason. Drugs should be used only when their value outweighs the side effects. Any prescribing physician should know all of the drugs you take.

The body has a way of adapting to drugs. After a while you might need a larger dose, or the drug might not work at all.

The last resort to treating pain is surgery. The dorsal rhizotomy is a procedure to cut nerves to simply turn off the pain impulse. More extreme is surgery to cut the spinal cord below the level of injury. This procedure is known as a cordotomy. Since it obviously can't be reversed, it would be performed in only the most severe cases. If injury to the spinal cord was not complete before the surgery, some function or useful sensation could be lost after the surgery.

Success rates are not high with these surgical procedures. Studies have found only half of people who underwent cordotomy experienced permanent relief. The percentage was 65 percent for people who had dorsal rhizotomy.[14]

Pressure sores

Perhaps the greatest scourge of wheelchair users is the danger of developing pressure sores from sitting for long periods of time or from being in bed. Sores—or decubitus ulcers—can take many months to heal, or require surgery or hospitalization. There was a time when insurance would pay for admission to a rehabilitation facility where you can remain active as you heal. But in the present health-delivery environment you are more likely find yourself spending your time at home in bed or in a nursing home.

Pressure sores can even be serious enough to cause death, if not cared for properly. Large sores present a great danger of infection with so much tissue exposed, often at deep levels below the skin. Ignoring smaller sores is a big mistake. They will inevitably become large if left untreated.

There are three stages of pressure sore development:

- Stage One: Redness of the skin. This stage might last for a short time, as circulation is restored to the area. The longer it lasts, the higher the risk of skin breakdown and the greater the need for caution. The area will be warm to the touch if it is approaching skin breakdown.

- Stage Two: An open area or blister appears. The skin might darken to a blackish color. This indicates cell death, and an open sore is inevitable. Remove all contact from the area to minimize any further cell death and to prevent the resulting sore from being any deeper than necessary.

- Stage Three: Open wound into deeper layers of the skin. Risk of infection is very high, particularly for sores close to the anal opening. Your doctor can prescribe medications to be applied to prevent infection and promote healing.

At its worst, a severe sore can progress into tendon, muscle, and even bone tissues. Such sores are likely to require surgery, either to stitch them closed (not always possible) or to perform a "flap" where a thin layer of skin is taken from another part of the body and grafted onto the sore. A long hospital stay will be necessary to allow the skin to integrate itself into the new location, and for the wound where the flap was taken to heal. Flaps do not always take, so all this time can be spent for naught. The need to limit your activity and stay in bed can produce additional sores in the process, trapping you in a downward spiral of skin breakdown. Be very serious about pressure sores. They are not worth the risk of these horrible possibilities.

Caring for a sore

Keep the sore clean so it can heal. Dead tissue or bacteria will slow the healing process and increase the chance of infection. Dead tissue and dried blood must be removed for healing to proceed effectively. You may be able to remove this yourself—for example, with wet-to-dry dressings. This process should not be painful. If it is, see your doctor. A doctor might need to remove the tissue with a process called debridement. Some people experience pain during the procedure, in which case your doctor could recommend pain medication.

The sore should be cleaned every time bandages are changed. Your doctor might recommend a cleaning solution, such as saline solution, to irrigate the sore. Saline solution can be purchased at the drugstore, or you can make it yourself by dissolving eight teaspoons of table salt in one gallon of distilled water. Make sure the salt is completely dissolved, and that you use clean utensils for measuring and stirring. Antiseptics such as hydrogen peroxide or iodine—although known for killing bacteria—are not recommended, as they can damage sensitive tissue.

Your doctor might recommend any of several measures to help the sore heal:

- **Wet-to-dry dressings.** Dead tissue adheres to this special dressing as it dries and comes off when the bandage is removed.

- **Hydrocolloid dressings.** These dressings retain oxygen and moisture. Sometimes they are left on for days at a time.

- **Enzyme medications.** These medications dissolve only dead tissues.

- **Gauze.** Often gauze is soaked with saline solution. It must be kept moist, or it could pull off new tissue when it is removed.

- **Hydroactive dressings.** Dressings such as DuoDerm are left on for days and allow the body's own enzymes to dissolve dead tissue.

- **Electrotherapy.** A recently developed approach that applies a very small current to the tissue to stimulate healing.

When there is infection present, dressings must be changed often, so hydrocolloid and hydroactive dressings are not used. Infection is potentially serious, as it can spread to tissues or bone. Report any redness or swelling to your physician.

Diet for healing pressure sores

When you are trying to get a pressure sore to heal, it is critical to support healing with diet. When you have a sore, good nutrition is important because the body is trying to rebuild a part of itself and needs proteins and nutrients as building materials.

When a sore occurs, a great deal of protein can be lost from the sore itself, depending on its size. Protein should be included in a healing diet. Good quality protein for healing comes from eating whole grains—brown rice, quinoa, bulgar wheat, and rye—and beans—lentils, peas, chickpeas, kidney, pinto, and lima. Vegetable and grain proteins are more effectively metabolized by the body than meat, and don't include other elements that place a load on the body such as fats or remnants of drugs used to fatten livestock. Use animal foods judiciously rather than relying on them as a primary protein source. Processed sugar—hidden in most commercially produced foods—uses up other nutrients when it is digested, robbing the areas that need them. White, processed flour has a similar effect.

Stress disrupts the process of healing, causing nutrients to be excreted from the body. B-vitamins and C can be supplemented in your diet to make up for loss from stress, but it is best to control stress. While it is upsetting to have a sore—with the possibility of having to limit yourself for weeks or more—giving in to fears hinders the process of healing. Do what you can to avoid falling into the trap of constant emotional—and therefore physical—stress which only interferes with your recovery.

Surgical treatments

Some people with chronic pressure sores opt for a surgical procedure known as an ischial shave. In an ischial shave, the ischial bones, or "sit bones," are flattened to spread the pressure across a wider area of the skin of the buttocks, reducing the risk of skin breakdown. The surgery is generally performed by a plastic surgeon and involves a minimum of three weeks for the surgery to heal, some or all of which will be spent in a hospital, rehab center, or nursing home until it is possible to place pressure on the area by sitting once again.

In rare cases, the tissue beneath the incision can heal improperly and break down quickly once you start to sit:

> Problems after my ischial shave meant another four weeks in rehab, basically starting back from scratch.

> In retrospect, I can't say for certain that I really needed the procedure. I chose it at an early stage of my disability when I was having repeated problems with skin breakdown. Problems were probably as much a result of sitting for too long on poor cushions, not doing push-ups often

enough, lifting myself up and down stairs sitting on carpeted steps, and because of my unhealthy diet.

Years later, I found that one side has calcified a bit more than the other. I no longer sit symmetrically and require a little extra support on the left side of my wheelchair cushion to balance myself.

It is typical to experience sores more often in early years after an injury while you are still adjusting and integrating self-protective habits into your daily lifestyle. Surgery should always be the last resort after thoroughly exploring noninvasive options.

Scoliosis

Excessive curvature of the spine is a serious problem. The spine supports you and allows you to bend and twist. The spine is meant to work in cooperation with the muscles of our trunk, whose job it is to balance and move us, and to maintain the intended shape of the spine.

The spine's gently curving shape is part of its flexibility. Because the curves are gentle, the spine's structural capacity remains strong. When the curves become severe—or when the spine curves to the side, out of its natural symmetry—the spine's ability to do its job of structural support is compromised. Muscles must start to do more of the work of carrying us, leading to fatigue, back pain, and continuing degradation of the spine. The further curvature and degradation progresses, the faster the damage happens.

Some people with disabilities have limited use of trunk muscles, particularly for high level quadriplegics from spinal cord injury and those with cerebral palsy, progressive stages of certain muscular dystrophies, multiple sclerosis, and amyotrophic lateral syndrome. Such people are at greater risk of scoliosis (as well as lordosis and kyphosis, which are curvatures in other directions), because muscles are too weak or paralyzed to help keep the spine in alignment.

Prevention

The spine—and the body in general—learns from how it is used. If you spend enough time in slumped and twisted postures, your body learns this state. Muscles, ligaments, and bones will begin to adapt, changing shape and adopting the curvature as normal. Your sitting habits—in or out of the wheelchair—and sleeping positions can either support the proper shape of the spine or teach it to go out of line.

Many chair users hook an arm behind them on a push handle to support the upper body while they reach with the other hand. If you have limited upper body balance, you are at risk of falling over unless you anchor yourself somehow. There is a tendency to reach with your dominant hand and always twist in the same direction, thus teaching the spine to adopt a curve in that direction.

For some people without sufficient upper body strength and balance, pushing a manual wheelchair puts deforming strains on the spine. This spinal cord quadriplegic in his early thirties found that using a manual wheelchair was not really appropriate for him:

> I used a manual chair for ten years. For me it was an ego thing. I really felt that people looked at me differently in a power chair than in a manual chair. The biomechanics of a quadriplegic or a paraplegic operating a manual chair are like the difference between night and day. I have a severe scoliosis from using a manual chair and also from hooking my arm around the back.

The proper specification of wheelchair and positioning systems—backs, cushions, stabilization accessories, etc.—along with vigilant postural management are crucial to preventing spinal curvature. Therapists often do not teach people enough about posture during the rehabilitation process. In the attempt to get comfortable, you might establish poor habits that can contribute to scoliosis. If spinal curvature has not progressed too far, it can be corrected by changing those habits. This man changed habits when he began to see a chiropractor:

> I used to sit in all kinds of curvy, slumping postures. Sitting in a wheelchair most of the day gets uncomfortable, so I was just trying to get some variety. No one ever talked to me about these issues. Then I went to see a chiropractor who took x-rays that showed my spine was very curvy. He taught me better posture, got me using a back cushion, and did regular adjustments to free up my spine to realign itself. After six months the difference in the x-rays was amazing, and now people comment on my good posture. Best of all, it's my natural posture now, even though at first it was an effort to sit straight. Now it's comfortable.

Wheelchair riders need a variety of posture because the body needs movement and comfort. Good posture is a matter of being conscious of how you hold your body, spending more time comfortably supported upright, and spending brief amounts of time in nonneutral postures. When you slouch to the right, next time do it to the left.

To the degree that you still have sufficient upper body balance and control, the risk of spinal curvature can be prevented by having the right equipment and knowing how you use your body. Being active, maintaining range of motion, and being aware of your posture are key to maintaining the health of your spine and avoiding the daunting impact of scoliosis.

What goes wrong?

A number of undesirable things happen when the spine goes out of shape. The muscles and ligaments around the spine get stretched out of shape, compromising their ability to support the spine and causing discomfort and pain. In the long term, it becomes difficult to sit for more than brief periods of time.

When the spine deforms, the rib cage also deforms; the lungs are compressed, compromising the ability to breathe fully.

As the spine deforms, the discs between the vertebrae get squeezed. Discs are gelatinous cushions, key to the flexibility of the spine. When the discs get compressed, they change their shape, get pushed out of position, and begin to lose some of their gelatinous fluid. It is very difficult for the discs to regain their shape, and once fluid is lost, it cannot be replaced. Damage is permanent.

Discs also help maintain the space where nerves extend from the spinal cord to the rest of the body. When the space between vertebrae gets smaller, nerves are pressed, causing damage and pain. This compression might cost you the ability to use parts of the body previously unaffected by your disability. Ultimately, neighboring vertebrae come into contact and begin to fuse. The flexibility of that "joint" in the spine is lost. If the curvature is severe enough, the spinal cord itself can be at risk of a compression injury.

Surgery

When scoliosis is allowed to progress, surgery becomes necessary. The typical approach is the installation of Harrington rods, steel bars attached to the straightened spine. Harrington rods maintain the shape of the spine without relying on muscles of the back. The surgery is very involved, and the rods limit the freedom of the spine to move, imposing a rigid upright posture on the person. In rare instances, there is a risk of injury to the spinal cord from the surgery.

When scoliosis has become progressive, the surgery can be lifesaving. Many people feel a great relief to have an upright, symmetrical posture again, despite the rigidity. For people born with cerebral palsy, certain muscular dystrophies, or other childhood disabilities that affect the back, this surgery is often necessary early in life, and can make a significant difference in the quality of life.

Spasticity

Spasticity is an issue for people with spastic cerebral palsy, spinal cord injuries in the thoracic and cervical regions, multiple sclerosis, ALS, and other conditions involving the spinal cord and brain. Spasticity can be a daily event—painful and significant enough to interfere with functional ability. Spasticity is particularly common for people with cerebral palsy, many of whom are able to walk, but greatly limited by spasticity. Many with CP choose to use wheels rather than invite spasms by the effort of walking.

There are distinct differences between spasticity in spinal and cerebral forms of disability. After spinal cord injury, spasticity doesn't begin immediately, but can take weeks or months to develop. In cerebral palsy or TBI, spasticity is less a matter of a loop trapped beneath the thoracic spinal level, and instead is a matter of how the messages get mixed in the brain.

How seriously spasms affect someone's life varies. They can be extremely painful and severely limit your ability to function. Or they can be an aggravating, occasional event, as this woman with a spinal cord injury reports:

> Generally spasms aren't terribly painful, just terribly bothersome. They make it hard to transfer and keep me awake sometimes at night. I have had a decrease in spasms since my release from rehab in 1996. I attribute the decrease to better medications. One kind of spasm has never changed: every time I lie down flat on my back, I get terrific extensor spasms (my legs become stiff as boards and my feet and toes curl outward). This usually subsides within a few seconds. But sometimes when I try to get up, it happens all over again.

Contracting a muscle is not a simple, one-way communication, where the brain sends a message and the muscle contracts. Instead, the communication between brain and muscle is two-way and more complex. The brain is getting immediate feedback from the muscle, about how much it has contracted, whether it is fatigued, and if there is pain, for instance. The communication is a loop of nerve impulses going back and forth.

Not all impulses to a muscle originate in the brain. Direct stimulation of the muscle causes a reflex response. This is what happens when a doctor taps you on the elbow with that little rubber hammer. The muscle responds with a contraction. With a central nervous system disruption, this loop of communication between brain and muscle can get interrupted. Reflexes run amuck, resulting in spasms; the brain is unable to sense the muscle contracting, and then send the appropriate messages to the muscle to calm the reflex. Spasms could be a brief episode in which parts of your body would suddenly move, sometimes in a repetitive, vibrating manner. The legs can extend or flex. High quadriplegics can also experience spasms in the arms.

Spasticity can also be chronic, pulling the body into positions which can lead to scoliosis, digestive problems, or resistance to making movements because of shortened muscles. In the past, chronic muscle contracture was treated only with physical therapy by stretching muscles or by cutting them surgically to release them.

Not all bad news

Spasticity is not always a bad thing. Spasms exercise your muscles since they are contracting; the only other way to exercise paralyzed muscles is with direct electrical stimulation. By maintaining muscle tone, you can be protected from pressure sores that are more likely with atrophied muscles. For quadriplegics, this muscle tone can play a role in maintaining postural integrity—the increased muscle bulk provides better trunk support. Many people find they are able to wear shorts, being less self-conscious of their legs, which remain muscular. Some who are counting on the future results of spinal cord cure research feel that keeping muscle tone improves their chances of being able to benefit from possible advances.

Increases in spasticity can serve as an early warning system for other changes in health, such as infections, an over-full bladder, a pressure sore, the presence of an injury you cannot feel, or more serious conditions such as the development of a spinal cyst (known as syringomyelia), spinal tumors, transverse myelitis, or Guillain-Barre syndrome, for example. Any changes in the general pattern of your spasticity should not be ignored—it might be an important sign.

Some people take advantage of spasticity to help them make transfers to and from their wheels, or to assist in emptying their bladder. However, spasms can also interfere with transfers, when they are more likely to occur. Spasms can force you constantly out of position in your chair, adding to the challenge of anyone assisting you who must manage your posture throughout the day.

There are three approaches to spasticity, depending on how it affects you: managing it on your own, pharmaceutical, and surgical. Doctors will often not treat spasticity unless it is disrupting the ability to make transfers, the ability to sleep, or is a substantial source of pain. Other times, you might be treated by a doctor who considers spasticity something to always prevent:

> I use spasticity. I work out my legs by inducing spasms. I just know how to do it.

> It was another irony of rehab that they put me on Baclofen to get rid of my spasms. When my leg extends in a spasm, I can feel it and it feels good. They wanted to get rid of that. To the extent where spasticity gets in the way of function, I would say yes, that needs to be controlled. I've known people who've had spasms where they almost fall out of their chair. But they didn't really consider me well enough to gauge that.

Managing it on your own

Some people manage their moderate spasticity on their own, learning how to avoid stimulations that cause spasms and knowing how to respond to calm the response if it occurs. For others, the spasticity is too strong a response and needs more significant measures to manage.

Stress increases spasticity, so relaxation methods are valuable. Simple breathing exercises and self-hypnosis can help moderate spasms. If you sense spasms coming and they are painful for you, you are more likely to become tense and upset, which actually promotes the spasms. Learning how to relax in response to the onset of spasms is a useful skill.

This woman with SCI has found a gentle approach to managing her spasticity:

> Warm water and massage are definitely helpful. I'm fortunate that one of my former rehab nurses has a massage certificate and comes to my home twice a month for massage sessions. She also does range-of-motion [exercises] and I can ask her questions about SCI-related topics. She is a gem! I highly recommend massage to anyone with SCI. It is so beneficial, not only with spasticity and pain management, but it gives such a feeling of well-being and relaxation.

Certain postures are known to promote or inhibit specific reflex patterns. Lying in the prone position, face down, tends to inhibit flexion, in which the body would close toward the fetal position. Standing also inhibits flexion, which would interfere with walking. Sitting promotes flexion. Lying on your side or face up (supine) tends to inhibit extension in which the arms, legs, and hips open up.

Spasticity promotes contracture—in which muscles are trained into chronically shortened positions. It is important to counteract spastic muscles with stretching and range-of-motion exercises, to prevent the body from becoming restricted in its ability to move and achieve comfortable postures.

Stimulants like coffee and caffeinated tea generate more nervous system activity, so can increase spasms. Relaxing drinks like chamomile tea have a calming effect. Kava kava is an herb which some people have found helps them manage symptoms:

> I read about kava kava online. I use it at night when my spasms are worse. They would keep me up at night. Using kava kava I have been getting the best night sleep in years. I have tried both baclofen and Robaxen, and the kava kava works better than either for me.

Your general health has an impact on spasticity. Being overweight and eating a poor diet—especially with too much sugar, which is a stimulant—adds stress to your nervous system.

Pharmaceutical management

The most well-known drug for managing spasticity is baclofen, known commercially as Lioresal. Baclofen is similar in chemical structure to GABA, a neurotransmitter deficient in people with spasticity. In some cases, baclofen has also been found to improve bladder control. In rare instances, reversible coma occurred from toxic levels of baclofen.

Baclofen is available as an oral medication, but if taken orally, little of the drug actually reaches the spinal fluid where it must do its work. The oral form only lasts in the bloodstream for eight hours.

Baclofen is more commonly used with an intrathecal pump which supplies a continuous stream of the drug directly to the spinal fluid. With this method of distribution, only 1/100th of the typical oral dose need be taken. The baclofen pump is surgically implanted underneath the skin and needs to be replaced every four to five years. The pump must be refilled every month or two by means of an injection.

The next most common medication is diazepam, sold as Valium. Diazepam is a muscle relaxant and sedative. It is absorbed quickly by the body and stays in the system longer than baclofen when taken orally. Still, diazepam needs to be taken two to three times per day. Diazepam works on the brain, causes drowsiness, and can lead to dependence.

The medication dantrolene—sold as Dantrium—weakens the muscles themselves, so is less likely to cause drowsiness or other central nervous system side effects common with sedatives. Dantrolene is more preferred for cerebral forms of spasticity. It is considered helpful for spasticity in multiple sclerosis which is predominately spinal. In a small percentage of users the drug has caused slight liver damage. There is some concern that it could exacerbate seizures in people with cerebral palsy.

Several other drugs are also used for spasticity, including tizanidine (Zanaflex) and vigabatrin (Sabril). As with all medications, be sure to ask your doctor specifically how the drugs function in your body, why she recommends it in your case, and what possible side effects could occur. For example, the medications might affect memory, emotional state, concentration, and energy level.

Drugs can also be injected directly into muscles, selectively impeding the spastic response. Alcohol and phenol have commonly been used for this purpose over the last twenty years, but are painful to people with sensation. Botulinum toxin (Botox) is a purified form of the toxin that causes botulism or food poisoning. It is safely injected into muscle and is now frequently used, particularly with children with CP. Botox injections are also found useful for abnormal facial contractions in multiple sclerosis. Botox usually takes two to three days to take effect, and can last for as long as two to four months. With the advent of the baclofen pump, Botox injections are used far less frequently.

> We tried Valium during rehab and I cried for three days—not a good choice. Baclofen definitely helps (I take 100 mg/day). Another beneficial drug is dantrium. I have had good luck with it, but unfortunately it is extremely expensive and sort of hard on your liver. I'm trying to decrease it (from 300 mg/day to 200 mg/day).

> I have a quadriplegic friend who had a baclofen pump installed and he said it changed his life.

Surgical treatment

The baclofen pump has also supplanted surgical measures which were once widespread. Aside from the aforementioned cutting of tendons—known as a tenotomy—the most typical surgery was the dorsal rhizotomy, still an option in some cases. In a dorsal rhizotomy the surgeon operates on the nerves in the spinal canal which branch out to the areas where a person experiences spasms. Under general anesthesia, he will literally test each nerve branch for abnormal responses to stimulation, and then cut, burn, or chemically injure those peripheral nerves to interrupt the spastic response.

For people who are functionally impaired by spasticity, experience considerable pain, and have no expectation of recovering use of the muscles fed by those nerves, a dorsal rhizotomy might remain a valid option which could make a great difference in quality of life. It is generally reserved for severe cases.

Tendon transfer is another option a surgeon might consider. This procedure moves the tendon attached to a spastic muscle to another connection where its force can be used. For example, it could use a spastic response to aid in the movement of a hand or elbow, or the ability to lift a foot while walking, a common issue for stroke survivors. This operation is very complex, and requires a surgeon to identify very specifically what muscles are impaired and which ones have a controllable spastic response in order to determine if a transfer could be of rehabilitative value.

Spasticity and aging

Getting older might itself lessen the effects of spasticity. Nerve conduction slows as we age and muscle mass and blood flow to the spinal cord become reduced.

At the same time, as you age your body also gets more sensitive, and your ability to be patient with spasms or pain might be reduced. If you experience overuse injuries with age, this also might cause spasms to be painful, which in the past could be better endured.

Stress

The human body's stress reaction is referred to as the "fight or flight" response. To help you fight with your arms or run away from danger, the body increases its heart rate and sends blood to the outer extremities. When you are experiencing stress reaction, blood is taken away from your digestive tract. While you are under stress you are not absorbing nutrients effectively; they are instead excreted through your bodily wastes. Vitamin C is lost in large amounts to the stress response.

Under stress there is a tendency to limit the breath and the amount of fresh oxygen you take into your body. Shallow breathing also involves holding muscles of the trunk, abdomen, and often the shoulders and neck in constant, low-level exertion. For people with pulmonary limitations as a factor of their disability, stress only decreases their respiratory efficiency.

There are a number of unique stresses you might experience as a wheelchair user:

- The effort of pushing a wheelchair raises your body's metabolic processes in ways that mimic a continual stress response.

- Awkwardness in handling your body while wheeling, transferring, or performing daily tasks such as work or cooking that preclude the relaxed state.

- Some daily tasks such as dressing or using the bathroom could be strenuous for you.

- You might experience psychological stresses from worrying how others see you, particularly at stages of disability when you are adapting to your new identity as a chair rider.

- You might experience discrimination, such as being denied access to jobs or transportation.
- You might face stresses with bureaucracies such as Social Security, Vocational Rehabilitation, Medicare, or other systems which you must rely on for support.

The simple act of breathing is an extremely valuable stress manager. When you take a couple of deep breaths and close your eyes, you can discover where you are holding physical tension in your muscles. Breathing allows you to notice that your belly is tight, your shoulders slightly raised, or that you are holding your head in a limited range. If you don't have the use of your trunk muscles, keeping the area around the lungs relaxed is all the more important.

You already know how to breathe, of course, but you might be in the habit of breathing only in your chest. Even if your disability precludes the use of your abdominal muscles, you can imagine your breath starting from that lower part of your body. Imagine that the air you are breathing first goes all the way down to the very bottom of your lungs and out to the farthest small branches of the brachial "trees" that make up your lungs. As you practice this method, you will find that you are able to take in more air comfortably. This ability to breathe deeply will help you counteract the stress response.

Another important technique for stress management is your own thinking. When there are parts of your life that are upsetting, staying focused on those problems increases the negative impact of the resulting stress. In time, you lose perspective and the ability to think objectively. Certainly it is healthy to experience emotions about events and challenges in your life, but not to be continually overwhelmed by them. You can minimize the effect of stress by doing your best to relax, giving your attention to other activities and allowing your mind to have a rest from what is troubling you. When you come back to thinking about a problem you will likely have a fresh perspective, and your body will not suffer so much from the tension, loss of nutrients, and other detrimental effects of excessive stress.

Meditation might sound like something that only Buddhist monks or Californians do, but it is a simple and powerful tool available to anyone, anywhere. Meditation is not about going into a trance, nor is it about superhuman concentration. To meditate, all you do is sit comfortably and pay attention to your breath. That's all. Your thoughts will continue, but each time you notice getting caught up in a certain thought, just put your attention back to your breathing. Decide that for the fifteen minutes you will spend in meditation that any thought that comes to you will still be around later, and you don't have to stop and explore it. The simple act of observing the breath will allow you to gain a fresh perspective, and help to moderate physical tension and emotions. Try it once a day for a week, without judgment, and see what happens.

Urinary tract infections

Urinary tract infections or bladder infections are a constant risk for those with a neurogenic bladder. If not cared for promptly, urinary tract infection (UTI) can make you severely ill with high fever, spread to the kidneys, and ultimately kill you. However, the only reason an infection would reach these proportions is if you don't take care of yourself.

Multiple sclerosis is often treated with immunosuppressive drugs that increase the risk of infection. Urinary complications are common with multiple sclerosis. Women more frequently have neurogenic bladders with MS than men do, and so have more UTI. When men with MS get infections, however, they tend to be more severe.

Some people with disabilities experience low-grade bladder infections two or three times a year without the infections being a major problem. Many other people find they constantly struggle with more severe UTIs. They find it difficult to hold a job or make social commitments because of the frequency of occurrence.

Despite a good bladder program, some people continue to struggle with urinary tract infections. It has been a chronic problem for this thirty-five-year-old woman with L5 paraplegia from a spinal cord injury:

> I've been plagued by UTIs. I've been getting them every month. They've been associated with my period. It's been like clockwork, when my period's ending. I've tried almost everything. Drinking a lot. Cranberry juice and pills. I've tried herbal remedies. Anticholinergics. Vitamin C. Irrigation. The only thing I haven't tried is prophylactic antibiotics.

> When I get them, it tires me. I fatigue fast. I have to go to the bathroom a lot more. I become more incontinent so have to wear more padding. It's a drag, and it can't be good for my kidneys.

The three most common sources of UTI are:

- Failing to drink enough and empty the bladder often
- Picking up infection from a sexual partner
- Bacteria carried into the bladder on a catheter

The answer to the first is obvious—drink enough and commit to a regular bladder program appropriate to your needs. The second is solved by using condoms, urinating after sex, and paying attention to signs of infection which indicate that you should employ sexual options other than intercourse until the condition clears. People who use catheters have a harder time preventing infections completely because they are regularly inserting a foreign object into their body. No matter how well you clean the catheter, some bacteria is going to get in. Nonetheless, practice the cleanest habits you can.

Signs of a urinary infection include:

- Fever
- Sweating and chills
- Nausea and vomiting
- Increased spasticity
- Difficulty urinating
- Pain during urination
- Cloudy or foul smelling urine
- Bloody urine (pink, red, or rusty in color)
- Change in volume of urine—either more or less
- Sudden onset of leaking between catheterizations

When you have a UTI you need to drink two to three additional glasses of water each day to help flush out the bacteria and prevent the infection from multiplying and spreading. Visit your urologist who will take a culture from your urine to determine an appropriate antibiotic, if necessary. People with chronic infections need to be careful with antibiotics. Overuse allows the body to build a resistance to antibiotics, rendering them ineffective for treating future infections.

Stones are another risk with a neurogenic bladder. Excessive calcium can collect in the bladder, kidney, or the ureters which pass between them. The formation of stones is encouraged by residual urine, chronic infections, incorrect catheterization, lack of fluids, or lack of physical activity. The ureters can become blocked by stones, increasing backup into the kidneys. Symptoms include sweating, severe pain, blood in the urine, increased spasticity, or pain in the lower back or abdomen. Stones are usually removed surgically, though there are new techniques being developed such as using sound to crush the stones.

As a diagnostic test, a urologist might perform:

- A renal scan or ultrasound, in which a dye is injected into the body which is flushed through the kidneys. An x-ray is then able to reveal the condition of the urinary tract.

- An intravenous pyleogram (IVP), similar to the above, although it is necessary to also empty the bowels.

- A cystoscopy, which is a visual examination inside the urinary tract with a cystoscope, inserted by catheter through the urethra, to inspect for stones.

Many physiatrists recommend that a renal scan or IVP be routinely performed every two years for people with neurogenic bladders as a preventative management measure.

CHAPTER 4

Staying Healthy

Your level of independence and function depends in large part on good health maintenance. Your energy, strength, weight, and the prevention of any potential complications particular to your disability all need regular attention. The more you build healthy routines into your life, the more they become simple habit and the less they seem like work.

Health maintenance is admittedly more work for some than for others. If your bladder routine requires catheterization, you have to commit more time and pay extra attention to diet and cleanliness. If you are limited in upper body strength, exercise options are more limited and weight gain is a greater risk.

This chapter addresses general health practices. We first talk about exercise—how to get enough, and approaches to cardiovascular health, strength building, and stretching. Next, we examine how diet impacts your health and discuss particular concerns for those using a wheelchair. We then look at bladder and bowel programs.

Many people with disabilities incorporate alternative therapies into their health maintenance programs; we describe some of those most often used. We next examine how aging will impact your general health, and what you can do to prepare for or ameliorate its effects. We close the chapter with a look at using personal assistance.

Exercise

If you use your body, you will live longer and more happily. It is especially important for chair riders to exercise to the degree possible. An inactive, sedentary lifestyle is an invitation to a variety of undesirable results:

- **Weak muscles.** The parts of the body you can control need exercise to stay strong and vibrant.

- **Cardiovascular loss.** Your ability to function depends on the heart's ability to get healthy blood out to your muscles. A weak heart means early fatigue and long-term decline in your level of activity and independence.

- **Osteoporosis.** Your bones lose density from lack of use.

- **Weight gain.** Calories turn to fat when you don't burn them off with activity. The heavier you get, the harder it is to exercise and so to lose weight. Extra weight adds to the strain on your heart and muscles.

Strength-building exercise

You don't have to be a bodybuilder to maintain strength. Muscle strength is as much a matter of softness and elasticity as it is of bulk. Flexible muscles can travel further when they contract, which translates to additional strength.

Whatever muscles you have voluntary control of can be exercised and kept at an optimal level of mass and elasticity. You can do this without an extreme amount of exertion. It is a myth that to exercise a muscle you have to strain it to exhaustion. Gentle and slow repetitions with little weight will maintain muscle tone, at least, and gradually build strength, at best. Exercising moderately two or three times a week will take you a long way toward attaining the strength, stamina, and general health you desire.

> *I find that a very simple routine of exercising doing push-ups in my wheelchair, using moderate free weights, and other resistance types of workout really makes a big difference. Once after an extended illness I lost some of that tone and really noticed the change in strength.*

Aerobic exercise

Heart disease is a widespread problem in Western culture. Heart disease is a greater risk to many whose mobility is limited. In the mid 1990s, heart disease accounted for almost 20 percent of deaths following spinal cord injury. Persons with cerebral palsy are at somewhat greater risk of cardiopulmonary dysfunction than the general population, accounting for the majority of deaths of adults with CP.

Difficult as exercise may be for some people with a disability, it benefits your quality of life. Aerobic exercise has a number of important benefits:

- It makes the heart stronger and improves circulatory efficiency. The heart is, after all, a muscle too.

- It helps reduce blood pressure and heart rate.

- It helps control your weight.

- It increases endurance for physical activity by helping more blood and oxygen to reach muscles.

Only some manual chair riders are active enough that pushing the chair alone is adequate aerobic exercise to benefit the heart and general fitness. Most manual wheelers do not push enough in the course of an average day to provide for optimal health, nor do they work up a sweat or increase their heart rate in the process, indicators of productive aerobic exercise.

Exercise programs

Unfortunately, medical schools do not teach much about exercise physiology or the preventive values of exercise. Your doctor will encourage you to be active to the degree you are able, and might refer you to physical therapy, but usually for practical purposes like activities of daily living. You should directly ask your doctor and therapists to develop an exercise program specific to your needs. Exercise needs to be a continuing program—not just short-term therapy.

Keeping to an exercise program might seem like an unwanted burden on top of everything else required of you by your disability. But even small amounts of regular exercise make a remarkable difference in a short period of time and more than compensate for whatever inconvenience the exercise entails.

After extensive exercise and training in rehab, this person noticed a decrease in physical abilities as he exercised less:

> I became very busy with my new business out of an office at home. This meant that I was not wheeling around the place where I used to work, not commuting back and forth, and not traveling or going to meetings as I used to. I think all of that physical activity helped keep me in shape. I especially noticed that it was becoming more difficult to transfer into and out of my chair. Suddenly I seemed to be throwing my body more than lifting it. So I started doing simple upper body exercises a few times each week for about fifteen or twenty minutes, and was amazed by how quickly I started to feel the difference. Now my exercise routine is important to me because I know it really works.

The type and duration of exercise appropriate for you is a matter of experimentation and building endurance. You will need to design a program for yourself working with the best qualified doctor and therapist you can find. Any professional who develops an exercise plan for you must clearly understand the physiology of your disability as well as your personal experience. For example, people with MS are sensitive to being overheated and must not let body temperature rise much. People with paraplegia need to take care not to overstrain their shoulders. For people with post-polio syndrome, certain types of exercise can be exactly the wrong thing to do.

> For a long time I pushed and forced myself to exercise, to use a stationary bike, etc., to help my respiratory system and to get myself "fit" after my daughter was born. I didn't know it then, but that was the worst thing that I could have done. Yes, I did need exercise, but I was modeling my exercise program on one that healthy people use. I overtaxed my respiratory system. I made the muscles that had taken over for those that were atrophied work even harder.

Even if you are a high quadriplegic or experience fatigue easily, you can be physically active in ways that benefit your general fitness. Aerobic exercise is very good for the heart, but just being outside enjoying even modest activity is worthwhile. It helps you maintain a more positive attitude and higher spirit.

An exercise program doesn't have to mean lifting weights, pulling on rubber straps, or using some exercise machine. There is a tremendous array of athletic options available. Almost anyone can participate in some form of sport. Many can swim or exercise in water. Bowling, shooting, or archery can be performed by even high quadriplegics with the use of newly developed adaptive devices. Those with higher degrees of function can participate in sports like wheelchair basketball or quad rugby. Accessible sports are discussed in Chapter 11, *Getting Out There*.

Health clubs

Of the vast number of health facilities, few are well equipped for wheelchair access, and staff is rarely trained in issues that relate to disability. Most weight trainers come from a body-building point of view. They are interested in building muscle mass to give your body a bulkier, sculpted look. Building muscle mass is generally not appropriate for a wheelchair user, although those wheelchair users involved in weight lifting or certain other wheelchair sports can benefit from this approach.

Ask whether your physical therapist can visit the health facility with you. She can review the various exercise machines, discuss whether swimming would be an option and how you would actually do it, and help you prepare a program. Asking for such consultation is not an unreasonable request on your part. Therapists are often given approval to make such visits. Your needs are specialized, and health club staff who offer personal training services are unlikely to be able to determine what is right for you. It is especially important that your program is balanced among the various muscle groups.

Some people go to health clubs to show off their bodies, their strength, and to check other people out. As a wheelchair user, you might find yourself uncomfortably conspicuous at first.

> I'd really like to go someplace where I can swim and use the exercise equipment, but it's important to me to have a place to dress and shower in private. I'd rather not be in public with my skinny legs or revealing my catheter. A few newer places are starting to include private dressing rooms with showers, but nothing close enough to where I live at the moment.

> The weight room in my building is all men. For the first six months I took the free weights into the hallway. All these men are grunting and I'm lifting these four-pound weights. But I got over that. I loved it. I saw the change in my body right away.

Standing frames

Two health risks of wheelchair users are softer leg bones and poorer circulation. When legs do not have to carry the weight of the upper body, they begin to lose calcium and become soft. Bones then break more easily on heavy impact.

The act of walking is a pumping action that moves blood through the body. Legs that are inactive have less efficient circulation since their muscles are not helping the process. Always sitting also limits circulation to the legs because of the angles that veins and arteries must pass at the hips and knees. Standing lets gravity help circulation, as blood passes straight down the body without having to turn corners. Circulation is also a matter of hydraulics—the assistance of gravity to bring blood down to your legs also helps it flow upward in the closed pressure system of the body.

The risks of softer leg bones and poorer circulation can be addressed with standing frames, which comprise a growing segment of the medical supply industry. There are three types of standing frames:

- **Fixed.** The frame remains in one place, and does not have a seated position.

- **Movable.** The frame includes wheels within reach, linked by a chain or belt to smaller wheels at the bottom so you can move within a room. Some frames are motorized and move by means of a joystick control like a power wheelchair.

- **Integrated.** Another kind of product is a wheelchair with the capacity to transform into a standing frame. Such a frame is intended for people at work, such as a mechanic who would need to stand beneath an elevated car, or for situations where an extended reach is needed, such as at a supermarket. There are both manual and power models.

Other benefits of standing frames pointed to by manufacturers are reduction of spasms and muscle shortening, less chance of pressure sores, and improved urinary and bowel function since the colon and intestines are constrained in the sitting position (although some physicians do not subscribe to this view). If you have shortened muscles from sitting for many years, a standing frame can be a means of getting your body straightened out again. A product which is able to be set at intermediate angles can allow you to therapeutically stretch in the frame and gradually lengthen your muscles out to a normal posture.

Getting into the standing position is achieved in various ways with different products. Some products have a well-engineered leverage system that allows you to manually lift your own body weight into the standing position with minimal effort. Some products are motorized. Still others may require you to have assistance, particularly if you have insufficient arm strength.

Standing frames support you with a surface behind you which generally contacts the buttocks and might extend as far as down to behind the knees or as far up as the lower back. While it is true that there is still some pressure on the buttocks, it is much less than if you were sitting directly on them. The knees are braced in front, and another support is generally located at the abdomen. All supports are padded for the prevention of pressure sores. Since there will be continual contact while standing, you would need to limit the time spent in any one standing session. Some frames include adjustable footplates. Frames are available with various options, such as a desk platform for writing or reading, storage compartments, and drink holders. Some come in a range of colors.

People with very brittle bones, cardiac disorders, or significant shortening of hip and knee flexor muscles might need to avoid standing frames, but might be able to work their way toward using them with stretching and therapy. You may require a prescription to purchase one.

Diet

The human organism is a biochemical machine. The body relies on water, vitamins, proteins, carbohydrates, fats, and minerals from a balanced diet of pure and healthy foods. There are also some issues to keep in mind as a chair user or because of particular features of your disability.

Manual and power chair users have some difference in dietary needs. A manual chair rider burns more calories in the act of pushing the chair, whereas a power chair user does not exert himself in the same way while using a joystick. Manual riders need more usable calories, while power chair riders should take extra care not to gain unnecessary weight.

High quadriplegics are particularly at risk of weight gain because their ability to perform aerobic activity is very limited, and because the muscles that have atrophied throughout the body require fewer calories. High quadriplegics are well advised to work closely with a dietitian to develop a dietary plan which includes foods they enjoy, but defines appropriate amounts for the sake of weight management.

All chair users need to take extra care of their skin, already at risk from the pressure of sitting for long periods. Power chair users have a more difficult time shifting their position if they have limited arm strength, so added weight gain only increases the potential for more pressure where they sit. Healthy skin can be promoted by a balanced diet with a complete range of nutrients.

> In the early years after my injury, I had a lot of problems with pressure sores. Looking back, I'm convinced that part of the problem was the

meat and potatoes diet I grew up with, not to mention my sugar addiction! A few years after my accident I switched to whole foods, no red meat, and a lot less sugar, and now I don't get pressure sores. Of course I also learned how to take care of my skin better, do push-ups, and use cushions properly, but the diet was definitely a big part of getting it under control.

Some important nutrients

A variety of whole foods with minimal processing is the best source of nutrients needed by the body. A few examples:

- Vitamin A helps in the growth and repair of body tissues, and maintenance of healthy skin. It is derived by the body from carotene, which is abundant in carrots, green leafy vegetables, and broccoli.

- Vitamin B Complex is a group of B vitamins which work together to produce energy by helping the body to convert carbohydrates to glucose. They are also crucial to the nervous system. They are found in whole grains, liver, and brewer's yeast. Some antibiotics limit the ability of the body to produce B vitamins in the intestines.

- Vitamin C, or ascorbic acid, plays a role in the healing of wounds by maintaining collagen, the protein that forms connective tissue in the body. It also helps fight bacterial infections. It is found in fresh fruits and vegetables.

- Calcium is the most abundant mineral in the body. It must be accompanied by vitamins A, C, and D, as well as magnesium and phosphorus. It is crucial to bones and teeth, as well as the proper function of muscles, which cannot contract and release without calcium. The best known source is in dairy products, but calcium is also found in many fruits, vegetables, and grains, particularly in figs, greens, and soy products.

- Iron exists in every living cell. It works with protein and copper to carry oxygen from the lungs to the tissues of the body. It is found in liver, oysters, lean meats, molasses, and green leafy vegetables.

- Potassium is involved in maintaining the water balance of cells, which is necessary for cell growth and to stimulate nerve impulses to muscles. It also stimulates the kidneys to eliminate toxins from the body. Potassium

is found in all vegetables, oranges, whole grains, sunflower seeds, potatoes, and bananas.

- Zinc is a crucial nutrient for chair users because of its importance to blood formation and the skin, particularly the healing of wounds.

The behaviors of nutrients in the body is a complex set of interactions. Certain vitamins, proteins, or minerals do not work on their own, but rely on
the presence of others to accomplish their task. Supplements are poorly
absorbed unless accompanied by a balanced diet; they are not food and
should not be relied upon to provide the basic needs of your body. However, a good vitamin-mineral supplement is a worthwhile addition to support a balanced, whole foods diet.

Vegetarian diets

You are probably aware of many of the general health risks from a diet rich
in animal foods. For people with disabilities who are unable to be physically
active, and therefore at risk of gaining weight, the health benefits of a vegetarian diet can be even more compelling. The saturated fats in animal meats
are extremely high in calories, and more likely to be held in the tissues
which leads to weight gain. Sufficient nutrients for optimal health can be
derived from a vegetarian diet that is lower in calories.

If you decide to switch to a vegetarian diet, it is recommended that you
remove animal food gradually and take time to experiment with new foods
and recipes. A vegetarian diet does not need to be bland and unexciting.
When you learn how to cook with whole, natural foods and seasonings, and
when you reduce sugar, salt, fats, and processed foods, your taste buds
reawaken, and even simple vegetables take on surprising qualities of flavor.
There are many excellent vegetarian cookbooks available.

Skin care

Pressure sores form because oxygen and blood are restricted in skin tissue by
the weight of the body pressed continuously on a small area of skin. For
people unable to use the gluteus maximus muscles, pressure is increased as
those muscles atrophy (thin from disuse). The skin comes in closer contact
with the bone, limiting circulation further. Two bony areas of particular concern are the ischial bones of the pelvis, which are somewhat pointed and
apply direct pressure to a small area, and the sacrum at the base of the spine.

Most pressure sores happen when a person is new to managing his condition, before good skin care becomes habitual. You can prevent pressure sores by vigilant skin care every day:

- Avoid unnecessary areas of pressure, noting contact at the knees, buttocks, and sacral bone, ensuring proper fit and contact with braces, catheters, and clothing.

- Regularly inspect areas that receive pressure.

- Use the appropriate wheelchair cushion, and maintain it well.

- Do push-ups often in your wheelchair for pressure relief.

- Shift your position and weight in your wheelchair if you are unable to use your arms to fully lift your body.

- Use a tilt or recline system with your wheelchair if you are completely unable to accomplish posture shifts.

- Do not wear rough or irritating undergarments.

- Do not wear loose undergarments—wrinkles can cause increased pressure in small areas.

- Keep your buttocks clean, particularly after your bowel program.

- If your skin is dry, use moisturizers in area of regular contact.

- Eat a balanced diet rich in nutrients needed for skin health—protein, vitamins C and A, B-complex, and zinc. Drink plenty of water to keep tissues moist and flexible.

Inspecting the skin

You or a personal assistant should observe your skin daily for any indications of pressure sore development, such as any open area or blister or redness of the skin, particularly if warm to the touch. Use a mirror to check areas where contact normally occurs—the ischium, the sacrum at the bottom of the spine, hips, elbows, heels, insides of the knees, and so on. Inspection mirrors are available which include a strap for the convenience of people with limited grip.

Skin breakdown can also occur from infection. The ischial area where you sit is at high risk because of its regular exposure to bacteria from your stool during bowel movements. It is possible for a microscopic invasion of the skin to occur, and an infection to develop beneath the surface. A pocket of pus can form which will result in skin breakdown, sometimes a significant enough area to require months for recovery. Prevention is simple. Keep the area very clean with good habits in your bowel program. Also pay attention to fevers or increases in spasticity, which can be indicators of infection.

> *I got a sore in the emergency room when I was injured. They didn't turn me since they were afraid of doing damage. It needed surgery. I spent two months going side to side because the sore was on my back, so I couldn't lay back. It was on my sacrum. It was very rough. And it delayed my ability to start rehab.*
>
> *Since then I've had no problems with sores. Since I've had a lot of luck, I realize that I get a little complacent. I don't inspect my skin enough.*

Ventilator users run some risk of developing skin breakdown at the tracheal opening in the neck. The tracheal opening is already an open wound, and so can attract bacteria. When using a cuffed tracheostomy tube to create a more effective vacuum for air flow, the area needs to be inspected daily. An area of skin will be in contact with the cuff, but is not generally visible. It is usually the goal to wean such a user from the cuff, since it also interferes with the ability to speak.

Cushions

The design of wheelchair cushions to minimize sores has become a large and technically advanced industry. It is critical for people who sit for long periods of time or who have reduced ischial muscle mass to sit on an appropriate surface that properly spreads and reduces pressure and to practice good pressure relief habits. The basic types of cushions are air flotation, gel, foam, and urethane. Cushions are described in more detail in Chapter 6, *Wheelchair Selection*.

For people less mobile in their chair, cushioning is also important for wheelchair backs. Quadriplegics who make more continuous contact with the back of the chair are at risk of developing scapular sores in the shoulder area. There are wheelchair back options that have scapular cutouts to prevent this from happening.

When you spend more time in bed than in your chair—for example, after surgery or during an extended illness—this a high-risk period for developing sores. Cushioning products are also available for beds. "Egg-crate" pads for the bed are commonly used in hospitals and are moderately priced for home use; the foam surface spreads and reduces pressure by means of peaks and valleys. Some sophisticated bed cushioning products include an air or water pump which maintains pressure throughout the pad, or alters it gradually, alternating pressure changes across the body to provide relief to one part while the other is more supported.

> *Even though my mattress is extra soft, it still needs something to help spread the pressure more evenly. An egg-crate pad has worked perfectly. I rotate it every so often, and at some point have to get a new one because it gets sort of compressed. I also like it because when my girlfriend spends the night, it's comfortable for her too, and as it's under the sheet, it doesn't make my bed seem like a hospital bed.*

Sheepskins are also popular bed cushioning. The wool is trimmed and the sheepskins laid under the bottom sheet. They are soft, comfortable, and minimize pressure points, particularly on the hips, elbows, and knee joints which tend to get the most contact while laying down. Some sheepskins cannot be laundered; the skin tends to become hard and brittle. Sheepskins tanned using glutaraldehyde-chrome hold up better in the wash.

Preventing osteoporosis

Without the regular loading of weight from walking, bones begin to lose calcium. This leads to osteoporosis, in which bones become more brittle and prone to fracture. The hips are a common site of fracture, as are the legs, spine, and arms.

Osteoporosis occurs with aging in some people, particularly in post-menopausal women. Risk is increased with diabetes, vitamin D deficiencies, or diets low in calcium. Smoking and alcohol abuse aggravate the condition, as do lack of activity and sunlight. If you are able to stand or walk, it is a good idea to do it as much as you can—with safety your first priority—to help your bones remain strong. People with traumatic disabilities such as traumatic brain injury, spinal cord injury, or amputation tend to spend an extended initial period in bed, which invites osteoporosis to begin.

Apparently spinal cord injury has its own biochemical effect on osteoporosis, although the mechanism is not clear. It has been observed that calcium and other minerals from the bones are lost through the urine at a more rapid pace after spinal cord injury. Even compared to people on extended bed rest—who are not standing much—the sequence of this mineral loss is different in people with SCI. The loss continues for one to two years after injury, is inevitable, and is believed not to be reversible.

If you have osteoporosis or are at high risk for brittle bones, avoid stresses to your bones. To help prevent breaks, remove your feet from heel loops or restraining straps first when you make transfers to and from your wheels, and straighten your legs before rolling over in bed to minimize excessive strain to your bones. A fracture could occur more easily than you might imagine.

If you don't have sensation in your lower body, you might incur a fracture and not know it—for example, a hairline fracture which produces only moderate symptoms. Pay attention to changes in spasticity or occurrences of autonomic dysreflexia. These could indicate a fracture that might not otherwise be apparent. If you hear a snap or other unusual sound, don't ignore it. A bruise from internal bleeding is another potential sign, which you could mistakenly assume is from an impact you didn't feel during the day.

Spasticity has a mixed impact on osteoporosis. When muscles spasm, they place a load on bones that help maintain their density. But severe spasms can break osteoporitic bones. For people who never stand, managing extreme spasticity is all the more important.

Standing frames are promoted as a means of preventing osteoporosis, but physicians are not in agreement that spending a little time each day in a standing frame is sufficient to duplicate the loads your bones would experience in walking. Standing frames clearly benefit circulation and range of motion, but it is less clear that they are a solution for avoiding brittle bones.

Bowel and bladder management

The ability to evacuate your bowels and bladder depends on the particular disability. For example, the ability depends on the level of a condition which otherwise affects your nervous system, such as a brain injury, MS, or ALS; the level of a spinal cord disability; or the strength of surrounding muscles of the bladder, such as the urinary sphincter.

Normal, reflexive emptying happens when the bowels or bladder become full and send a message to a particular area of the spinal cord. The message then goes to the brain, which can send back the instruction to relax the sphincter muscle or to hold on until later.

Injury or disease can interfere with this communication process. For example, in a spinal cord injury, if the spinal cord is damaged above T12, the message will reach the reflex arc, but not the brain. This is known as a reflex or spastic bladder or bowel; you will not be able to control when they will empty. If the cord obstruction is below L2, the message will not reach the cord at all, and your body does not know it is time to respond. This is known as a nonreflex or flaccid condition, sometimes referred to as a frozen bladder.

Management of these neurogenic conditions is central to the degree of independence possible in your life. Tremendous amounts of time can be spent dealing with your bowels and bladder. A poor bladder program can invite nearly constant infections. Surgeries could become necessary, such as installation of a suprapubic catheter through the abdomen, or cutting the sphincter muscle to allow urine to flow. Hospital stays for severe infections can compromise your independence and your ability to make commitments to a job.

A poor bowel program can allow constipation, making evacuation very difficult. You might spend hours dealing with evoking a bowel movement, inserting suppositories, stimulating the area, manually cleaning out the stool with a gloved hand, or relying on a personal assistant to do so. For some, bowel management unavoidably takes some time, but you have some control over how much time it takes, depending on your habits and discipline. Severe constipation, impaction, or diarrhea will certainly occupy your time.

Soft stool and constipation

A good bowel program starts with avoiding constipation and maintaining a good consistency in your stool. When your feces becomes too dry and firm, not only will you have more difficulty in emptying your bowels, but you are allowing bacteria to remain in your body for a longer period of time. Bacteria can multiply and become the cause of infections and other problems.

Firm stool is irritating to the colon and can cause hemorrhoids. It might also require you to apply more aggressive manual stimulation in your bowel program which can further irritate those delicate tissues. Diarrhea can be an indication of constipation, since the runny stool can be from the water lost from the fecal matter farther up the intestines. The more severe the diarrhea becomes, the more likely you can become impacted. You need to drink more water to replace the fluids lost with diarrhea.

Avoid becoming reliant on laxatives, which dull the nerves of the bowel and compromise whatever reflex activity you might have retained. If you continue to have chronic constipation, there might be another medical issue involved, and you should see your doctor. Enemas are also a poor standard method. They stretch the colon and compromise its tone. Your body can develop a dependency on these measures if they are overused.

Start with food

Diet plays an important role in managing stool softness. Before relying on drugs to manage your bowels, start with food. Foods that prevent or cure constipation include fluids, wheat bran, rice bran, vegetables, and fruits—especially prunes, figs, and dates.

The advice you have heard for years is true: include fiber and bulk in your diet. Fibrous food absorbs and retains water, keeping your stool at an appropriate softness. Fiber remains in the intestines because it is not digested, being too coarse to either be broken down by digestive enzymes or absorbed into the body. Fiber helps stimulate the nerve reflexes in the colon wall which trigger bowel movement. Fiber also reduces your chances of developing hemorrhoids, varicose veins, or diverticulitis, which results from the formation of small pockets in the intestines where stool becomes trapped, allowing bacteria to grow.

Fiber can be overdone. Add fiber gradually, making note of how it affects your stool, and work your way up to a consistent level, allowing the body to adapt. Because fiber absorbs water, you must increase fluid intake as you increase bulk in your diet. Too much fiber without enough fluid can cause hard stools—and eventually impaction. Diuretic medicines, designed to remove fluid from the body, will also affect the amount of fiber you can accommodate.

The modern diet in general is much lower in fiber than in the past. To add fiber to your diet, choose whole grain, coarse breads, or use a bread machine to make high-fiber breads. Miller's bran and rice bran are available in powdered form to sprinkle on cereals, salads, and other creative alternatives. Whole fresh fruits and vegetables provide bulk and fiber.

The age-old belief in prunes is true. Prunes are high in fiber and Vitamin A, have no cholesterol or fat, and have a laxative effect. A glass of prune juice each day can help manage your bowels. Or keep a supply of pitted prunes around to pop one in your mouth now and then during the day.

Don't use coffee as a tool to manage your bowels or health. For some people, a cup of coffee has a laxative effect, but not because of the caffeine, which can be a cause of constipation. If you have chronic problems, either with constipation or diarrhea, look at your coffee habits. Too much coffee also amplifies stress.

Dairy foods, by virtue of their calcium content, contribute to constipation. Milk should not be too large a part of your diet.

Medications influence your diet and how you process foods. Ask your physician how drugs he prescribes for you will affect your stool consistency and bowel program.

Have a program

Most of you will have received guidance in a rehabilitation program or been advised by your physician on what bowel and bladder management program will work best for you. However, sometimes a doctor or program will simply apply a given model that doesn't take individual abilities and needs into account. Experience will show what your individual capabilities are and guide you in determining the best management program. Many brain or spinal cord traumas—whether from injury, infection, birth defect, or disease—are not complete, so some messages from the nerves might be getting through. Although you might be diagnosed as having no control or sensation, you might retain some manual control of the sphincter muscles or have some capacity to sense when your bowel or bladder is full.

> *Rehab had me use a leg bag attached to a condom to continuously collect drips from my weak bladder. I found that I had enough control to only need to put a cap in the condom, assuming I used the bathroom before my bladder would fill. That is when I experience involuntary urination. This continues to surprise doctors, given my level of spinal cord injury.*

The bladder program

A neurogenic bladder has a difficult time emptying itself completely. Urine left behind in the bladder will stagnate and cause infection. A very full bladder eventually backs up into the kidneys, disrupting the important filtration task they perform, and leading to infection and disease.

You must drink plenty of water, as much as three quarts per day or a glass every hour. All of this fresh fluid keeps flushing you out, and reduces the risk of bacteria remaining in place long enough to cause trouble. But chair users face a contradiction in drinking extra fluids. For many chair riders, using the bathroom is time consuming, and involves a lot of mechanical or physical effort. You must find a balance for yourself, putting a priority on your safety and health, while reducing inconvenience.

> *I was avoiding going to the bathroom because I didn't want to have to do all the work of getting my pants off and back on. I have some control, but it is not a reflex. That means I have to push continuously to urinate, and it can be tiring. But I discovered that I wasn't drinking enough and so got infections more often. Or else I would delay going, and my external catheter would slip and get me all wet. Now I know I have to drink enough. I do my best to stay calm in the bathroom and do the whole routine with the least possible strain. It turns out I didn't have to push as hard to urinate after all.*

With a flaccid bladder, some ability is lost to know when it is time to empty. The bladder cannot develop enough pressure to overcome the resistance of the sphincter muscle, so urine is held in. If the bladder fills too much, it begins to stretch, known as "overdistention," and urine begins to back into the kidneys. Remaining muscle tone will be damaged, and what bladder function you have can be lost. Since your body is not giving you the sensations to know when these events are happening, you must practice a regular bladder program and be very conscious of how much fluid you take into your body and how it determines when you need to void.

It might be possible to empty a flaccid bladder if you use the *Credé* technique—pressing against your bladder with your fist to overcome the resistance of the sphincter. Discuss this method with your doctor to ensure that it is safe for you. This technique is likely to leave behind residual urine, but depending on your fluid intake this does not have to be a problem. It might be necessary on occasion to catheterize yourself.

A spastic bladder might try to void itself at any time; the amount can be small, leaving behind residual urine. The reflex is most likely when the bladder is full, but can also be triggered by contractions from muscle spasticity in your legs, if that is an issue for you. Spasms in the bladder will increase with the presence of an infection or stones. The spastic bladder can be triggered by massaging the abdomen, by leaning forward or doing pushups from the sitting position, or by stimulating the rectum with a gloved finger. Once the reflex begins, it will continue so you need either to be sitting on a toilet or commode or have an appropriate collection system in place. Many women rely on medication, urine absorbing pads or, as a last resort, bladder augmentation surgery.

With either a flaccid or spastic bladder, you will want to limit your fluid intake in the evening to reduce your need for emptying during the night.

Catheterization

Catheters are used to empty the bladder. A catheter is a narrow tube inserted through the urethra, beyond the sphincter muscle, and into the bladder, allowing it to drain. There are two kinds of catheterization, indwelling and intermittent. Which kind you use depends on the bladder condition you have and other considerations such as convenience, lifestyle, and cost. An indwelling catheter is usually attached to a drainage bag which straps onto the leg and collects urine. With intermittent catheterization, urine is emptied into a plastic urinal or container or directly into a standard urinal.

A flaccid bladder typically must be emptied with an indwelling catheter, since the sphincter muscle is frozen and cannot be relaxed consciously. A spastic bladder might not be capable of emptying itself completely, so occasional use of a catheter might be necessary to remove residual urine. Males with spastic bladders or some control of the urinary sphincter can often manage well with male urinary condoms.

This woman who uses intermittent catheterization describes her routine:

> I prefer to cath in bed, because it's easier for me to pull my pants up and down. I do clean cath, I don't do sterile. I don't use gloves or Betadyne. I boil my catheters to clean them. I use a mirror which makes it easier for me to find the spot. I don't want to be poking around because I'm so prone to UTIs [urinary tract infections], and I don't want to chance causing irritation.

Catheters come in various sizes, identified in French units, which indicate the outside circumference—16 and 18 Fr. are common sizes. The overall size does not indicate the size of the inside channel, so it is important to learn more about the design of the product you choose. You might want to cut open a used catheter to become familiar with its design. The size of the inside channel will determine how quickly the catheter might become clogged. A larger catheter is not always a good solution, as it can still plug up and cause complications in the urethra.

Catheters are made of latex or silicone. Some latex catheters are coated with Teflon to ease their passage. However, latex catheters will generally be smaller inside because of the extra surface layer. Some people develop latex sensitivity and so must use the more costly silicone type.

Either intermittent or indwelling catheters entail a risk of chronic infection.

Indwelling or Foley catheters

An indwelling or Foley catheter remains in place for up to a month, allowing the bladder to empty continuously into a leg or bedside drainage bag. Indwelling catheters include a small balloon at the internal end which is filled with water and keeps the catheter from pulling out. An indwelling catheter is also the solution for quadriplegics who cannot perform intermittent catheterization for lack of hand dexterity.

A suprapubic catheter is a type of indwelling catheter inserted surgically through the abdomen into the bladder because of conditions that prevent entry through the urethra. Some people experience leakage around the opening where the catheter enters. There is a chance of having to relocate a suprapubic catheter after some years; the previous opening could take a while to close, leaving you to deal with leaking from the opening until it heals.

With indwelling and suprapubic catheters, there is an increased risk of infection from the continuing presence of a foreign object in the body. Catheters can become clogged in time if the urine contains sediment or is cloudy from a persistent infection.

Indwelling and suprapubic catheters empty the bladder continuously. As a result, the bladder shrinks and loses muscle tone. Eventually, bladder walls can become firm. Carefully consider whether to go ahead with either of these two options, since they can result in a change to your bladder which might not be reversible. Consult with your physician on the reasons to use them. Despite these permanent changes, one of these options might be the right thing for you to do. In particular, those without the hand dexterity for self-catheterization benefit from continuous drainage. The logistics of getting assistance or the difficulty of trying to do it alone when it challenges your ability might not be worth the effort to avoid the possible complications. If you will continue to use an indwelling approach, a smaller bladder might not matter to you.

Spasms can cause leakage around a catheter, since the strength of the muscular contraction may force more urine into the tube than it can accommodate. The excess will flow around the tube instead. Some spasms can be powerful enough to force out an indwelling catheter even with its balloon inflated, which can stretch the bladder and cause damage to the urethra. This is more of an issue for women, whose urethras are shorter than in men. There are two commonly recommended anti-cholinergic medications for this problem, Probanthine and Ditropan, which relax the bladder to minimize spasms.

If you are having to change your catheter more often than usual, take time to find out why. Not drinking enough fluid is the most common reason for a catheter to become prematurely clogged. Water is the best fluid to drink. Tea, lemonade, and fruit juices are also good. Cranberry juice has long been thought to be healthy for the bladder and even part of a treatment program for infections, although there is no hard research to support it. Do not choose products that rely heavily on sugar, corn syrup, or artificial flavors and sweeteners.

A clogged catheter might also be an indication that you are developing stones. Stones do not develop when your urine maintains a sufficient acid level, rather than becoming too alkaline. Carbonated drinks and certain foods make the urine more alkaline, noticeable by a stronger odor. The best way to get your urine back to an acid level is simply to drink more water. You can test this yourself with pH paper found at any pharmacy. A good pH level is from 5 to 6.5.

Intermittent catheterization

With intermittent catheterization, you insert a catheter when it is time to empty the bladder, performing the process several times per day. A nurse or therapist trains you in the proper techniques for self-catheterization. In the hospital, a fresh catheter is used each time. After discharge, the same catheter can be reused, assuming you practice very clean habits. If you use intermittent catheters, you would carry catheters and supplies for cleaning; these can be carried in a pack on the back of your wheelchair.

Historically, bladder catheterization programs have been based on a time model. Such a program encouraged you to empty your bladder every four to six hours. At times there would be a small amount of urine, meaning that the invasion of a catheter was an unnecessary act. In that interval between catheterizations, the bladder might also have become very full and distended, an even more undesirable state. Without sensation, there was no way to know how full the bladder was.

There are new catheterization products being developed. For example, Diagnostic Ultrasound Corporation has released a product based on volume-dependent catheterization. The BladderManager PCI 5000 is an ultrasound device which can be worn continuously and can warn you when your bladder reaches a selected percentage of fullness. The company's research found that 67 percent of timed intermittent catheterizations were performed prematurely and 16 percent were performed too late. The BladderManager is promoted as a means to limit infections, upper urinary tract damage, and costs for healthcare and supplies.

The O'Neil catheter is designed to limit urinary tract infections. It is a catheter already placed inside a sterile collection bag. The special tip is first inserted into the opening of the urethra. The manufacturer claims that its opening goes beyond the area where bacteria is most likely to invade. The sterile catheter is then extended from inside the drainage bag, and enters the urethra beyond the entry tip, supposedly bypassing the place where it could pick up bacteria from the urethral opening and carry it into the bladder. O'Neil catheters are portable and the integrated drainage bag is convenient. The company claims that it reduces the incidence of UTIs considerably. O'Neil catheters are a single-use product and cost more per unit. Such catheters might be insured by your private insurance carrier or Medicare/Medicaid.

Intermittent catheterization can be more costly than an indwelling catheter if you rely on additional personal assistance services to change them. Dr. Alex Barchuk of the Kentfield Rehabilitation Hospital in California observes:

> The difference in cost for a high quadriplegic on intermittent catheterization versus having an indwelling catheter is unbelievable. It's almost

triple the cost of an indwelling catheter because someone who can't cathe-
terize himself has to have either an attendant or a nurse. You have to
have someone around every four to six hours to do it, which costs a lot of
money. If you don't have the attendant—or if the attendant doesn't show
up, which happens a lot—you have to go through an agency. An agency
costs $35 an hour for a nurse to come out and do the catheterization. The
cost difference is astronomical.

For someone with sufficient hand dexterity to do the intermittent procedure themselves, the cost might not be a concern, particularly with good insurance coverage.

Male condoms or external catheters

Many men with spastic bladders or a degree of manual control of the urinary sphincter can manage well with a male urinary condom, also known as an external catheter. Men using condoms will need to catheterize only occasionally, if at all, to remove residual urine. The condom is changed or reapplied at least once a day to provide the skin a chance to breathe and be inspected for irritation. It is a good general practice to swab the penis for hygienic reasons.

There are three types of male urinary condoms:

- The Texas catheter is held in place with an external strap, either of sticky foam or with a Velcro tab at the end. The strap must be applied carefully. If it is too loose, the catheter will leak. If it is too tight, the skin of the penis can become irritated or break into a sore.

- Another design uses a two-sided sticky foam strap which is first applied to the penis, and then adheres to the condom as it is rolled over the strap.

- The third type is self-adhesive and adheres as it is rolled onto the penis.

Some urinary condoms are supplied with a small pad of skin protector. The skin protector is also available as a separate product you can order from a medical supply store or catalog.

Condoms are typically made of latex. Some men develop latex sensitivity, in which the skin of the penis becomes dry, red, and irritated.

*My latex sensitivity appeared twenty years after my injury. At first I
thought the condoms I used were defective, but instead I needed to switch
to the silicone condom which is available only in the self-adhesive type.*

Urinary condoms come out of the package rolled up, just as with condoms
for sexual use, although they include a tubed end for drainage of urine. The
tube might be an extension of the material of the condom or a separate plastic tube attached at the end of a latex catheter. Urinary condoms come in
several sizes, and the latex type are flexible enough to accommodate the
changes in size that some men experience throughout the day.

When a man has severe ongoing problems with bladder infections and other
complications, a urologist might recommend a sphincterotomy. Surgeons cut
the sphincter muscle and release its capacity to keep the bladder closed. The
bladder empties continuously, and a condom and leg bag system collect the
urine. This very invasive procedure should be considered a last resort. Take
care not to allow your physician to overly influence you. Consider him a
provider of information. Take time to understand the full implications of
such a measure, talking to others who have been through it. A sphincterotomy is not reversible.

The bowel program

A study reported in the *Archives of Physical Medicine and Rehabilitation* states:

> *An ineffective bowel program affects virtually every aspect of the
> patient's life, including physical, psychological, social, vocational, and
> sexual goals, as well as the ability to maintain an activity level, func-
> tional independence, and social interactions.*[1]

Your body systems can run your life, unless you take control and establish
regular habits to make your bowel routine predictable and manageable.

If you don't have a movement every day, this does not indicate constipation.
It can be normal to have a bowel movement every two to three days. What
counts is that you have a routine and that you manage your stool consistency. You need to establish a pattern in a managed bowel program that
depends on what kind of neurogenic bowel you have. Evacuate your bowels
often enough to ensure you do not become impacted, yet not so often that
you unnecessarily disrupt your schedule or risk the health of the tissues of
the rectum and colon. Without an effective bowel program, some people can

eventually require a colostomy after falling into patterns of constipation and impaction.

The less your nervous system allows you control of the sphincter muscles, the more you need to train it to prepare for defecation at a time when you can control and induce it by the use of one or more following techniques:

- **Digital stimulation.** Gentle massage of the area around the anal sphincter muscle encourages it to relax.

- **Manual removal.** Wearing a latex glove, stool is gently scooped out with a finger by yourself or a personal assistant.

- **Suppositories.** The two types are Dulcolax suppositories, which work by stimulating the nerve endings in the rectum, causing the bowel to contract, and glycerin suppositories, which draw water into the stool to stimulate evacuation. Overuse of suppositories or laxatives can cause deterioration of the tissue in the colon.

- **Mini-enema.** Softens, lubricates, and draws water into the stool.

A program which relies on the aid of suppositories or enemas can take from thirty to sixty minutes to complete. In a 1997 study of 100 people with spinal cord injuries, 23 percent of them took more than forty-five minutes with their bowel program.[2] Some of that time might be spent lying down waiting for the treatments to have their effect. You will develop a sense of when you would need to be on the toilet, though a protective bed pad is always a good precaution.

If you have sufficient balance to sit on a toilet or commode chair, gravity can help you along. Many people with high quadriplegia are unable to be stable sitting on a toilet or commode for a bowel program, so it must be performed by an assistant while lying down.

If you can push on your own, that is certainly more attractive than having to put on a glove and dig, or sit waiting for a suppository to act. If you have some manual control of the anal sphincter, beware of the inclination to push continuously to force the feces out. It seems reasonable to think that since the muscle is weakened you have to make up for it with more effort, but such a strategy is exhausting and stressful. The rectum actually works somewhat on its own. If you can make a contraction, you will achieve more effect by alternately pushing down and relaxing. Alternately pushing and relaxing allows the natural reflex of these muscles to work with you, and you will find that stool will evacuate more easily.

Take care not to irritate the delicate lining of the rectum, which can cause bleeding or development of hemorrhoids. Emphasize this with any personal assistant who aids you with your program.

> While I was in rehab, I remember a nurse's aide who seemed to be pretty rough doing my bowel program before I had been taught to do it myself. And then I noticed blood on her glove. I bled almost every time I moved my bowels for years, until I finally had hemorrhoid surgery to correct it.

Alternative health practices

More and more people are exploring so-called alternative healthcare options to maintain their health. Many have been in use for a very long time. Chinese acupuncture is thousands of years old. Herbal medicines are even more ancient.

One man, a polio survivor, reports:

> I've been on total disability since 1991 and the only thing that helps me stay fairly mobile is my chiropractic/acupuncture/massage treatments. Depending on how I feel, I may get one or all of the above treatments. Treatment is painless and very relaxing.

Using these health practices does not mean that modern medicine has no place or that you should eschew the use of drugs altogether. Modern medicine continues to uncover amazing discoveries and therapies that reduce suffering and promote quality of life. Those who use alternative health practices typically try to find a balance—partaking of more natural and less invasive (and costly) measures where they make sense, while relying on modern, technical medicine for the things it does best. Following is a brief description of some widely used alternative health practices you might be interested in exploring.

Yoga/stretching

Yoga derives from Hindu traditions, and has gained great popularity in Western culture. The most widely practiced form is Hatha Yoga, which involves adopting certain body positions and breathing techniques. The effect of these exercises is to stretch muscles, giving the body great agility.

Yoga might be one of the best activities for a person with a disability. The stretches that a physical therapist teaches you have essentially the same effect. Even if stretches are performed passively with assistance to improved and maintain your range of motion, the body benefits in much the same way.

When muscles are not used—whether paralyzed or due to a sedentary life-style—they shorten and get tight. This shortening of muscles is the reason that you feel stiff when you wake up in the morning and want to stretch. As muscles get short, they become weaker and begin to restrict movement, and eventually define and limit posture. Scoliosis, for example, sometimes involves muscles adapting into shorter lengths, pulling the spine into curvature.

Alex Barchuk, physiatrist at the Kentfield Rehabilitation Hospital in northern California, feels that yoga and stretching are some of the best habits a person with a disability can develop:

> *Strong, active wheelchair users are already getting aerobic exercise from how they get around. Stretching helps prevent trigger points from forming, which are painful and can limit muscle strength. Keeping muscles elastic is all the more important as you age.*

There are many books and videos offering yoga instruction and local studios offering classes. Most yoga exercises involve the whole body, but you can adapt them to your capabilities. If you can, get a consultation with your physical therapist to develop a set of yoga stretches that work for you. The therapist will advise you on how often to do the stretches, and guide you in subtle issues of how to move and where the stretches are having their effect.

General yoga material is still useful, with its discussions of breathing and overall health attitudes. Yoga has made a difference for this woman with an L5 spinal cord injury:

> *I was watching TV at five a.m. one day and saw this incredible woman doing yoga. They announced a video for people sitting down, and I ordered it sight unseen. It has two fifteen-minute stretching routines, and I love it. I have to be so limited in how I use my body, so the yoga helps me use muscles that I don't always use. It's like nirvana for me. It's sensual. It's a great feeling.*

Acupuncture/acupressure

Chinese medicine—which has developed over the last five thousand years—believes the body has a great capacity to heal itself and uses the body's own forces to accomplish healing. The basic life force is called Qi (pronounced "chee"). Pathways throughout the body—specifically mapped—relate to all systems of health and life. A practitioner working in this mode will activate points on these pathways to free up blockages and promote the movement of Qi to allow the body to regain its natural state of health. An acupuncturist activates these points by use of needles; acupressure involves pressing on the points with the fingertips.

If you have never tried acupuncture, you might fear that it is painful—the same as getting an injection with a syringe. This is not the case. Acupuncture needles are very thin and do not go in very deep; a skilled acupuncturist knows how to apply them in a way that is not noticed or that feels like a very small sting. There are some points on the body which are sensitive, so an acupuncture needle is sometimes briefly painful.

Acupuncture and acupressure have been found helpful for pain management, to promote healing, to level intense emotions, and to aid recovery from illness. Acupuncture has gained much in popularity. Increasingly, scientific study is bearing out the positive effects of this approach.

Feldenkrais/Alexander

Although the Feldenkrais and Alexander methods are two distinct disciplines, they have similarities. Each method involves an awareness of the body. Instruction/treatment in each discipline guides you to become attuned to your movements. Practitioners are certified in training programs that last for years and are often trained in other health fields as well.

Both methods are based on the observation that people use their bodies in an unconscious fashion, not fully aware of how they are moving, what muscles are involved, or their relationship to the environment, and missing the chance to use energy efficiently. Both methods seek to increase your awareness of subtlety. You are shown how to use small movements to renew your brain's awareness of its connection to your whole body. Large movements are not the goal. The act of thought is powerful; almost the exact same impulses are sent out through your nervous system when you imagine a movement as when you actually perform it. You can enhance the quality of how you use your body by employing small, subtle movements and by using your mind.

Frederick Matthias Alexander was an actor in the late nineteenth century who developed chronic laryngitis. Rather than give up his craft, he devised this method of body awareness to regain his voice. The Alexander Technique, as it is called, is commonly taught to actors today. You are taught to be aware of the spine, to imagine lengthening and opening it as you sit. You are taught to allow the rib cage to open and close with the breath, freeing the lungs to expand and receive more oxygen. By being aware of the forces at play in your movement, you increase the ability to move fluidly and naturally. There is a focus on how gravity affects how you move.

Moshe Feldenkrais was a scientist who saw that people suffered poor health because they were not integrated and because their life experience created "sensory motor amnesia" in which the brain is not fully in contact with the body. A person slumped over in pain, he saw, was suffering from chronic muscle tightness that could be relieved by teaching him to renew contact with the muscles so as to release them and regain control.

> *I learned that the arms are not just limbs that pivot at the shoulder joint, but involve one half of the entire trunk. Muscles in the chest and the back are very much involved with our arms. For those, like me, who have control of abdominal and pelvic muscles, there is tremendous power when those muscles are used integrally with the arms. When I open a door, rather than simply pulling from the shoulder, I employ my back muscles and turn my trunk as I pull. It is remarkable how much more power I can draw on this way, and how much less strain there is to my shoulders.*

> *The same thing is true for wheeling technique. Friends independently observed how my wheeling style changed after the Feldenkrais work. It was visibly evident that I was involving my entire body in a new way.*

There are Alexander and Feldenkrais practitioners all around the country, as well as books and tapes on the topic. These methods have a great deal to offer people with disabilities who can benefit from learning how to use their bodies efficiently, making the most of the strength and function at their disposal.

When I sit up in bed, move to the edge, and transfer to my wheelchair I find that the Alexander training has helped me to use the momentum of my movement, rather than moving entirely by means of muscular effort. Swinging my legs to the side helps draw my upper body around, and when I lift myself into the chair I am aware of how my body is pivoting on the arm I am pushing from. Feldenkrais helps here too, as I use the muscles in that arm to push more efficiently, twisting my pelvis into the chair rather than lifting myself entirely from the shoulders.

Chiropractic and Osteopathy

Chiropractors are fully trained in anatomy and physiology. The central skill they are taught is to make adjustments in your skeleton, usually the spine.

When I went through rehab in 1973, no one ever taught me anything about posture, and I found that I was comfortable in some pretty twisted looking positions! In 1986, someone recommended I see a chiropractor who took x-rays that showed my spine was getting very curved. So they taught me about posture, gave me a lumbar cushion, and I went for adjustments a couple of times each week. After six months they took another set of pictures and my spine was incredibly different, really straightened out. I have gone regularly ever since, and now a proper, upright posture is what's most comfortable for me. It was amazing to see how my body could adjust back to the right shape, but I know it was because we caught it in time.

Osteopathic physicians are fully trained medical doctors, but they take an extra level of study in what they call osteopathic manipulative treatment.

Both osteopathic and chiropractic practitioners are focused on the spine and overall skeleton, and tend to be holistic in their approaches. Osteopathic manipulation is gentle compared to the high-velocity method used by some chiropractors. Osteopathic physicians focus more on soft tissues than chiropractors. Each works well in conjunction with massage therapy and exercise to keep muscles well-conditioned.

You will also find differences within each field. Osteopathic manipulation is actually practiced by a minority of osteopaths these days, whose practices are closer to traditional—or allopathic—medical doctors. While there are chiropractors who perform spinal adjustment as their entire practice, many have begun to incorporate other disciplines. In both cases, you will often find practitioners who have studied for and become certified in subspecialties such as orthopedics, nutrition, or various holistic practices such as herbal medicine.

Osteopathic doctors are conscious of the movement of cerebrospinal fluid through the body. They are attuned to the four diaphragms in the body—the pelvis, the abdomen, the chest, and the brain. They are concerned with the freedom of movement of the ribs and practice a mode called cranio-sacral work, which senses the relative movement of the sections of the skull. (Cranio-sacral work is a method other types of physicians might also be trained in.)

Massage therapy

People's bodies absorb toxins from the environment and foods. Holding these elements in tissues can weaken the body or immune system. Metabolic waste from the contraction of muscles gets trapped between the muscle fibers, leading to stiffness, soreness, and limiting the full strength of those muscles.

The goal of massage therapists—no matter what style they employ—is to rub the muscles to release toxins and allow the bloodstream to carry them out. Massage therapists study anatomy, so they know what muscles they are working on, how they are connected to the skeleton, and how they should feel when they are normal and healthy. They will generally work toward the heart, to help the blood carry toxins into the kidneys and out in the urine. It is a good idea to drink plenty of water after a massage to help this process of elimination.

There are many types of massage. Some are very gentle. It is quite wonderful to be rubbed gently, in a peaceful, trusting setting. Touch is itself healing, as even traditional physicians increasingly recognize.

Other types of massage can be deep and intense. Many massage therapists will say that it is important to work deep, even if it is a bit painful, in order to release the locked tissues and clear the toxins. For example, the experience of being rolfed is a deep massage. Good rolfers are able to start gently and work down deeper. ("Rolfing" is the common term for a massage therapy called Structural Integration, developed by Dr. Ida Rolf.)

Homeopathy

Homeopathic doctors see illness as a message trying to tell you something about your life. Homeopathic doctors want to determine what your body is telling you. They believe the symptoms exist for a reason, and conventional treatment might not work if the root issues are not addressed. Even an injury can raise important questions about what led you to that moment.

At the initial visit, homeopathic doctors will do an extensive interview about your life. Practitioners treat with granules—very small doses of certain substances, usually herbal, but processed commercially. These granules are micro-doses of the disease you are suffering. According to the homeopathic view, homeopathic medications attempt to stimulate the body's own reaction to the illness, much in the same way that a vaccine works by putting a small amount of a disease into you.

Steve and Aviva Waldstein, homeopaths in the Denver area, write:

> These natural remedies are made from plants, minerals, and other natural substances. They are prepared by a process of step-by-step repeated dilution and shaking, which makes them capable of stimulating the body's own defense system. The remedy is usually given one time only, and then allowed to work for a long time. Homeopaths recognize the importance of intervening as little as possible. They know the body is intelligent and produces symptoms for a reason. Rather than giving a medicine which ignores the intelligence of the body, homeopaths choose the one homeopathic remedy which can strengthen the body and allow it to heal itself.[3]

Homeopathic medications are now widely found in health food markets and are extremely popular in Europe. Homeopathy is the primary approach to health in some countries.

Aging and disability

With medical advances, there is a growing population of people aging with disability. Urinary tract infections are less widespread because of safe catheterization products, drugs to control bacteria, and appropriate education. New bedding and cushion technology dramatically reduces the risk of pressure sores which had led to severe infection and mortality. People are able to live far more actively and maintain their health, rather than falling into poor health habits as a result of depression and hopelessness. Drugs now exist that help manage spasticity, reduce exacerbations of multiple sclerosis, or slow the progression of diseases like MS or ALS, among others.

Already survival statistics are better than they used to be. Those injured in the 1940s survived a median twenty-six years. For those injured in the 1960s, the median survival rate improved to thirty-three years. Researchers assume that survival rates for anyone injured in the 1990s will be further improved.

Now that the world has an aging population of people with various disabilities, there is much more research interest in how disability affects the normal aging process. This thirty-five-year-old woman with SCI thinks about what will happen to her as she ages:

> I think about the transition to a power chair. When will that happen, and how will it affect me. I worry about breaking an arm. I'm a single woman, and I'm very independent. How will I manage down the road if things change?

> I assume I will need assistance at some point, and I just want to be able to make the psychological adjustment. I'm already doing less than I used to. The process is already starting. I work with elderly people, so I'm really aware of aging issues.

What happens when you age?

Life itself is a degenerative process. But you still have considerable control over the quality of life as you age. When you understand the innate changes in your body over time, you are better able to craft a lifestyle to maintain optimal health and reduce the chances of catastrophic problems.

It is common to lose muscle mass, although this is largely the result of less activity. Range of motion becomes limited as muscles shorten, tendons and ligaments become less elastic. Some degree of arthritis might affect the bones of the joints. Muscles remain responsive to exercise and stretching, but require regular use to prevent significant, functional weakening.

The skin becomes less elastic and more thin, bringing with it increased risk of bruising, cuts, and skin breakdown from pressure.

Bones become more brittle. Osteoporosis is common in elderly people, particularly women. Being at higher risk for breaking bones as you age is not just because you become less stable and fall more, but because your bones have lost calcium and therefore break more easily.

As you age, your senses lose sensitivity, reflexes slow down, coordination is reduced. Ultimately your short-term memory becomes less acute, although longer-term memories typically remain intact. Energy levels get lower, and you need less sleep.

These facts of life are not inevitably limiting. For nondisabled people, quality of life can be maintained by keeping active.

Aging is a mix of psychological losses and gains. There can be sadness over the loss of youthful health, fear of approaching death, regret over certain life choices or missed opportunities, the loss of friends and loved ones, and increasing dependency on others. Aging also can bring increased maturity, wisdom, perspective, certainty of one's identity, joy in reaching a point of completion, and peace. Psychological benefits can help offset physical decline.

Increased risks with disability

The lost muscle mass that normally occurs with age becomes a greater issue when muscles are already weakened by paralysis or a genetic disorder such as a muscular dystrophy. As you age, you need to continue to exercise moderately to maintain relative strength as muscle mass declines, so that you can function as independently as possible. The ability to transfer to and from your wheelchair is probably the greatest concern. Loss of this ability is a key reason why a previously independent chair user might require the use of attendant services.

Chair riders are already at increased risk of skin breakdown from sitting. Skin that is thinner and more brittle with age increases this risk. You will need to take extra care as you age with keeping the skin clean, with doing pressure relief push-ups and changes of position, possibly change your cushioning strategy, and be vigilant about maintenance of your wheelchair and cushion to ensure proper support. Since aging increases susceptibility to other heath problems such as pneumonia and flu, you might find yourself spending more time in bed. If so, take extra care to change positions or consider using a different mattress or cushion.

As a chair rider, you must rely on the remaining parts of your body that you are able to control. The arms and shoulders take on a lot of the work once performed by the legs, whether pushing your chair, transferring yourself in and out of it, or adjusting yourself in bed or in a favorite recliner in the living room. The shoulders can be a significant weak point, as they are made to do much more than they were designed to do. Such stresses are cumulative. After enough years of extra work, there is a high risk of chronic pain or joint overstrain. A young chair rider able to push long distances over sloped or rough terrain might discover in his fifties that he overused his shoulders and has to switch to a power wheelchair.

For a person with a disability, it is vitally important to manage the aging process. Drs. Gale Whiteneck, Ph.D., and Robert Menter, M.D., write:

> Most of the changes and declines associated with aging might be prevented through awareness, vigilance, active health maintenance, and wellness strategies.[4]

How it's gone so far

There have been a number of studies of the effect of aging on disability, generally focused on the spinal cord population. Since issues such as shoulder strain, pressure sores, and bowel and bladder management are experienced in common by chair users across a wide range of disabilities, these results have something to inform anyone using a wheelchair.

Some subjects in these studies have been disabled for up to fifty years. Quite a lot has changed in that time. However, enough differences were found between disabled and nondisabled populations for this information to be telling about the impact of a disability over time.

A 1991 Craig Hospital study reviewed the records of 205 people with spinal cord injuries. It found a few notable patterns:

- Age at disability was a factor. Given the same levels of injury, older patients had more functional disability.

- The higher the injury level, the more significant the decline in health and independence with age.

- Medical and attendant care costs increased with age, particularly when combined with years post-injury, particularly for C4 quadriplegics.

- Daily activities took more time and effort to complete.

The study concluded:

> *While these declines of physical and psychosocial functioning might be expected to occur in older able-bodied individuals, they appear to occur much earlier in the SCI population.*[5]

Another study reviewed the records of the Model SCI system, a group of eighteen major rehab centers across the United States. As of 1994, looking at the population in terms of years post-injury, the study found that risks of urinary tract infections, pressure sores, and kidney stones rose as more time passed. The same study found that those in the population who were older reported more pain, fatigue, and needing help.[6]

Another Craig Hospital study published in 1993 looked more closely at what kinds of activities people needed more help with. In a group of 279 subjects—who had sustained their injuries anywhere from ten to forty-seven years ago—22 percent reported that they needed more physical assistance as they aged.The greatest need was in making transfers to and from their chairs, in some cases requiring the use of a mechanical lift. Other statistical leaders were getting dressed, toileting, and of course mobility, a greater concern for quadriplegics who were able to function with limited arm strength when they were younger, but could not maintain their capacity over time. Thirty-nine percent of the people who reported a need for increased help attributed it to weight gain. The study found that the average age when people needed more assistance was forty-nine years for quadriplegics, and fifty-four for paraplegics.[7]

The good news: in the same study, people who did not require more help rated their quality of life better as they aged. The bad news: those who became more reliant on help reported lesser quality of life. Although 78 percent of the study participants did not report needing more help, it remains up to you to maintain your health and ensure that you don't fall into the group whose lives become more limited and unhappy as they age.

How old and how long

Most aging studies look at both the age of onset of the disability and the length of time one is disabled. People who become disabled when they are older tend to recover and adapt less effectively than younger chair riders. When older people are injured, they are already dealing with some results of the aging process which make adjustments to disability more difficult. The length of time you are disabled is another factor that affects the degree of change you might encounter as you age. Dr. Robert Menter, in a speech on aging in 1993, noted:

> *Following the losses of function of spinal cord injury (SCI), it appears that the aging process is accelerated as a result of the impaired protection of various body systems compromised by SCI and increased demand and wear on limited resources.*[8]

These two factors sometimes have opposite effects. Pressure sores, for example, are found to increase with the age of the person, but decrease with the length of disability. The skin is more frail when people get older, but a more experienced chair user will have better skin care habits and skills.

Other conditions more closely related to an older age at onset are heart problems, pneumonia, respiratory infections, kidney stones, fainting and headaches. A longer period of time post-injury was more associated with musculoskeletal overuse strain, tendon and joint pain and stiffness, hemorrhoids, and urinary problems among men.

In general, signs of aging occur earlier in the disabled population than in able-bodied people.

It gets expensive

The less you take care of yourself and manage the decline of your health due to aging, the more it will cost. Increased costs are reflected in a variety of expenditures for:

- Power wheelchairs which require more maintenance and part replacement for batteries and heavier duty tires
- Additional architectural conversions to the home if forced to switch from a manual to a power chair
- Hoists and lifts for transfers in bed and bathroom
- A more elaborate and expensive vehicle, if you are able to afford an accessible van
- Attendant support in the home
- More hospital or nursing home stays to recover from bone breaks or pressure sores

Some added expense is probably inevitable with increased age; consider this in your financial planning.

Using personal assistance services

Your ability to stay healthy and have a full life might rely on being helped with certain tasks. The kind of support you might require could be as simple as some light cooking or running a few errands, or as involved as help with your bowel program, getting dressed, and getting into and out of your wheels. A personal assistant (PA) might also administer an injection or perform simple physical therapy tasks such as range-of-motion and stretching exercises. Certain tasks might need to be performed by a registered nurse; some states require this for catheterization, for instance.

The basic questions to ask are:

- How much support do you need?
- Who will do it?
- How do you find these people?
- Will it be a family member or friend?
- If necessary, how will they be paid?

How much support?

It might already be clear that you are unable to perform various personal functions. A high quadriplegic doesn't have to wonder if some personal assistance is necessary.

A lower quadriplegic or someone with MS experiencing a significant exacerbation *could* do many things for himself, but might quickly fatigue if he does. There is a point where personal assistance makes sense in order to preserve your energy for the rest of the day. No one likes to surrender independence, so people in this gray area will have more difficult decisions. For example, deciding to allow someone else to perform a very personal task like a bowel program can be a difficult line to cross.

> *In fact, when you come right down to the nitty-gritty, PAS (personal assistant services) is an interruption of the flow of my life. I'd really rather do it myself.*

A good goal is to find a balance that optimizes your energy so you can do what you want with each day. That could mean assistance from someone every morning and evening, or perhaps just an hour or two every other day. Some people perform their bowel programs on alternate days, but are able to dress and perform basic household tasks.

The assistant's role

Ideally, assistants are the means to gain control over your own life. Having assistance is a tool you can use to adapt to your disability. Having assistance allows you to make your own choices and pursue the level of activity you prefer, according to your ability.

The relationship between you and an assistant is a human relationship, with feelings on both sides. Many people avoid receiving assistance from someone they know, and prefer to hire someone or work through various agencies that provide these services. That way, the assistant is an employee, and his role is easier to define.

Many people develop a detailed job description for an assistant, with a list of specific tasks. The job description does not have to be cast in stone, preventing you from asking for other kinds of assistance. A job description lists what is needed and helps define what the relationship will be like, including:

- Clearly defined tasks such as dressing, administering medication, bowel and bladder programs, or cooking
- Hours to be worked
- Your requirements for notice of late arrival or non-arrival
- Provisions for vacation coverage or illness
- Payment

The personal assistant will benefit by having a detailed and clear description of what you need:

> As a PA, some kind of list of "must dos and don'ts" is imperative in some situations. At the very least, it prevents misunderstandings. For example, I cared for a paraplegic diabetic and needed to know specifically when his regular mealtimes were, what he could (or would) eat, what to do with regard to blood sugar and emergency insulin, and when and how to use the emergency insulin.

While working out the description of what a PA will be doing, you can discuss such tasks as running errands, house cleaning, or anything else you feel you need help with. Some of these things might not be acceptable to an assistant or might be precluded by the overseeing agency. This does not mean such requests are impossible—assistants might be willing to do things on their own time or make exceptions to policies in order to provide what you need.

Assistants are not there to be slaves, any more than they are there to tell you what to do. You must respect them and understand that they will be conscious of a boundary they should not cross, such as when you ask for something that would injure you. One PA describes this dilemma:

> *The only time this is a problem is if a person may want or is doing something I know is not necessarily good for their own physical or mental health. For example, my employer asked me to stop and get him some beer. He is diabetic, a stroke victim, and has heart problems. I had to take a deep breath, and decide that he knew the risks, and that it's his life. So I got him the beer. But only a six-pack, not a case. I don't know if this was right or wrong, probably wrong according to an agency.*

Some tasks have to be done at a certain time, such as catheterization or getting dressed. Other tasks, like house cleaning, can be scheduled more flexibly. These things get worked out over time in a flexible, working relationship. Doing a description up front gets this process off to the best possible start.

A working relationship can develop into a friendship, although still with clear boundaries. Hopefully you will work with compassionate people, who will inevitably come to care about you as a person, as any friend would. Two PAs talk about their jobs:

> *Sometimes all I did was have coffee with him and share the day's news from the paper, or come sit while he played online, especially when he was depressed. Or he would call at night, his wife not having come home, needing to be put to bed or just have someone with him. This was done on my own time because of the limitations the agencies have on hours. Certainly both parties need to know what the PA is comfortable with doing, especially regarding personal care. But the rest comes from getting to know each other and honesty on both sides.*

The majority of the people I have assisted require some personal care—hygiene, meal prep and feeding, transferring, etc. They also need help with day-to-day activities like walking the dog, changing kitty litter, rearranging furniture, shopping, gardening, etc. Yes, every person's situation is different. The only way I have managed to stay in this field that I love for seven years is to be flexible.

How to find a personal assistant

Start by checking with your medical funder, be it insurance or government healthcare. Medicare provides funds for home health, but has some restrictions on how much you can be out of the home.

Many local Independent Living Centers (ILCs) run personal care assistant (PCA) services programs. The center might be limited to offering you classes on using a PCA or be an actual provider of services with a database of assistants. Some ILCs have contracts with their respective state to run a program using government funds.

Your ILC is not the only possible administrator of PCA programs. The city of San Francisco, for instance, offers services with city money, and the state of California runs the IHSS (In Home Supportive Services) program.

One type of program is not necessarily better than another. Do your own research on what programs are well administered, provide the best range of services, and screen their workers well. The following man had a mixed experience with his agency:

I'm a thirty-four-year-old quad. I've been getting PCA care through an agency for fourteen years. I've always thought it would be nice to hire my own PCAs, but never followed up on it because the service I received from the agency has been good. However, the agency has been screwing up big time lately; PCAs not showing up at all, no one calling to tell me so, two PCAs showing up at the same time, etc.

You are, of course, free to hire people on your own. Many people advertise in local papers or list themselves at the local ILC looking for people to work. Other places you might advertise include the unemployment office, community agencies such as Catholic Community Services, grocery stores, senior centers, social service agencies, community colleges, or hospitals. Also spread the word to friends, acquaintances, and neighbors.

Don't rush the hiring process. You might feel you have an urgent need to hire someone, possibly because a personal relationship is being strained. But this is an important choice. Like any employer, you have to take the necessary time to find the right person that you will be comfortable with and can trust. Otherwise, you'll end up doing it all over again.

Family member or friend?

Many people who use personal assistants report that allowing someone already close to them to play this role is fraught with problems. That doesn't mean that a parent, child, or spouse taking the job guarantees problems, but it will influence the relationship. This is a complex relationship that requires patience and communication. There is a tendency to get caught up in power issues or just plain getting tired of too much contact. Sometimes the relationship changes for the better: deeper intimacy and trust, and increasing friendship and mutual appreciation. Working with someone already close to you should be handled carefully.

Even more complex are the dynamics with a spouse. The desire to be partners is a strong part of the marital relationship, and the person being cared for can struggle greatly with feelings of not carrying his share. When it comes to sexuality, it can be difficult to get in the mood when you have just shared the process of a bowel program.

But a spouse taking this role does not have to ruin the sexual relationship. If you can talk openly about how the roles are affecting you, and find ways to plan time so that personal tasks don't interfere with sensual times, you can make it work. Some people have even found ways to make something like catheterization a form of foreplay. Others have experimented with someone else performing assistant tasks specifically to help them prepare for sex.

It's a bureaucracy

If you are getting help through a medical funder or ILC program, there will be a process to evaluate your needs. Most programs have a formal requirement. The program balances making sure your needs are met and confirming that services are being used appropriately.

Some people with disabilities are concerned when the evaluation is performed by the funding source. They are afraid that the need to control a budget will override the priority of optimal assistance.

> *I have problems with the ILC workers—who are pressured to keep hours down and purse strings tight—being the people who assess. I think this kind of assessment needs to be done by a less biased party. Please don't misunderstand me. I know that the bias in an ILC tends to lean toward the consumer, but I also know how pressured they are to assess low.*

This man feels that the ILC that runs his assistant program is the best candidate for the evaluation:

> *First, some agency has to assess our needs. Otherwise, some disabled people would abuse the system. Second, I would rather have my ILC (whose bylaws direct that three-fourths of its board of directors be comprised of disabled people and whose director is a paraplegic) assess my needs than some other agency that might not be as attuned to my circumstances. Third, if the disabled person doesn't agree with the ILC decision, there is an advocacy agency where the person can bring a grievance.*

You are really the expert on what you need. Your needs are not limited to clinical services, but include being supported in a way that allows you to have enough energy to function in the world, rather than being exhausted by everything you can do alone, but that would fatigue you. Defining needs is tricky. Sometimes the process can leave you unsure you deserve assistance.

> *I've lived with post-polio residual all my life and now get the extra kickers post-polio syndrome throws my way. Suffice it to say that after four months of "doing it myself," my arms were giving me severe pain, and fatigue was robbing me of productive hours. The muscles that were barely allowing me to live without a personal assistant were weaker and their endurance had dropped to almost zilch.*

> *We're constantly guilt-tripped for needing assistance in order to live independently. I say, from wiping my butt to preparing the food for a dinner party to which I have invited friends, I deserve all the assistance I need, and only I can decide what I need.*

When you are working with government coverage or local programs—depending on how they are structured—there will be some amount of paperwork. Certainly you have to confirm time sheets for payment or might be asked to evaluate your care. Despite a clear ongoing disability, some people are made to repeatedly establish their need for support.

I have to continue to prove need even though it is very evident that my condition, cerebral palsy, will not improve and I will need the service for the rest of my life. This results in mounds of paperwork and requires calls and visits to see if I have indeed found the right snake oil and can walk again! My case manager has to come over and fill out extensive forms every two months. This takes at least three hours of our time. Sometimes this wall of paper blocks me from getting to work on time.

Who chooses to be a PA?

Those who do the work include students looking for some part-time work while in school, nurses and aides who work for home health agencies, and good-hearted people interested in helping who don't really need the money.

There is a wide range of possible motives for someone to choose this work. The Independent Living Service Center in Everett, Washington, has put together a manual on using PAs. It includes the following slightly tongue-in-cheek list of personality types to watch out for in people you interview:[9]

- Savior: Those who try to convert you to their brand of religious belief

- Rehabilitationist: Those who think you need to put on your own socks instead of being helped so you can go to work

- Condescender: Those who pat you on the head saying how courageous or what an inspiration you are for trying to live a normal life

- Do-gooder: Those who see you as a charity case

- Pitier: Those that look at you with that "poor you" expression

- Parent: Those who see people with disabilities as children needing to be supervised

- Healer: Those who think your life will have more meaning when there is a cure

Not everyone has some ulterior or misguided motivation. Some PAs find great meaning in helping people who need support to continue living at home.

I learned what a joy and how rewarding it is to be able to help a person live at home, where they want to be, and in most cases, can be. Whether permanently or temporarily handicapped or dying, it makes no sense to put a person in an institution that costs so much more than home care, and takes away dignity, self-worth, and freedom, not to mention loved ones and familiar surroundings.

Checking up on potential assistants

It is important to interview people carefully, to have others around if possible during the early stage of the working relationship, and even to do criminal background checks. Careful screening is standard procedure for some agencies and programs, and you should ask whether that is the case. You should request it. Even if it is refused, it is possible to hire a detective agency at nominal cost to do a simple background check.

Some people are simply desperate for work or unfortunately interested in taking advantage of someone who is vulnerable. Desperation might lead people to prey on you. There are reported instances of physical and other abuse.

> *My friend caught her PA with her hand in her purse—stealing not money but her prescription pain medications. Turns out meds were missing at a couple of the other homes too. The PA had a back injury a few years ago; she is addicted to pain meds and her own doctor won't prescribe as much as she wants.*

This employer of personal assistants found college students more reliable, and advertised in the college newspaper:

> *I hire college students almost exclusively. I find that only about one out of fifteen are no-shows for the interview. On the other hand, when I advertise in the local newspaper, no-shows are more than 50 percent. What does this mean? I guess it comes down to motivation. College students are motivated to study and earn money to put themselves through school.*

Payment

What does a job as a PCA pay? Not much. One of the great challenges of filling the needs of a disabled population is the limited supply of people who are able—or willing—to work for minimum wage.

> *Here in California, our IHSS system only allows us to pay minimum wage, presently $5.25. Most people are able to pad their hours a little bit, so they can pay a little more. That is to say, some people are able to be*

allocated a few more hours than they really need, allowing them more
flexibility in what they pay their PCAs. People like myself who need more
hours than the state pays for—283 hours per month—are put at a signif-
icant disadvantage because we don't have a "pad."

Your program might pay for your PCA, or simply be a service to provide referrals and training to help you find and use such services. Funding could come from sources such as Vocational Rehabilitation or the Veterans Administration.

Payment is usually provided by means of vouchers authorized for a specific number of hours. You typically fill out forms reporting hours, submit them properly signed for payment, and hope they go through. Payment is not always an efficient process, as a PCA describes:

I would receive a voucher to take to my employer who would have to
fill it out. Both of us sign. I mail it in. If I was lucky I would get my check
in two weeks. Usually it took at least a month—sometimes many phone
calls and a couple of months. I soon learned not to include my paycheck
in the monthly budget.

Restrictions

A Medicare regulation regarding payment for home care only pays when your absences from home are "infrequent and for periods of relatively short duration" which "require a considerable and taxing effort." Otherwise they will not cover visiting aides and certainly not at a place of work.

An article in the September 1997 issue of *New Mobility* magazine describes the experience of two people, needing assistance in the morning and evening to get into and out of their wheels, who found themselves cut off from coverage when it was discovered that one of them was volunteering at the local school, and the other was driving a modified van once his elderly parents were unable to do so.[10] A worker provided by an agency blew the whistle, because the agency is forced to protect its status as a provider of Medicare-covered services. The choice of these two people was to either stay at home or to surrender coverage.

The article explains that the Health Care Financing Administration (HCFA), which runs Medicare, is aware of the problem. The HCFA explains that when home health coverage was established, it was meant as a short-term solution. It was progressive coverage at the time. There are legislative attempts underway to correct the problem. The restrictions on home care have become obsolete as the ability to function outside of the home with basic levels of support is more possible—and more demanded by people with disabilities.

An agency you work with who provides and funds a PA might have a variety of specific restrictions, often based on the criteria of "medical necessity." Many times, such services are designed for people thought to be sick or bedridden, not as support services to allow someone to be active.

> *Is it medically necessary for me to go with my personal care worker to a conference on health promotion and safe sex? My agency says no. Are short vacations medically necessary with your personal care worker? "No!" my agency exclaims. Can my personal care worker take me to visit the chiropractor three times a week, regardless of medical outcome? My agency says yes. These are deemed medically necessary. My case manager cannot come to my work environment and do her paperwork because I am supposed to be sick in bed or something. I'm a square peg that doesn't fit into the round hole.*

Keeping them happy

Al DeGraff, in *Home Health Aides: How to Manage the People Who Help You*, lists ten reasons PAs quit their jobs:[11]

1. Their initial job description was incomplete or keeps changing.

2. The method and order in which they must perform their duties are illogical, inefficient, and waste time.

3. Their working environment is messy, unpleasant, disorganized, etc.

4. They're not paid enough, don't get appropriate raises, or don't feel their work is appreciated.

5. The employer (you) is either too passive or too aggressive in his/her style of interaction.

6. They feel another PA is favored over them.

7. The employer is dishonest about the hours worked, the salary owed, or has inappropriate expectations such as monetary loans or sexual favors.

8. There are unreasonable duties—those the employer is able to perform alone, those which cannot be performed in the allotted time, or those which are too tightly supervised.

9. The employer is intolerant of honest mistakes, the need for sick time, etc.

10. The employer doesn't respect the PA's personal life and expects that his or her needs should take priority over all else in the PA's life.

Service animals

You might be able to get some help from service animals, using programs that train animals and place them. A dog can learn to open a door, turn on a light, answer the phone, push elevator buttons, or pull you over a curb in your chair. In the bargain, you also get a loyal companion.

There is cost involved. The training is expensive, and animals do have to be fed regularly. Programs that train and provide service dogs do their best to raise money to help cover the costs to make them available to more people.

Boston-based Helping Hands provides capuchin monkeys, the type usually depicted with an organ grinder, to quadriplegic clients. They are raised in foster homes and placed at the age of four years. A key requirement, says program director Jody Zazula, when she brings a monkey to meet someone for the first time, is that "they fall in love with each other."

Your choice

Whatever your disability, whether stable or progressive, you have a tremendous amount of control over the quality of your health and life. There is an optimal level of health that is possible for you—and a much lower level if you neglect yourself and elect not to practice at least some of the concepts discussed in this chapter.

You may well struggle with depression, disappointment, frustration with cultural attitudes, financial limitations, or many other difficulties that you can face in the disability experience. But none of that needs to stop you from eating well, doing simple exercises, getting into the sun from time to time, and following basic medical principles to protect yourself from skin breakdown, infections, and other risks inherent in being a wheelchair rider. There is always something new to try, and there are many people out there who are true healers in many different modes with their skills—and hearts—to offer, not to mention a vast offering of information on the Internet.

On the other hand, if you are really out there, working, traveling, playing, raising a family, engaged in a fully active life, then you must be conscious of your limits—as everyone must be, disability or no. Your lifestyle is simply more strenuous, so you must take more care with your health.

Trying to make too many changes at once is a recipe for failure. Take one change at a time. Wait until the change becomes integrated into your daily life before adding another. Maybe you start with a little stretching or add a new food to your diet—like eating a couple of prunes every day. The benefits in improved health and energy will be so precious that you will come to enjoy and value health management habits that might have seemed unappealing at first glance.

Taking care of yourself is a lifelong process. Good health habits are crucial for your life on wheels.

CHAPTER 5

The Experience of Disability

Each of us experiences disability in his or her own way. No one can tell you how disability is supposed to feel or how you are going to respond to yours. There are, however, common patterns in the emotions and beliefs experienced by people with disabilities.

This chapter explores some of the dynamics of what disability feels like from the inside. We start by discussing identity issues: how cultural views of disability color your sense of self, how a sudden disability can foster a far-reaching self-evaluation, how lawsuits over injuries can be a barrier to adapting, and the sometimes subtle urge to "pass" for able-bodied. We look at issues common to the newly disabled, then examine a range of emotional responses to disability and adaptation to changed circumstances. Next, we look at issues that have to do with other people: interacting with your family, dependency, and asking for help. We close by discussing public attitudes toward disability and advocacy in modern society.

Hopefully, considering the issues discussed in this chapter will help you better identify and understand feelings you might have and support the process of maintaining your sense of self even though your body has changed dramatically.

Change of identity

Major life changes often require adjusting your sense of identity. According to disability psychologist Carol Gill, a polio survivor, reconciling your identity as a disabled person with previously held notions about what being disabled means is a common hurdle:

> *When you become a member of the group that you have previously felt fear or pity for, you can't help but turn those feelings on yourself.*

A traumatic injury or diagnosis of disease that suddenly makes you a member of the disabled community is a shock to your sense of self. Whatever image you had of disability will be the image you first apply to yourself. Before you were disabled, what were your reactions to people you saw or heard about who had a disability? How did you react when you saw a person in a wheelchair? Did you feel pity? Did the notion of it happening to you fill you with dread? What was your image of what their lives must be like? Could you imagine them with careers, families, being creative or athletic, having sex? Or was the only image you could conjure one of sadness, dependency, pain, and loss?

Even if you know someone who has lived an active life with a disability, you might doubt you could do it. Despite the increasing public visibility of active chair riders, U.S. culture still tends to promote negative beliefs about the experience of disability.

In his book *Missing Pieces*, the late sociologist and disability researcher Irving Zola—himself a polio survivor—wrote:

> *The very vocabulary we use to describe ourselves is borrowed from that society. We are de-formed, dis-eased, dis-abled, dis-ordered, abnormal, and, most telling of all, called an in-valid.*[1]

For most people, the onset of disability heralds an intensive self-evaluation, the beginning of a process that never actually reaches conclusion. You are now a member of a minority foreign to most nondisabled people you will meet. You will remember your previous identity and always retain a sense of it. In the case of a traumatic disability, a part of you will resist accepting membership in the society of chair riders.

Most chair users eventually accept the internal contradiction between their disabled and nondisabled identities. But this adaptation takes time. The early years are marked by a series of adjustments which are deep and sometimes troubling. But life after the adjustment can eventually be meaningful and rich—if you let it.

Notes Carol Gill:

> *We all differ in the degree of "equipment" we have to even look at such things as our values. But the people who can do that end up with different values. They redefine important aspects of living. They redefine roles, for example. Mothers and fathers redefine what being mothers and*

fathers means. What being lovers means. What being productive and contributing members of society means. This is how they adapt.

If you think your self-esteem relies on whether or not you can walk, you limit yourself. Your self-esteem is more truly related to your compassion, generosity, and doing your best in any situation. You don't have to be able to walk to take pride in yourself, or to be recognized and appreciated by the people you care about and who care about you.

You are still yourself

In the ways that really matter, disability does not change you. Rather, disability threatens concepts you have held about who you are. You bring to your disability whatever mix of attitudes, beliefs, fears, talents, charisma, or social skills you have—or have the capacity to develop. Who you are impacts your adjustment to disability.

Notes a man who has been on wheels for years:

> *The most common question I've been asked by people who know someone who was recently disabled is, "What can I do to help?" My answer has always been, "First, understand that they are the same person they were before their disability. Don't treat them any differently, don't expect them to be any stronger or weaker than before, but don't be surprised if they discover new qualities in themselves that never came to the surface before."*

A disability forces the issue of "finding yourself." Some people take pride in what they learn about themselves through their disability experience, and appreciate the way in which it helps define their values.

Many psychological adjustments have little to do with your disability, and more to do with issues common to all of us. For example, you might be frustrated by the difficulty of finding a mate and think that your disability is the central cause of your loneliness. But this issue is part of many people's lives—disabled or not. Don't make your disability a scapegoat for issues that may well have come up in your life anyway. A disability in and of itself does not preclude finding a mate, as many people have proven.

For most people, disabilities do not define them but are something to deal with when necessary:

> My name is not cerebral palsy. There's a lot more to me than my disability and the problems surrounding it. That's what I call the disability trap. This country has a telethon mentality toward disability that thinks disabled people are not supposed to talk about anything but their disabilities.

> I had a girlfriend back in the '60s. One day we discussed the idea that the whole human race is disabled because we can't live in peace with each other. This was always so and it will continue that way in the future. So who is "normal"?

Sexual identity

You might believe that you are not entitled to a sexual identity, that no one could possibly see you as a sexual being, or that you don't have sexual "performance" options. These conclusions are not true. Exploring your sexual identity can be a valuable part of your adjustment, whether you acquired your disability later in life or are making adjustments in teen or adult years with a disability since birth or childhood.

Irving Zola wrote:

> While I agree that sex involves many skills, it seems to me limited and foolish to focus on one organ, one ability, one sensation, to the neglect and exclusion of all others. The loss of bodily sensation and function associated with many disorders, and its replacement with a physical as well as psychological numbness, has made sexuality a natural place to begin the process of reclaiming some of one's selfhood.[2]

Chapter 8, *Intimacy, Sex, and Babies,* discusses sexuality in detail.

Lawsuits

If you were injured in a way that has led to a personal injury lawsuit, you face another complication in adjusting to your self image with a disability. Typically, attorneys will urge you not to work during the case, because working reduces the apparent impact of your disability on your life, and so reduces the amount of money you are likely to win.

Deborah Kaplan is an attorney at the World Institute on Disability in Oakland, California, and a wheelchair rider. She is concerned about the message people get during the extended process of the lawsuit:

> The legal system and the personal injury system—and I think the lawyers aid and abet it—are premised on the same notion: that disability equals inability to work. One of my concerns is the impact on somebody who has just gone through a huge shift in their life, a huge shift in their self respect and self image. They sit through a trial where all they hear, over and over and over, even from their own advocates, is how worthless their lives are. I think it's difficult for someone who's had all that negativity instilled in them to then go out with self respect, get an education, get a job, and be productive.

Passing

In U.S. culture—so imbued with fear of disability—it's probably fair to say that anyone with a recent disability will, to some degree, resist fully adopting the identity of disability. One of the most common ways to deny disability identity is to try as hard as possible to function in the culture as if your disability did not exist. This is known in the disability community as passing.

What's the problem with passing? After all, the disability movement is working hard for inclusion in the society and for removing barriers to the ability to function as independently and fully as possible. However, passing is *not* about interacting in the world, being involved with able-bodied people, having a non-disability-related career, or dancing at your cousin's wedding. If you can be an auto mechanic or a dance instructor because you found a way to adapt to the task and you have some real expertise to offer, what could be wrong with that?

Passing is crossing some line where the acting as if you are not disabled causes a problem. For example, perhaps you resist using an adaptive device necessary for your safety. Perhaps you are a quadriplegic with use of your arms, but you exhaust yourself using a manual chair because you resist the image of being a person using a power wheelchair. There is a borderline between challenging yourself within reasonable boundaries and acting against your self-interest because you don't want to define yourself as a person with a disability.

Passing is effectively denying the truth of who you are and the real possibilities in your life. Disabled psychologist Carol Gill describes passing in this way:

> I think passing is trying to convince society that we're more like non-disabled people. We just happen to have this disability. I think a lot of people want to be assimilated into the mainstream and try to act the part of what they think people in the mainstream are like. "Passing" to me implies some dishonesty.
>
> Trying to pass as something you're not is always bad, unless you can carry it off so well and you have an emotional makeup that doesn't require honesty and authenticity. It's true! Some people can be happy playing a role all their lives. They'd be playing one role or another even if they weren't disabled—playing a role rather than looking inside and being at peace with who they really are.

The cultural pressure to pass is great, as this deaf woman observes:

> When I was growing up, adults made it very clear that bringing up my deafness would signify that I was slacking—if I "tried hard enough" I could get by. The message was clear: Shut up about it, and look like you're doing okay. I think that as long as "overcoming" disability is such a cherished cultural myth, social pressure to engage in passing behavior will be part of the disability experience. When people manage to pass, they're seen as successfully overcoming their disabilities by most nondisabled and some disabled people.

If you can be free from having to prove yourself, your choices will not be tainted by this skewed motivation. If you are able to look at yourself honestly and with acceptance, you can see this motivation and not allow it to affect your choice.

Passing doesn't have to be only about how you are viewed by the broader culture. It can be an attempt to make up for your losses: being athletic, seductive, capable of robust physical work, and so on. People with disabilities are driven to substitute. Irving Zola wrote:

> An uncomfortable assessment of my last twenty years was that they represented a continuing effort to reclaim what I had lost.[3]

Thinking about where your motivations are coming from and what you're trying to prove can be complicated:

> I have felt some satisfaction in having my disability disappear in the eyes of colleagues and friends, but does that mean I was necessarily passing? Or was my desire to minimize the social impact of my disability a motivating force that helped me accomplish what I have with my life?

The boundary between making the most of your abilities and trying to pass as not disabled is a fine line. Some of the more radical disabled might accuse you of passing, but only you can know what drives you. A man with SCI recalls:

> A man I used to work for, impressed with my level of activity and work, once said to me, "You're not really disabled!" He thought he was complimenting me. He didn't realize he was exposing his belief that it was a bad thing to be disabled. It is something to "overcome."
>
> I remember mixed feelings. On one hand I took some pride in having participated fully in my career and being accepted as an equal—in having "passed," though I wouldn't have used that word. On the other hand, his comment was upsetting because it denied an essential part of who I am—a person with a disability. I wish he could have said, "Through knowing you I now understand that a physical disability is not necessarily the limiting, tragic experience I had believed it to be."
>
> I want to explore my own limits on my own terms. My inner discomforts with my disability identity will probably always be around. My task is to observe and learn.

A woman who got polio at the age of five observes:

> For those of us who grew up with disability, that is a very common crossroads we face—the moment where we discover we were trying to pass and it just is not worth the effort. "Wait a minute! This is costing us too much!" It's much more fun to be a disabled person if we just relax into it. Then we'll save ourselves a lot of energy.

The dividing lines take time to sort out. Figuring out the subtleties might not be a priority for you now. Whatever choices you make are basically driven by a desire for comfort and security. If you're at peace with yourself, no one can fairly accuse you of trying to pass.

The newly disabled

Most able-bodied people imagine disability to be a far more negative and difficult experience than it is. At first, you have no conception of how someone functions with a wheelchair, so it appears to be a life of complete dependency and endless difficulty.

When you've suddenly become disabled by injury or diagnosis of a degenerative disease, you bring your previous notions of disability to it. It is no surprise that many people find themselves experiencing depression, anger, anxiety, fear, and a very deep sense of loss in the early stages of the disability experience. Regardless of how well-adjusted, mature, or emotionally strong you are, this is a catastrophic event that shakes many of your basic beliefs about life. It also asks you to draw upon coping skills you might never have needed before.

Strong emotions are a natural response to this shock. A woman who has made her own adjustment to disability counsels someone raw from the experience:

> You have every right to those feelings that threaten to drown you, but you will learn that they will not drown you, and that things will get easier, and that there are things that make life worth living. But you don't want to hear that now, so just keep howling at the moon, and most important of all, keep breathing.

You will have many questions floating around in your mind about your life with a disability. Will I be able to work? How will my friends and family feel about me? Can I be loved? Can I make love? How will I get around? Can I travel? Where will I live? Why did this happen?

Your future can seem so uncertain, with no way to grasp an image of where your life can go from here. According to Jeri Morris, Ph.D., of the Northwestern University Medical School in Chicago, this uncertainty of the future can be so extensive that you "feel virtually without a lifestyle."[4]

There is a wide range of disability and experience. You might be a low level spinal cord injured paraplegic highly capable of independence. Or you might have suffered a traumatic brain injury or broken neck which has paralyzed you almost completely. Each situation entails its own set of adjustments, some admittedly more challenging than others. Yet what all such people have in common are the tasks of separating their misconceptions from reality, discovering over time what adjustments can be made, and learning that even the most severe disability need not preclude a meaningful life.

Being a person who uses a wheelchair is not an easy experience. But it can be an opportunity. Carol Gill is a disability psychologist who contracted polio at the age of five. She has worked directly with people as a therapist and performed research. She knows from her own experience how large a challenge a disability is. However, Gill notes:

> When you go through any crisis, any experience that tests you, in which you feel you may fail, but you triumph instead and come out on the other side, I think that deepens you. I think it gives you a lot of perspective on life.

Gill carries an image in her mind of:

> ...a piece of pottery going through a kiln. The temperature is very hot. If it's too hot the piece can melt down and break, but if it's just right the piece comes out stronger with lots of color, a beautiful piece of art. I think that's what happens with most people with a disability.

Just the fact of getting through the rehabilitation process is the first proof for people of what might be possible, as this quadriplegic woman says:

> I remember toward the end of my rehab, thinking, well I broke my neck and I got through it, I can do anything.

While your experience might be marked by negative emotions, fatigue, confusion, or a sense of powerlessness, you also have the chance to experience hope and confidence as you witness your ability to deal with such a challenging situation. The fact is that most people who acquire a disability make the adjustment in ways they never dreamed possible. Plenty of people before you had similar feelings and could not imagine how they would adjust.

Notes Carol Gill:

> The overwhelming majority of people can and will adjust, given proper social support, meaning not just family and friends, but society at large. I worked in rehab for many years, and it's just amazing how people can take this in stride, given adequate social support. People I never would have predicted would have the inner resources to deal with a disability, just do!

Emotional responses

Regardless of how well-adjusted, mature, or emotionally strong you are, powerful emotions are a natural reaction to a crisis and part of the recovery and adaptive process. Emotions are neither positive nor negative (although you sometimes experience them that way—most people would rather feel happy than angry). They are a natural part of your being human.

It's important to realize that the emotions related to your disability experience will rise and fall, come and go. Keep in mind—especially when you are feeling emotionally overwhelmed—that these reactions are not lasting. Most of all, when you are troubled, remember it is because of what happened to you, not because there is anything wrong with your mind.

Following are common emotional responses experienced by those with a disability. Whether you experience some or all of them, and to what degree, depends on a number of factors, including your individual situation and temperament. Those who are newly disabled—when the shock is new and the future uncertain—are apt to feel a sense of tragedy or grief, or protect themselves with denial to some extent.

Sense of tragedy

No one can say your disability isn't tragic, but whether or not you think of it as a tragedy depends on how you believe it will affect your life. Society ascribes images of dependency, pain, isolation, and fear to disability. These qualities are not true of the experience for many people with a disability, or may not be present to the degree you might imagine. Your sense of tragedy may be amplified by these assumptions. Such exaggerated beliefs about disability are a source of unnecessary suffering.

That is not to say that you should be expected to just "get over it." Carol Gill says:

> As a therapist I would select a tone with people who are dealing with a new disability which says, "Yeah, this is a crisis that is catastrophic for you." I would not try to minimize that. After all, who wants to become disabled?

In *Sexual Adjustment*, Martha Gregory writes:

> *For healthy persons, the thought of spending the future [with a disability] may be so completely endowed with tragic overtones that they assume no one could be stable and happy.*[5]

If you consistently project only the negative aspects of your experience of your disability to your family, friends, and the public, they are more likely to reflect negativity back to you. The way you feel about yourself and your disability affects others' reactions to you. You might also feel negative messages about your disability from others. It goes both ways. Self-confidence is no guarantee of not being seen in tragic terms, but revealing your positive side will often overcome discomfort some people have with your disability.

Your sense of tragedy about the experience of disability is important to face. Are you willing to consider that it's *not* as horrible as you always imagined?

Once you can discover that the impact on your life options is less than you feared, the sense of tragedy is reduced. Tragedy is really the beginning of the process. As a man who has spent years on wheels observes:

> *Those of us with a disability who have made our significant adjustments do not think of ourselves as tragic. Nor do we want to, having gone beyond it to get on with our lives. The tragic part is history—old news.*

New people you meet who find out what led to your using a wheelchair will experience your story as tragic and respond with sympathy. This is natural on first contact. They need to feel the tragedy of it themselves, and make their own adjustment, especially if they are people you will have a continuing relationship with. Just as you adapt beyond the initial sense of tragedy, so will the significant people in your life.

Denial

When reality is too hard to bear all at once, the mind protects itself by using defense mechanisms, one of which is denial. In the short term, denial can help you get through difficult situations. Denial buys you time to gradually come to terms with what has happened. It gives you some control over the pace of psychological adjustment. A disabling injury is so powerful an experience that people just can't take it all in right away. The first tendency is to believe that it's not serious. This is one of our miraculous, self-adjusting "design features."

Lying on the ground, having fallen twenty-five feet, unable to move my legs, I remember very clearly thinking that they would take me to the hospital, and I would be home that afternoon. Walking and fine.

There are a number of ways in which denial can manifest itself. A person might:

- Forget what the doctor has said about his condition

- Disagree with the doctor's prognosis, perhaps insisting that he will recover fully after being told his condition is permanent

- Grant the facts about his condition, but resist the idea that his life will need to change

According to psychologist Ann Marie Fleming:

Some people will say, "Well, I'm the same me I've always been, so I should be able to do all the same things I used to—let me at it." They want to go back to their normal life, regardless of what kind or degree of disability. But once they get through their hospitalization and rehab and get back home, once they get out there and try everything, at some point they're going to hit a wall and say, "Ouch. Omigod, this is hard!" It is a big shock, but that's when the real adjustment begins.

Denial gets to be a problem when it continues well past the initial shock of a crisis and is so pervasive it keeps you from acting in your own best interest. For instance, someone in denial:

- Might not take recommended medication or participate fully in a treatment or rehab program

- Might not arrange for needed support at home, thereby risking injury

- Might not make necessary home-access adjustments, risking injury

- Might not speak honestly to family and friends so they know what support is needed

- Might be careless about health maintenance, for example, not responding to early signs of a pressure sore or infection

Staying stuck in denial about your condition can also drive you to over-achieve, unnecessarily trying to prove that you *aren't* disabled. That can be a great waste of energy and put your health at risk.

It's so strange that for most of my life after polio, all I could think about was to keep going as fast as I could. Never did I want to think about polio. I would also ignore my physical discomfort and limitations completely—unless, of course, they had me flat on my back or hospitalized. Even then, as soon as I was back on my feet, I'd be back on that treadmill. Now after all these years, I realize the need to heal all of the wounds inside.

If others—medical professionals, family, friends—tell you you're in denial, it's worth asking yourself if they might be right and to what degree it might be hurting you. But no one else can know what you are experiencing, and you have to find your way the best you can. Psychologist Carol Gill has respect for the help denial can offer individuals:

If a person stays in denial but it insulates them from pain, who are we to decide it is a bad adjustment? I've met people who've used denial all their lives, and although I might get frustrated, if it gets them through, who am I to judge?

Grief

Some people say that when they became disabled, they died. The person they were was gone. The natural response to loss is grief. You grieve for the loss of your former self—lost plans, lost capacities, lost relationships.

Ann Marie Fleming, a rehabilitation psychologist, observes:

When you become disabled, you lose some part of yourself that you knew and cherished. Everybody goes through multiple, major adjustments which affect their career, marriage, and relationships.

There are a number of stages in being newly disabled which can elicit more feelings of loss and grief. After dealing with the injury itself, you might face disappointment about how much recovery you accomplish in the initial months. When you are released, you will face losing certain abilities in the outside world, such as easily going wherever you want. Relationships will change. Until you get through these milestones, and face these losses, it will be more difficult to redefine yourself and replace those lost parts of your life with new activities, interests, and relationships.

Grief is part of the healing process and diminishes over time. With a new disability you might well experience a deep, immobilizing grief over being injured or discovering you have a degenerative condition of some kind. But it will pass, if you allow yourself to mourn. In time you might continue to feel a sense of loss about your disability, but says Carol Gill:

> People are complex. We're capable of feeling loss and remembering a sense of grief, but also of pursuing our lives and feeling real joy about other facets of our lives.

There is great social pressure not to grieve, or at least not for long. Society does not encourage vulnerability, particularly for men. You may already be feeling dependent on family or friends because of your disability, so to also need emotional support can feel like you are demanding even more. Because you care about how your disability has affected loved ones, you naturally want to be strong for them, to not cause them more pain by having to watch you suffer more. Seeing you cry can raise great fear—that you are not adjusting well, or that you will continue to be dependent, maybe increasingly so. But if you need to cry, do.

Irving Zola wrote about people's fear of crying:

> [They believe] once started, it, like self-pity, will never stop. My own observation is that those people with an oversupply of tears are ones who have been unable to mourn their losses fully, especially when they first occurred. As a result they "leak" and mourn a little bit at a time.[6]

Anger

Some features of early disability and rehab can understandably lead to angry feelings. The future can seem ruined, you have to submit to the care of strangers, who often must perform invasive medical or personal care procedures—sometimes with a cavalier attitude. This can be experienced as a loss of control and dignity. These feelings need not necessarily occur, but you might have thoughts such as:

- This isn't fair.

- Why did this happen to me?

- It was my fault. How could I have been so stupid to let this happen?

- It was their fault, and I will hate them forever for what they did to me— or didn't do to protect me.

- I will never have the life I wanted, so nothing can be okay now.

You have the power to decide how to express the anger, and how to face the source of it so that you can move on with your life. It's exhausting to go through life angry.

> *I'm a C4-5 quadriplegic. It takes way too much energy to get through the typical day living with my disability to be spending the bulk of that energy on hostility, denial, and rebellion.*

You will also find yourself in situations that will likely arouse anger. There will be people who will speak to your companions on your behalf rather than directly addressing you. You might be left waiting for the wheelchair you need because Medicare or your HMO is refusing to pay. You might be unable to get down the aisle of a store because of advertising displays. You might be trying to find an apartment to rent and discover how few meet your access needs. The list goes on.

If you use a wheelchair, your anger—no matter what its source—is often seen as bitterness about your disability. Carol Gill explains:

> *I think anger is one of those emotions that gets interpreted by outsiders in the context of what they think about us in general. It's been said that when a man is aggressive in his profession he's considered a go-getter, but when a woman is aggressive she's a bitch. I think those same contextual interpretations exist for people with disabilities. If a nondisabled person was told, "You can't get into this store, we're not going to move this box so you can get down this aisle," they would become angry and leave the store in a huff. That would be considered justified. But if a disabled person got equally angry about not having access to that store, he would be viewed as having a chip on his shoulder.*

Even if you never see people from these encounters again, they might interpret your behavior as bitter—the "rude cripple." Learning to manage anger will not only save you a lot of trouble, it will help forward the perception of people with disabilities in the broader community. Managing anger does not mean keeping quiet. It means recognizing you are angry before your anger gets out of control, and taking charge of what to do about it.

When you are angry—for whatever reason—you might feel like screaming, flailing about, throwing things, or hurting yourself or others. These are the actions most people associate with anger. Since these expressions are not socially acceptable, many people will instead suffer in silence, repressing their emotions. But anger that is held in has a way of finding its way out, often in subtle ways you may not notice. You might begin to be more cynical or sarcastic, or more of a tease—which can be a disguised form of attack. You might begin to drive more aggressively or start hitting the keys of your computer keyboard harder. Your wheelchair can become the object of your anger, as you handle it heavily, being less than gentle as you put it in and out of the car or when you open or close it. Many people with disabilities throw their legs—such as while getting into or out of bed—or fail to be as gentle as necessary in bowel and bladder management. These subtle ways of venting pent-up anger can be harmful to you. Anger can fester and grow, and maybe lead you to say or do something you ultimately regret.

Fortunately, there are healthful ways of expressing anger, although they may take practice. For instance, you can talk about your anger with people you trust. If you think they won't believe you unless you *act* angry, tell them, "I know I don't seem like it, but I'm really angry." Then tell them what's bothering you. This paraplegic man in his twenties, now a social worker in a major rehab center, describes learning that lesson:

> I was really into being a tough guy at the time I was injured, so felt that I couldn't let people run my life once I broke my back. I really put my family through a lot of hell, but then I realized I was just stuck in a trap. One day I got on the phone and called a lot of people and apologized. They let me know that it sure wasn't fun to be treated badly when I was rude to them, but they tried their best to understand. It helped clear the air, and we're all the closer now for having talked about it.

When you're feeling explosive—and not in the mood for a heart-to-heart chat with anyone—you can channel your anger into some physical activity. If you're able to exercise, that can release a lot of angry tension. Even if you are very limited physically, there are ways to express your anger so that it doesn't hurt anyone, especially yourself. Other ways to physically release anger are to throw darts, or blow up balloons and then pop them, all the while reciting the reasons for your wrath. Sometimes your only outlet is your voice. If it helps you feel better, go ahead and yell, but make sure anyone in hearing range knows that you're not in danger—nor is anyone else. Or you can sing. As strange as it sounds, singing when you're angry not only releases energy, but makes you feel better. You can even make up your own angry words to popular melodies. Use your creativity to come up with an outlet for anger that works for you.

Anger doesn't have to be full-blown. Having a disability can make your life harder at times, and being frustrated is a logical reaction.

> If I'm having problems transferring [to and from my chair] and I'm exhausted and it's hard for me, it means I'm having a bad day like anyone can. People with disabilities have those day-to-day frustrations too.

> When I feel angry and most frustrated about being disabled, it is almost invariably when I'm trying to be too nondisabled. Say I'm putting on a dinner party, which is pretty difficult for a quadriplegic to do. If something goes wrong, I get pretty frustrated. Now, someone might say that it means I really hate being disabled, but I say, "What was I trying to do!?" It's frustrating when you get caught up in the expectations of what you think you're supposed to be able to do. When I'm having a bad day it's not because I hate having a disability. I just don't attach it to this greater thing.

It's not always enough to express anger. If you are being treated poorly or unjustly, you can use your anger as redirected energy to try to resolve the problem. For example, if your insurer won't pay for something you need and you believe you have a right to it, hitting pillows isn't going to change things. You need to do some research, write letters, and make phone calls to make a difference. Righteous anger has moved many a mountain, especially if you take the time to find out the best methods to make your case, and enlist the help of the right people.

Feelings of resentment and rage toward society's misconceptions of the disabled drive many people to become involved in disability activism. Anger played a part in the motivation of trailblazers like Judy Heumann, Justin Dart, Ed Roberts, Bob Kafka, Evan Kemp, and Mary Lou Breslin—among many others—to get out and work for the kinds of changes that have already been accomplished. Despite the passage of the Rehabilitation Act of 1973, the ADA, and other victories, there is a great deal to be done. Anger will, and should, stoke that fire. Chapter 10, *Politics and Legislation*, talks more about the changes being made by and on behalf of the disabled community.

Depression

There are basically two kinds of depression: the kind almost everyone experiences from time-to-time, often called "the blues," and chronic, clinical depression. There is a distinct difference in the effects each kind has on the depressed person, how long the depression lasts, and how it is treated.

Common depression

Few people get through life without ever feeling down. Common depression always has a reason that triggers it. The trigger can be something significant—like dealing with a disability—or more mundane, like a week of rainy weather. During a common depression, brain chemistry is altered, which is why you don't feel like your normal self. The chemical alteration usually rights itself after a few days, when the trigger has either dissipated or you have had enough time to begin to cope with it.

When you are newly disabled, it's normal to feel sad and disappointed, maybe even a little hopeless. You recognize what has happened and are troubled by it. You may wonder, "Will I feel like this forever? How much worse will my life get? Who could ever love me with this disability? Is it my fault that I'm disabled?" These are normal things to worry about and they can foster feelings of depression.

When you are depressed, it is hard to separate problems associated with your disability from those problems you would have anyway. Be careful not to make your disability the scapegoat for feeling that life is a struggle. Blaming everything on your disability means missing the chance to review other aspects of your life that need attention, and it means defining your disability as an unendurable state which you can never rise above. That can be a lifelong sentence for unhappiness.

Common depression can last from a few hours to a couple of weeks. You might feel unmotivated, sluggish, or distracted as well as blue. You might be tempted to retreat into yourself, spend more time sleeping, and be as passive as possible, maybe watching television a lot more than you usually do. However, you will still be able to function well enough to maintain necessary daily activities, and you will be able to acknowledge that there can be solutions to your problems, even though you might not be able to imagine what the solutions are. Although you may not laugh as readily as when you're not depressed, you'll still have a sense of humor. Most important, you will retain a sense of being in control of your life. You just won't feel like working very hard at it.

Most of the time, depression of this kind runs its course, and you begin to feel better about yourself and your life. You can help yourself feel better sooner, though, and possibly ward off a more serious depression by taking some small steps, even if you have to push a bit to get started.

One of the most common pieces of advice is to simply do *something*. The simplest activity can give your mind another perspective, and provide the opportunity to become engaged and interested in something other than your problems. It's also important to maintain human contact, since loneliness tends to amplify depression, but try to include other topics of conversation besides your woes. Finally, take especially good care of yourself.

The following list offers ideas that can help lift you out of a common depression.

- Listen to your favorite music. Music has a way of bringing feelings to the surface so you can explore them rather than just being miserable.

- Play with or read to a child. It will help you get out of your world and see things from a simpler perspective.

- Work—or just spend some time—in the garden.

- Straighten up a room or a table, or bring in some flowers.

- Try to distinguish between what you really are unable to do and what you just don't feel like doing. For the latter, try to apply yourself if only for a couple of minutes. You might discover you are able to do what you thought you couldn't.

- Divide big jobs into small ones. They add up quickly that way and will give you a sense of accomplishment.

- If you can, exercise. Physical activity is stimulating, and can change the chemistry of your brain to lift your spirits.

- Play a game—athletic or otherwise. It will help you focus on the moment. You might even have fun.

- Go out with a friend, perhaps to a funny movie.

- Hug someone or have someone hug you.

- Do something unexpectedly nice for someone.

- Do something unexpectedly nice for yourself.

- Remember to eat—as healthfully as possible. Keeping your body well-nourished will speed your return to your happier self.

- Observe good hygiene and grooming. You're less likely to feel depressed when you look your best.

One thing *not* to do when you're feeling depressed is make major life decisions. Postponing decisions does not mean you surrender faith in yourself. It means you have the good sense to know you'll make better decisions when you can think more objectively—when your emotions are in better balance. This day will arrive soon.

Clinical depression

When mental health professionals speak of depression, they are usually referring to a condition much more severe than common depression. Clinical depression affects about one in twenty people in the United States each year. Whereas common depression is a temporary emotional downswing, clinical depression is an illness that can last as long as three years and be completely debilitating—although this is a worst-case scenario. Unlike common depression, clinical depression doesn't necessarily have a trigger. Even if there is a reason, the depression lasts long beyond the time it normally takes to start coping with a trigger event. Clinical depression is more about the alteration of brain chemistry that doesn't right itself than about logical reasons for feeling blue.

Although modern research is learning much about brain chemistry and depression, it remains a chicken and egg question. It is not clear whether the chemical change is a cause or a symptom of depression. This means that one must be careful of simply taking anti-depressant drugs to curtail depression when at the same time it might be important to engage in the deep personal and spiritual work of self-evaluation such feelings often elicit.

A person ill with clinical depression needs medical intervention. If you have any of the following symptoms that last more than a couple of weeks, tell your doctor:

- Persistent sadness, hopelessness, or pessimism

- Feelings of guilt or worthlessness

- Lack of emotion; a feeling of emptiness

- A sense of helplessness

- Lack of interest in activities you would normally enjoy; inability to find pleasure or humor in anything

- Marked change in sleeping or eating patterns

- Chronic fatigue; exhaustion

- Restlessness or irritability
- Cognitive difficulties: remembering, concentrating, making even simple decisions
- Preoccupation with death or suicide

In the darkest moments of clinical depression, there can seem to be no options remaining for happiness or meaning in one's life. Feeling like nothing can ever be better is part of the insidious nature of the illness. Some people might tell you to "snap out of it!" They might as well tell you to snap out of pneumonia.

If you suspect you are clinically depressed, remember it is not your fault. It is not a sign of weakness. Eighty to ninety percent of people with clinical depression can be treated effectively. Almost everyone benefits to some extent from treatment, which usually involves a combination of drug therapy and psychotherapy—exploring your feelings and life events with a trained therapist.

Long-term depression is an empty place to be, but things are never as hopeless as you think they are when you're depressed. Don't be afraid to reach out for help.

Suicide

Having a disability—regardless of the physical severity—sometimes leads even those who are not clinically depressed to the point where they feel their situation is unchangeable and hopeless. They see themselves as having no options, no place to move, no resources for change, and no one to turn to who could make a difference. Perhaps the thought of adapting to a life with disability seems unacceptable, too far out of line with their understanding of what it means to have a full, rich life. In a moment of utter despair and darkness, a person may consider that he would be better off ending his life.

The serious consideration of suicide should not be kept secret. If you find yourself thinking that death is the best solution for you, tell someone right away. Many cities have a twenty-four-hour hotline (look in the yellow pages under "crisis intervention"—if there is no agency specific to your need, any of the listed numbers should be able to help you). No matter how hopeless or ruined you believe your life to be, one phone call can save it.

If you are worried that someone you love might be thinking about suicide, don't be afraid to say, "I'm concerned you are thinking about taking your life." It can be a great relief for the person to know someone is willing to listen. Encourage him or her to get immediate professional counseling.

Following are warning signs to watch for:

- Withdrawing from friends and family
- Changes in appetite, weight, behavior, level of activity, or sleep patterns
- Making self-deprecating comments
- Talking, writing, or hinting about suicide
- Purposefully putting personal affairs in order, such as tending to a will or life insurance
- Giving away possessions
- Sudden change from extreme depression to being "at peace" (may indicate a decision to attempt suicide)

It is the nature of suicidal feelings that the world appears very small. It doesn't occur to a suicidal person that there may be options he is not aware of, or that he could ever feel differently about the quality of his life.

Unfortunately for people with severe disability, some professionals have dangerous misconceptions about what level of quality of life is possible for their patients.

Yet there is ample evidence that people with even the most severe disabilities—including those who are mostly paralyzed and ventilator-dependent—consider the value of their lives to be very high. Make sure whoever is helping you is committed to uncovering every conceivable possibility to enrich your life and make it worth living for you.

In *No Pity*, Joseph Shapiro describes Larry McAfee, a thirty-four-year-old engineering student who became quadriplegic from a motorcycle accident and was in an intensive care unit for three months. McAfee was the subject of a high-profile assisted suicide case. He asked to have a switch installed on his ventilator so that he could turn it off; a court granted permission. After a dizzying series of bureaucratic battles regarding where he could live and access to computer equipment, McAfee's outlook changed. Thanks to the efforts of his family, other individuals, and disability groups, Larry McAfee finally returned to the community in a group home. According to Shapiro:

> *His mood bounced up and down, but on the whole, he pronounced himself happy to be alive, living a "good" life that had given him "Hope."*[7]

The current debate on assisted suicide is discussed in more detail in Chapter 10.

Hope

Hope is powerful, giving you strength to overcome grief, denial, and depression. Even a small ray of hope can help to keep you moving forward. Sometimes, hope is all you have. It is only natural to hope for a significant recovery after a disabling injury or diagnosis of a chronic or progressive disease.

After an injury or diagnosis, medical professionals are cautious about encouraging what they fear could be false hope. Every one of them has seen people suffer heartbreak when their hopes didn't come true. Yet doctors, nurses, and others don't want to rob you of a positive outlook, or make themselves your adversary. It is a difficult balance for them to achieve. They want to foster your motivation as much as possible while at the same time protecting you from the potential for psychological trauma.

How you discuss your hopes with the medical professionals who care for you makes a difference in how you are perceived and responded to. If they perceive you as being stuck on expecting a complete recovery or cure, to the exclusion of all other possibilities, they might not want to encourage your hopes. On the other hand, if you are asking questions about possible outcomes, and what active measures you can take to bring about the best possible result, they'll be more comfortable supporting your hope for a degree of improvement even if they personally doubt you might achieve it.

At its best, hope will spur you to do whatever is necessary to make life as good as possible for yourself, including participation in the rehabilitation process. Embracing rehabilitation or other adaptations doesn't mean you surrender hope of recovery. It means you recognize that it is the best you can do right now. Should the hoped-for recovery be on its way, full participation in therapy will ensure you are in optimal health and in the best position to take advantage of it.

Sometimes, what people call hope is really denial. Some disabled people seem to use potential cure as an excuse to not acknowledge their disabilities or adapt to them, and to allow themselves to be unnecessarily dependent.

Real hope isn't limited to the hope for a full recovery. You might hope you will still be able to pursue the career you want, hope you'll still be able to participate in some of the activities you love, hope you'll find a really great personal care assistant, or hope you can learn to pop wheelies as well as some experienced riders you've seen. Your hopes can help bring into focus what is truly important to you, and therefore help you make it happen. The ancient Roman poet Ovid had the right idea, "My hopes are not always realized, but I always hope."

Acceptance

There will be people who will try to get you to "accept" your disability, as if it is just a simple decision that you make and then are done with it. It is not so easy, and not just an intellectual choice. Not only is there a complex set of inner forces at play, but acceptance is *supposed* to take time. What you learn along the way is worthwhile.

Well-trained medical staff know that people need to be allowed their natural emotional responses, and will try to help family members understand this as well. That response might include a refusal to initially accept a new disability.

Attitudes do change. You can reach a balance appropriate for you, as happened for this spinal cord injured man:

> More than seventeen years ago I remember saying I would not accept my disability. But by investing my life in positive activities my attitude slowly changed to one of tolerance. Don't believe I have fully accepted it—or want to—because, for me, that would diminish hope. You don't need to accept this situation, but you must learn to deal with it. You have a life you might as well live.

Acceptance doesn't have to mean you're happy about having a disability. It means you accommodate its needs so it won't compromise the quality of your life any more than necessary, if at all.

Many people say that they just need to know what is really happening. For example, multiple sclerosis used to be much more difficult to diagnose, before the advent of magnetic resonance imaging (MRI). People could go for years experiencing the weakness of MS exacerbations and remissions before knowing what was happening. Once people have a diagnosis, it becomes possible to adapt.

Resisting acceptance implies there is some preferred state, other than the one you are in, or some way to resolve your situation. Buddhist nun Pema Chödrön describes seeking resolution this way:

> We don't deserve resolution; we deserve something better than that. We deserve our birthright, which is the middle way, an open state of mind that can relax with paradox and ambiguity. To the degree that we've been avoiding uncertainty, we're naturally going to have withdrawal symptoms—withdrawal from always thinking that there's a problem and that someone, somewhere needs to fix it.[8]

Acceptance includes the willingness to let go of always having answers and wanting things to be "solved." It is possible to recognize that things are out of control and still find a way to relax in the face of chaos.

Humor

You might be surprised at being able to laugh about your disability experience. The more comfortable you are with your disability, the easier it is to have a little fun with it. Even tentative humor in the initial stages of adapting can reassure you that things are going to get better. Laughter is healing. Humor can affirm that your ability to see the funny side of life is unaffected by disability.

> We had a lot of fun at the therapy gym where I went for rehab. It added to the spirit of the hard work, increasing my motivation.

Joking about disability makes some people uncomfortable. They are so used to thinking of disability as tragic that to joke about it seems cruel. You will undoubtedly feel more at ease with such humor than the nondisabled people around you. For instance, John Callahan is a spinal cord injured paraplegic who is well known for his sometimes skewed humor about disability. He has drawn many published cartoons now collected in several books, and also written a book on his own disability experience, *Don't Worry, He Won't Get Far on Foot*. Another rider collects disability one-liners to use in various situations:

> *I have built a repertoire of lines over the years of using a wheelchair. When the opportunity presents itself, I can joke with someone that "I'll never set wheel in here again!" or that I need to "take a sit" on a certain issue.*

You can find plenty of examples of humor in daily life:

> *There was the man in a movie theater who thought that the Americans with Disabilities Act entitled me to go ahead of him in the popcorn line. Or the time I took a spill after trying to show off a bit too much with wheelies.*

Reynolds Price is a writer who faced an extended experience fighting cancer, which included paralysis. In his book *A Whole New Life*, he writes:

> *Best of all, with the help of friends, I managed to laugh a few times most days. Sometimes the rusty sound of my out-of-practice chuckle reminded me of how a gift as big as the tendency to laugh in the face of disaster is a literally biological endowment.*[9]

Your disability should not be off limits to humor. Your friends can become comfortable with where the boundaries are on jokes at the expense of your disability. Spend time with friends you enjoy, and let them know they don't need to restrain themselves on your behalf.

> *I consider it a proof of intimacy when friends demonstrate they know I won't break down and cry if something truly funny comes up around being a chair user.*

Emotional support

The need for medical treatment and therapy for a newly disabled person is obvious. Ongoing support to help maintain good health is also expected. Your inner self is equally deserving of support. Support can help see you through the initial emotional trauma of injury or diagnosis, and help you gain increasingly deeper insight as you live with disability. Common sources of emotional support include family and friends, support groups, and psychological counseling.

The emotional support of family and friends is a tremendous comfort. If you are lucky enough to have strong support from the people closest to you, don't be reluctant to let them help. Because they know you so well, you can get to the heart of what you are feeling without having to explain a lot of background about who you are. Trust is already there, so you don't have to worry about exposing your deepest emotions.

This man with C5 quadriplegia recalls:

> All my friends were super-supportive. I remember going out to dinner when I was still wearing my halo! We were sitting in a crowded restaurant on a Friday night where all the beautiful people come out. Here I am wearing a halo, so for them to do that for me, and take me to bars— we were all learning things together. My family and friends are the single most important thing. I can give myself credit, but they totally changed how it went.

Unfortunately, not all families and friends are able to offer ideal emotional support, especially not at first. They might be having their own difficulty coping with what has happened to you and need emotional support, too. It's important that you don't feel responsible for their emotional needs. That can be a temptation—and a drain. Sometimes family or friends will have to take time away from you in order to make their own emotional adjustments.

> I had some friends who just didn't know how to deal with my injury. They couldn't come to the hospital. It was too much. Some were honest enough to say they needed time, and were sorry they couldn't be there for me. One of my best friends just cut off all contact. I found out later that he was overwhelmed, and didn't know how to even approach me. It took a few years, but once I was back out in the world, we were able to resume our friendship, which was very deep. Now he is like family to me. I could have been angry and chosen not to forgive him, but I realize how painful the whole thing was for him, and would rather not sacrifice what he means to me now.

Another source of emotional support is a support group. There are many different kinds of groups; the common denominator is that people in them share the experience of disability. Group members can honestly say, "We know how you feel." You don't have to be falling apart emotionally to benefit from a support group. It is a chance to meet with people who share your experience. Whether you need someone to understand and relieve your fears about the future, recommend a helpful product, or share ideas for dealing with insensitive strangers, group support can be a wonderful resource. You can find support groups in your city or on the Internet. Many rehab hospitals have support programs that include peer volunteers.

Professional counseling is another option for getting help dealing with disability. Long gone are the days when going to a psychologist meant there was something seriously wrong with your head, or that you weren't smart or strong enough to get through rough times on your own. A professional counselor can save you unnecessary distress by helping you understand yourself better and see a disability as a part of your life that offers opportunity as well as challenge. (You may have to shop around a bit to find someone with whom you feel comfortable. Don't be discouraged if the first counselor you visit doesn't seem right for you—it's worth it to keep looking.) Counseling is confidential, so you can feel safe revealing your thoughts and feelings. So well-recognized is the importance of giving newly disabled people adequate emotional support that psychologists are now commonly included as part of the rehab team.

Whether you choose to work with a counselor when you first become disabled or at some point later on is, of course, entirely up to you. You may find that your other sources of support are all you need. There are circumstances, however, when it is extremely important to seek out the services of a psychology professional. If you are suffering from chronic depression or having thoughts of suicide, the sooner you talk to a professional counselor, the better. In these situations, human beings are too emotionally distraught to be of much help to themselves, and non-professionals don't have the necessary training. Being depressed or suicidal is nothing to be ashamed of—although it will probably feel that way. Don't hesitate to contact a counselor. Your physician can recommend someone.

Adaptability

Change is the one constant in life. A disability—whether acquired at birth or later in life—is one heck of an exercise in adapting to change. Being injured means instant and intense adaptation. Being disabled at birth means adapting throughout development, with changing issues in adolescence and as you become increasingly socialized outside of the family. A progressive condition like MS, ALS, or one of the muscular dystrophies means a continuing process of adapting as the effects of the disability progress, sometimes very slowly. Even people with spinal cord injuries, once thought to be a stable condition after the rehabilitation process, face changes in levels of impairment as they age.

This quadriplegic woman in her forties is finding that she is being called upon to make new adaptations she didn't expect to face:

> It's depressing. Is this a change? Is this just one step and I get used to it and it's going to stay like that for a while? Or is it going to be something that's more limiting over time and I'm going to have to get used to more and more limitations?

Part of adaptability is the ability to create an environment for yourself in which your disability does not unduly limit you. In many ways, the disability itself is not what "handicaps" you. It is when you can't get up the steps or through the door that you become disabled. You can create more psychological security for yourself by creating an environment which does not unnecessarily limit you.

In *Missing Pieces*, Irving Zola asks:

> What happens to all those without sufficient money or power to alter their environment, without resources to have railings built or clothes custom-made or sufficient influence to have meetings take place in more physically accessible locations? I suspect that they ultimately give up. Unable to change or manipulate the world, they simply cut out that part of their life which requires such encounters, which contributes to a real, as well as social, invisibility and isolation.[10]

Self-advocacy is a critical skill in this process of finding your place in a life on wheels. The very act of pursuing your needs and asserting your rights is in itself psychologically supportive. While Professor Zola's suspicion that some people give up may be true, it need not be. Your resolution of anger, comfort with your identity, gradual release of denial, and the entire process of adaptation—your emotional reality—relies on addressing your physical environment, as well as remaining intellectually stimulated and spiritually curious.

If there is one central lesson that the experience of disability has to teach you, it is how remarkably adaptive human beings are. Some people might have fewer obstacles than others, but chances are you can do more than you might think you can.

> *After becoming disabled, I got a college education, accomplished a great deal professionally, traveled, made close friends, loved and lost and loved some more—what I consider the ingredients of a pretty full life. I wouldn't tell you that my disability has been neutral in all of this, or that there aren't things I would have loved to do that I can't. I'm telling you that at the time of my injury I could not conceive of doing the things I ultimately did.*

The capacity to adapt seems to be related to age. Rehab psychologist Ann Marie Fleming sees that children tend to make relatively easy adjustments. Their lives are all about constant change and their adaptation skills are well practiced. The older people are, the more difficult it can be for some of them to accept a major change such as disability.

> *As we age, it becomes harder and harder to accommodate major lifestyle changes. We become more fixed in our ways, and we just plain get tired out with the weight of our lives behind us.*

For some people, the shock of disability can jolt them from a self-destructive path. Fleming states:

> *For someone who maybe used drugs or had trouble holding down responsibilities, that brush with death is a spiritual crisis. All of a sudden they want to be alive, they want to be straight, they want to be conscious, they want to be clear. They say, "I don't want to die. I don't want to medicate any more."*

Disability is a chance to be reminded of the universal truth of the frailty of being human. The struggle to adapt to the many demands of disability can increase your empathy for all people, as is the experience of this woman with Charcot-Marie Tooth disease, a form of muscular dystrophy:

> *I believe, too, that having CMT has definitely given me the sense of being more accepting of others, whether they are "disabled" in some way or not. We are each so individual, thank goodness! How boring it would be if not! I try to see people's insides more than their outsides.*

You will inevitably consider how you previously felt about people with disabilities. You get to revisit your attitudes, now that you have joined the club. Carol Gill sees an advantage in this, saying:

> You learn a lot about being human from the way you once looked at people with disabilities and the way you now look at yourself and others with disabilities. You go through a values overhaul.

Family

The experience happens to family, too. Family members will have intense emotions and struggles evoked by your disability. They have adjustments to make and your relationship with them will need to adjust.

> I know my disability was very painful for my parents. Their son had been seriously injured. On the day I was admitted to rehab, after weeks in another hospital recovering from back surgery, my doctor told them point-blank that my condition would stay just as it was on that day. Having gone to rehab with hope that I might walk out, they found themselves sitting in the lobby, crying together. This was a powerful experience for them, too.

Family members could be afraid to bring up certain topics, for fear of upsetting you. Let them know how open you want them to be with you. It might fall to you to draw them out, to start the ball rolling on discussing a sensitive topic related to your disability.

Professionals tell families not to withhold what they feel. If their injured relative makes them angry or very sad, they might fear that revealing these feelings could overwhelm their loved one.

Social worker Joan Anderson of the Santa Clara Valley Medical Center in California writes:

> Families seem to believe that if a person has a disability he or she is too fragile to withstand normal human interactions. Such an attitude dehumanizes the disabled person and robs him or her of the normal exchange of feelings that keep our relationships mutual and balanced.[11]

Family members, especially parents, often feel they need to exercise some control, to make sure that you are being taken care of. It might be that they need to feel the need to accomplish *something*, since they can't make you well. But this can be disempowering:

> There was a time in the hospital when my mom was running down the hall saying, "My son hasn't had a shave in three days! Somebody shave this guy!" If I could have moved as fast as her I probably could have killed her, but I couldn't. I was too slow, so it was very frustrating for me to feel so powerless about them trying to baby me.

Family members who express doubts about your ability to function or pursue certain goals might unwittingly weigh you down. Doubt is particularly dangerous when it comes in the form of loving, presumably protective concern. You can be drawn into self-doubt, giving too much consideration to others' opinions. Or you might feel you have to prove your family wrong, overexerting yourself by ignoring your own realistic limits and capacities.

Just as serious a trap is over-optimism, where a family member denies the seriousness of your disability and promotes unrealistic expectations. It is easy for you to want to play along, especially in the early stages when the urge is to remain as "normal" as possible. You usually want to please the ones you love, so you might want to match their expectations, pleased that they see you as someone capable of their proposal—whether it is an aggressive schedule of education, travel, starting a business, or returning quickly to a job.

It is natural for you to care about what your family is going through, at the same time as you face your own feelings. You might feel the need to be strong for them or protect them, but in the process you risk hiding your own true experience and denying them the chance to know you.

Families usually have a lot to learn about disability. To the degree that you bring unrealistic attitudes about disability into your own experience, you might well have picked them up from your family. You will all have to revisit these assumptions, and reconsider how you have allowed society to influence your reactions and views. Many rehab centers offer family support groups for this very purpose.

If family members resist understanding, or if conflict arises, it might be necessary to seek assistance from a counselor to help you work things out. It is not an admission of failure to ask for professional support. When so many changes need to be made at once, it is a hard process for any family, no matter how strong or well-adjusted. Your family relationships are one of the most important supportive elements in your success at adapting with a disability. It is worth any effort to reach a balanced understanding with your family, to allow them to work through their own needs, and to welcome their support and guidance. Then you can all direct your energies in positive ways and accomplish the best quality of life for all family members.

When you and your family find a balance, there is less strain on your relationships and you have a better opportunity to discover your limits and abilities.

> *My mother never imagined that I would not be active and independent. She did not try to do things for me that I could do myself, and she was not negative or doubtful about my plans to return to school, drive, or any other goal. It was not a matter of blind ambition, but a balanced view of what was possible. On the whole she did exactly the right thing. She believed in my capacity to have a normal life, but did not push me to be heroic.*

Letting go

As you progress through the acute stage of an injury or illness, or grow into maturity after a childhood with a disability, your family and friends will need to gradually let go of their roles as caregivers. This is an especially hard task for parents, who feel more secure being able to care for you, relieving them of the worry of your being out on your own. Fleming states:

> *After a while the injured relative will start to say to the family members who continue to help him, "Get out of my face. You're driving me crazy!" It's like an adolescent who starts to test his wings to see how much he can fly on his own. Parents have to be willing to let their children fall once in awhile. I tell the parent, "You've done it before, you can do it again."*

You need to let go, too. You might be surprised at how accustomed you had become to people taking care of you during the early stages of a disability or your childhood with a disability. It is like a repeat of the young adult experience, when you can't wait to get out of the family home and have the freedom to do as you please—until you find out that includes washing the dishes and doing the laundry! Home starts to look pretty good at that point.

The same process of growth happens with your disability. As you embrace adjustment, you might continue to face moments that make you wish your family was still pitching in. Your need to reach for optimal independence is not about your family; it is about defining your needs and the best way to meet them. If you need assistance dressing or transferring, a family member could continue to play that role if you are able to maintain a balanced relationship.

But Carol Gill warns that:

> The deck is stacked against you if you use a family member or an intimate partner as a personal assistant. It sets the stage for confusing various aspects of the relationship. It's hard for family members to just see themselves as providing assistance and not being caretakers. Using outside support is also easier for the family. It makes it easier for them to establish more balanced relationships with the disabled family member.

Letting go might be a matter of identifying how your needs get met, and that could mean deciding that someone other than a family member should perform certain tasks.

Family backgrounds

Different families respond differently to disability. Response is based on a family's previous experiences, including how society tells them to respond. Your family's reaction might be colored by what once happened to Grandpa Joe or cultural expectations from the media or from a country of origin.

- Some families have very close family structures, perhaps all living in the same town or living in extended families with several generations living together. Such a household is accustomed to supporting each other and sharing key life experiences.

- Some families view a physical disability as a "loss of face." The injured relative might face a family attitude that does not believe he can or should have an active lifestyle.

- Some families have a very deep work ethic which can encourage an optimal recovery and hard work in therapy.

- Some families place a high value on privacy. Letting someone into their home is akin to making them a member of the family. This might lead them to refuse help from outside agencies.

- Language barriers can make communication with medical staff difficult. Doctors, nurses, therapists, and peer support volunteers may find it hard to communicate complex medical and social issues effectively.

- If you're aware of assumptions, expectations, or language barriers that stand in the way of optimal treatment and independence, talk about them with rehab staff and other professionals.

Dependency

When an experience is difficult, you might feel pressure to give up. You get tired, or the scale of the task seems overwhelming. Maybe life was already tough prior to your disability, and now you have the perfect excuse to surrender.

There are several possible outlets to spare you all the trouble—or so it seems: reliance on others, over-reliance on government support, or substance abuse. Each is a trap, a downward spiral which only produces more grief and pain, less personal freedom, less self-esteem. Each is more likely to alter your experience from simply being disabled to being truly unable.

Letting others take care of you

A person with a disability who is unable to transcend the stages of trauma, tragedy, fear, and depression will commonly resort to dependency. Having failed to address the psychological dynamics of the situation, putting yourself into the hands of family or institutions whom you expect to take care of you can be tempting.

You might just find it is easier to let someone else care for you. Perhaps your parents are in that role. Perhaps they have fallen into the trap of feeling more secure if they are taking care of you, rather than having to relive the worry they experienced when you grew up and began going out on your own. But your parents will get old before you do. Many people who relied on parents are finding it hard to adjust as their parents age and are no longer able to help with chair transfers or other physical tasks.

People who perform necessary tasks which allow you to function are not "taking care of you." They are assisting you. You decide what they do and how and when. It only becomes dependency when you surrender decision-making and allow others to determine what your life will be like.

Living on the government

Some people don't have any choice about taking government assistance. They are unable to work, unable to find work (all too often because of discrimination), or the disincentives are so strong that they can't work, lest they lose their medical coverage, for instance.

However, if you are thinking that you can't work and don't bother to find out what is possible, you might well be underestimating your abilities. Plenty of people with significant disabilities have good jobs or businesses of their own. Corporations are increasingly learning that making accommodations and hiring people with disabilities is profitable for all parties. Computer technology makes it possible to work by voice command or with limited hand and arm capacity. Computers also make home-based businesses more viable.

Relying on the government often means reduced quality of life. People with disabilities can tell many nightmare stories of struggles with the bureaucracy, having to fight for benefits, and getting trapped by arcane regulations or incompetent workers. Living on Social Security disability benefits earns you the right to medical coverage under Medicare, but Medicare has strict limits on what it will cover. The power wheelchair that might be ideal for you could be refused. You could need home healthcare assistance, but a rule that says you must be unable to leave the home could mean that volunteering at a local school two days a week might cost you your coverage. It's a mistake to assume your only option for financial support is government assistance or that relying on this aid is the best means for adapting to your disability. For many, this decision carries a high price, including the missed potential to be more financially self-sufficient.

Substance abuse

Perhaps your inclination is to depend on substances to get you through, to protect yourself from the internal strife your disability seems to foster. Maybe you received a legal judgment, and accepted a lump sum which put a lot of money in your pocket. Maybe you don't need to work. Sitting at home drinking or smoking pot might be an option, and a hard one to resist.

Substance abuse, be it alcohol, drugs, or food, will compromise your health, and hugely amplify the limiting effects of your disability. You will lose strength, and need more assistance pushing a chair or making transfers. You will likely gain weight, increasing the risk of pressure sores, and again, be more likely to need help in transfers. Changes in your health and strength might force you across that boundary of needing personal assistance or even having to move into a "care" facility.

Many other health risks accompany substance abuse, including heart attacks, liver problems, and even cancer, especially if you smoke. You are compromising your immune system when you abuse substances. Drugs and alcohol also compromise your ability to absorb and metabolize nutrients from your food. This lowers your body's defenses and affects your ability to maintain healthy skin and good circulation, recover from an illness, and heal an injury.

Scientists now understand that good feelings relate to chemicals known as endorphins. In effect, your body makes its own drugs—a natural high. When you habitually abuse substances, your body ceases to produce endorphins on its own. After a time, the only way to feel good is to generate endorphins artificially with drugs or alcohol.

Alcohol and drugs affect your judgment and ability to make decisions. At worst, your family might come to believe you are no longer able to make responsible decisions for yourself, and consider taking control of your life. They might even get legal guardian status and have you placed in a nursing facility.

Independence, not heroism

Independence does not mean that you have to push yourself too hard and become the stereotypical "supercrip." Independence means using the capacity you have, whether it's your physical ability or your ability to manage resources such as benefits and personal assistance services. Independence is about being willing to take some risks, more than might be comfortable at first. Just like going into a pool of cool water, you'll be surprised at how quickly you'll get used to it.

If your fears of facing life with a disability lead you to escape through various forms of dependency, think again. The results of dependencies are far worse than if you jump in, test your capacity to adapt, and seek support for the process. Yes, this can be very tough to do. There are many people out there willing to help, be it the local independent living center, free community counseling, support groups, or friends and family. Fight hard for optimal health and independence rather than accepting a downward spiral into increased suffering and dependency.

Being helped

Thanks, at least in part, to the Boy Scouts and the March of Dimes, people have a desire to help those "in need." Unfortunately, such well-meaning gestures can be more of a hindrance than a help. Your disability does not entitle people to make you the involuntary object of their "good deed for the day."

There is an art to giving and receiving help. One of the most interesting and never-ending features of life on wheels is to find the balance: to learn to ask for and graciously accept help when it is truly needed, and to teach those close to you how to help appropriately—which often means *not* helping.

> *I have no problem with people wanting to help me, but on the other hand I need to live my life, so there are certain things that I'm going to have to do by myself.*

How it feels

The emotions around being helped are amplified for wheelchair users. It is a fact of life that there are now a variety of situations beyond your capacity to handle alone or which are awkward or difficult. An object may be too heavy or awkward to pick up from the floor or put on a shelf. You may need to get down a flight of stairs. No one wants to be dependent on others, but at times accepting help is a fact of life for people with disabilities.

> *I remember my own notion of disability before my injury. I imagined that these people must be used to being helped. Now that I know better, I continue to get the sense that nondisabled people think the same thing. Why would we resist help? Isn't it part of the disability experience and accepted as such?*

Because you must accept some degree of help, the level of independence still available becomes that much more precious. It is sometimes worth a little extra effort or strain to avoid having to surrender control. But going it alone is not worth the extra effort when it wastes precious energy or risks injury.

The line between doing it yourself and asking for help is a hard line to straddle. As Irving Zola wrote about his own experience:

> *Hardest of all was to ask for something that I knew I could do. In fact, if I could do it, there was a moral imperative to do it, no matter how*

tired I was or what risk it demanded. I did not want to be put into a position of always asking favors and thus having to feel obligated. The key was what not doing something communicated about me. It confessed to all a weakness. But just because an individual can do something doesn't mean that he should. By spending so much time and energy on basic tasks, we eliminate the chance of realizing other possibilities.[12]

The experience of being helped is inevitably charged on both sides. Carol Gill observes:

> *You have to look at the realistic consequences of being a disabled person who accepts assistance. One study found that every time you ask for help, there can be consequences. For some people we meet there will be no consequences. They'll just help us matter of factly and see us as the same person they did before. But for the majority of people in our culture right now, if you ask for help as a disabled person and they give you that help, there is the risk that they will see you as dependent, incapable, needy.*

Do you actually need help?

Particularly in the early days of a disability, the boundary is not clear about when to ask for or accept help. For example, it can be easy to fall into the trap of trying to prove to the world that you are not disabled. "No thanks, I can do it" can become a habitual response to any offer of help simply because the identity of being disabled may be very uncomfortable.

> *It is extremely common to fall into the habit of trying to "prove that you're not disabled." I certainly did this, being the hotshot speedster in my wheelchair as a young paraplegic. I hated letting anyone do things for me. It was very uncomfortable for me to imagine that they felt I couldn't do things like open a door or push myself up a ramp.*

Many times you will turn down offers of help because you can easily do the task yourself. The person trying to help actually gets in your way! You will have gained many skills from your experience of using wheels, but most people you encounter in public will not know how you adapt. They can only react according to what they imagine it would be like if they were in your position. Opening a door from a wheelchair looks very difficult to them. They don't know how easily you might be able to do it. So they assume it is hard, and they try to help.

In the first year after my injury, I was getting into a car, assisted by the father of a friend who I had known since before my injury. I opened the door, maneuvered my chair in place, and lifted myself into the car—all easy for me, and best done without any help. All I needed from him was to fold the chair and stow it in the trunk. But during the transfer he kept trying to move me in the chair, lean over me to open the door, and insert himself in the process. After I fended him off a few times to do it myself, he finally sputtered in frustration, "Why do you have to be so damn independent!"

No one needs help until they truly need it. Plain and simple.

Who is in control?

The best-intentioned helper risks crossing a line where his desire to contribute actually robs you of control. A helper who helps without asking or who doesn't take no for an answer is invading your independence. Experienced wheelchair users know very well what they need and how it should be done. When someone imposes his will on you it implies that you cannot decide for yourself. This is frustrating and insulting. For a wheelchair user, the experience is an almost daily event.

You will develop techniques for dealing with common events:

I notice where people are as I approach a door, and will vary my speed depending on whether or not I want them to hold the door for me. Often I will hang back and wait until I can have the door to myself. It is usually easier to do it myself.

As time goes on, I'm finding it easier to let people open the door, and just say thank you as I go through. Once in a while I have to ask them not to stand in the doorway as they hold the door, but then I can joke about running over their toes, and the tension is released.

At those moments when it is necessary to essentially "fight" for control, it becomes necessary to explain:

"No thanks, it's the only exercise I get," is just the most reliable way I've found to keep someone from pushing me. It's the loss of control that bothers me the most. I tend to lose my temper if someone tries to push me without my permission, and that's another loss of control.

I find myself using the "It's easier if you don't help, thank you"
approach. At my car, that's actually true. People try to lift my wheelchair
which makes it harder to bring into the car. I try to let them know that
their desire to "make it easier for me" is actually fulfilled by not helping!

Being helped does not mean surrendering control, unless you let it. Whenever someone is helping you—whether grabbing an item from a shelf or performing an intimate, clinical task—the assistance should be done on your terms. Their actions are an extension of your own intent—the means of acting on your choices. That does not mean ordering them around. It means letting them know how they can best help you. It means knowing your own needs and being informed, especially about clinical tasks. It means you remain aware of what is happening and teach them how to help you properly, safely, and with dignity for you both. And it means respecting the good intentions of others while you educate them.

Being pushed around

Perhaps the most common offer of help to a manual wheelchair user is a push. To the able-bodied, pushing a wheelchair looks like a lot of work. For them it may be, but most manual chair users have gained enough strength and skill so that wheeling a chair is almost as natural as walking. Modern chairs are well designed and wheel easily.

The offer to push is very charged:

For a long time it was like an insult to me when people wanted to
push me. I felt like they were saying, "You can't make it by yourself so I
will help you." For me, I think it has to do with trying to be as indepen-
dent as I can. To have someone push me was losing hard-fought-for
independence.

Once I was crossing some distance with a friend on a fairly level side-
walk. She—more than a little casually—offered to push saying, "Why
waste so much effort?" It made me really think about what it was she
didn't understand.

Partly, it's about that difference in perception about how much work
it is. She offered because she thought it took much more effort than it does.
If she had to do it, it would be hard. It is not hard for me. Given that
wheeling is to me much as walking is to her, offering to push me is not

much different—emotionally—from my offering to carry her. "Why waste the effort?" indeed.

Being pushed also changes the nature of the interaction between two people. Now, rather than walking abreast where you can see each other and enjoy eye contact during the conversation, one person is behind the other in "helper/helped" mode. The nature of the relationship is changed.

If you are being pushed, your public appearance also is affected. Now, rather than being two friends strolling down the sidewalk, you can become self-conscious of being seen as someone getting—and therefore needing—help.

Irving Zola observed this problem of social interaction in his book *Missing Pieces*.[13] As a man who wore a brace and walked with a cane, he walked to the left of people so they wouldn't accidentally kick his cane. This meant he could not always obey the socialized model of men walking on the outer street side. This example—apart from any question of equality between men and women—illustrates how a disability sometimes forces you into contradiction with social convention.

Perhaps most important, the very act of wheeling yourself maintains your strength and stamina to be able to continue to do it—the "use it or lose it" principle. It can be a satisfying test of limits and a reassuring reminder that you have the strength to control your own mobility. You might be willing to work a bit harder to push up a gentle slope or even a movie theater aisle. However, there are times it makes sense to let someone push for a while when it is a long distance. This is a choice you will often face. You need to remember that your long-term health is your first priority.

Apart from perceptual, social, and health issues, there are issues of comfort and security. There is much more subtlety and skill involved in handling a wheelchair than a helper realizes. A skilled rider is constantly modulating the ride for all of the little bumps and changes along the way. A helper pushing the chair is not sensitive to this, so the ride is not as comfortable or secure. A bump in the pavement—and there are lots of them on any paved surface—can be very dangerous if someone is not paying close attention. A wheeler will simply give a little extra push to lift the front casters over a slight rise in surface. A helper who is pushing might wheel right into it, bringing matters to a sudden and surprising halt—possibly even throwing the "beneficiary" of the help out of the chair!

The people who spend the most time with you will develop a sense of where it is appropriate to help, if you take the time to discuss it, and give accurate feedback when they offer help. If you accept when you don't need it, or resist it when it would be valued, they can never learn the appropriate boundary.

> My best friend has a great sense of when I prefer help with push-
> ing—often one hand on a handle as he continues to walk next to me. It is
> clear enough that he doesn't have to ask. And he knows when to stop as
> well as to start.

Reacting to offers of help

You have three choices in how you react to people during the offer to help: passivity, aggression, and assertion. If you modify how you respond, you can modify the interaction.

When you are passive, you surrender your own point of view and priorities in favor of another person. Passively accepting what you don't want means that their feelings matter more than yours do. You violate your own rights, often because you are so concerned with that person's acceptance, that you err on the side of caution rather than risk upsetting them. Ironically, passivity is a form of disrespect for other people; it implies that they are unable to handle your disagreement or assertion. By being passive, you will not get what you need, and you will deny other people the opportunity to know you for your own views and feelings.

Aggression does not serve your purpose well either. It is a way of standing up for your rights, but denying others their rights in the process. Aggression is a way of overwhelming others, not of fostering cooperation and understanding. Aggressive behavior often means humiliating, degrading, or just plain overpowering other people. It will not make them want to be in contact with you, much less care about your views and needs.

The middle-ground, being assertive, involves expressing your ideas and feelings honestly as well as being attuned to other people's feelings. Being assertive is a matter of mutual respect. It avoids both the body language of passivity—moving away from the person, nervous gestures, covering the face, a quiet voice—and the body language of aggression—finger pointing, a raised voice, an intense stare. You speak plainly, making eye contact without challenge, and listen as much as you speak. Acting assertively is how you can develop comfortable relationships with people. It gives you the chance to increase your confidence in your own view of the world and to communicate it effectively. You express and protect your personal rights, but at no one else's expense.

Public attitude

A significant aspect of being a wheelchair user is the conspicuous quality of it. People with disabilities are aware of being looked at and set apart as wheelchair users and are often self-conscious about their bodies. For this woman with Charcot-Marie Tooth muscular dystrophy:

> *A big part of me wants to say "screw it" to others and what they see and think so I can wear whatever I want. A bigger part of me, though, is very affected by the way others see the outer me, and hates negative scrutiny. I thought I'd be past that at thirty-three years, but I'm not. So, to keep me more comfortable inside, I wear my sandals, high tops, long skirts, dresses, and jeans, and only sunbathe in the privacy of my back yard. I really have no desire, anymore, to wear shorts or a swimsuit around others, so I will continue to keep my skinny bird-legs hidden out of the sight of others, except myself, my husband, and our cats and dogs!*

You face all of the attitudes people have about disability whenever you go out in public. People hold doors for you, offer to carry your groceries, grab their children from your path, try to relate to you with stories of other disabled people they know, or speak to your companions on your behalf rather than directly to you. In daily life, these issues are a constant presence, and as a chair user you need to develop your own style of dealing with these attitudes.

As noted in the summary of the 1998 National Organization on Disability/ Harris Survey of Americans with Disabilities:

> *Many people with disabilities continue to feel that the rest of the population treats them as if they are different, and to have a strong sense of common identity with other people with disabilities. Fewer than half (45%) of adults with disabilities say that people generally treat them as an equal after they learn they have a disability.*[14]

There is work to do to get beyond the emotions these public contacts can bring up. You may not want others to see you as disabled—at least not in the negative image so many people associate with disability. You may want them to know you are really one of them and perhaps to know that you were once able-bodied too. You may be angered by the sometimes patronizing attitudes you encounter and by being suddenly treated as needy, unable, and tragic.

First encountering prejudices

There are many new feelings to confront in your early forays into public. What may seem overwhelming at first—potentially to the point of making you not want to go out—becomes familiar. You will learn how to let people have their beliefs and find you don't need to care how they see you. You can demonstrate through your attitude that they don't need to pity you—or make a hero of you. You will learn to check up on accessibility, and become familiar with what entrances to use at common locations like movie theaters or shops. These adaptive tools will help you level your emotions so that your attention can return to the primary tasks of your life—work, play, family, community, love, and spirit.

Teen and early adult years can be very difficult for people disabled since birth or with a disability acquired as a child. As children they may have been very well supported by their families in how to face the attitudes that the wider culture feels about disability. Disability psychologist Carol Gill notes:

> I think that a lot of us who were disabled early in life grew up thinking of ourselves as pretty okay and pretty normal. At some point in our lives we get disabused of that notion. Our peers and others in society begin to treat us abnormally. When we are school age, we don't get picked for the team, people make fun of us. For example, it intensifies in the teen years when dating begins.

Attitudes are learned

The unfortunate truth is that there are many deeply embedded attitudes in the culture about people with disabilities. People will usually be uncomfortable unless they have already had direct experience with a disabled person. Your presence might make them nervous at first. They'll be wondering if there's some special way to treat you or if they'll be expected to help in some way. They might have an association with someone else, perhaps a parent or grandparent, who used a wheelchair at a time when they were very ill. They might be projecting themselves into your experience, imagining it as a horrible way to live. All of these attitudes are significant obstacles to your ability to make a connection with that person. Once they come to know you well, and witness the kind of life that is possible, they find out that your personality shines through even the most severe disability.

Beliefs about disability are planted very early in life. It's evident from the experience of any chair rider in any shopping mall in America. As you wheel through the crowd, parents frantically pull their children out of your path. Of course, parents naturally want to protect their child from a collision and are likely trying to be considerate so you don't have to maneuver around the child. But the child gets the message to stay away from you.

Another scenario is more telling. Many children will innocently come up to you and ask why you are in a wheelchair. They don't yet know that it is "rude" to ask. The child's interest makes the parent very uncomfortable, and that gets communicated. Irving Zola wrote:

> The wheelchair is quite visible and of great interest to the child, but he or she is taught to ignore it. A near universal complaint is, "Why can't people see me as someone who has a handicap rather than someone who is handicapped?" Young children first perceive it that way but are quickly socialized out of it. [15]

Children are not mature enough to understand these boundaries, and there is a danger of communicating through your actions that people with disabilities are unapproachable. You can be in the delicate position of wanting to demonstrate that disability is a feature of many people's lives and does not preclude a full life, while at the same time being entitled to your privacy and dignity.

> A child can't distinguish whether I'm in a bad mood, so I am never bothered by a child's questions. I have a "spinal cord is like a telephone system" story that I use. An adult needs to use some judgment, but most of the time I am happy to have an adult approach me in public and ask why I wheel. I'm glad to explain it, but I also try to give a picture of my life as a whole.

Sometimes parents will give the child their own answers:

> I cannot count the times I have been in public and have heard a parent telling their children ridiculous things to explain why I am in a

wheelchair. Things like "Her legs are tired," "She is taking a break from walking," or "She's resting by sitting down." I always would rather have the parents have their kids approach me in these situations with their questions so I could tell them the truth.

How you respond to being asked about your disability is a case-by-case question. You will have to find your own balance. You can decline politely, by saying that it is a private matter, and that you reserve discussions about such things to people you know better. The more someone gets to know you, the more appropriate it becomes to ask such questions. As Carol Gill says, "If you have an intimate relationship, you're allowed to ask more intimate questions."

Just as often, people will delay or avoid asking about your disability:

> *In a company where I worked for eight years, there were people who never knew why I wheeled. They never had the courage to ask. Many, I expect, assumed I was disabled since birth, or had been in the Vietnam war, neither of which is true.*

Attorney Deborah Kaplan is quadriplegic, but is able to stand, has full sensation, and is a mother. She also has more than twenty-five years of disability activism behind her. She says:

> *By and large, it isn't so much a stereotype as the fact that we just really scare people. People don't want to have to think about disability. It's very personal. It's very deep-rooted, I think almost cellular. We remind people that we exist in a soft, vulnerable body, and that they're vulnerable. People don't like to be reminded of that. That shows up when somebody looks at my résumé and they go, "Oh!" What are they so surprised about? I've been on every commission in the world and I travel all the time. They're telling me something about what their expectations are.*

The more severe or visible the disability, the larger the attitudinal obstacle you're likely to encounter. Notes Carol Gill:

> *If there is going to be a person with a disability who is accepted by society first, it's going to be the young white male who is okay from the chest up. But that's not the majority of the disabled population.*
>
> *I really feel I have made a contribution. Not only to the disability community, but to society and to my neighbors and everybody else. The*

work that I do. My son that I raised. I am a valuable person, but I think that the average person who sees me would think my life is not tenable. I use a ventilator, I need help with all activities of daily living, and I feel that if I hit a significant medical crisis I am much less likely to receive aggressive measures to protect my life than someone else.

Professor Zola granted the value of his family and support system in adapting to polio and subsequent auto accident injuries, while at the same time condemning societal attitudes:

Had my family been poorer, less assertive, my friends fewer and less caring, my champions less willing to fight the system, then all my personal strengths would have been for naught. On the other hand, if we lived in a less healthist, capitalist, and hierarchical society which spent less time finding ways to exclude and disenfranchise people and more time finding ways to include and enhance the potentialities of everyone, then there wouldn't have been so much for me to overcome.[16]

But appearances are not the only thing that count. Says psychologist Gill:

A lot of the people we do hit it off with in the nondisabled community tend to be people who are more open. Sometimes they have what I would consider deeper values, and are people who would critique the same superficial American values that our community does. It gives us a common bond.

Perhaps your interaction with the nondisabled is a chance for them to change as they learn from the experience. Perhaps, as they encounter the truth of a person living with a disability, they can adjust their beliefs after seeing the evidence.

I've heard from many people who say that after getting to know me their fears about people with disabilities subsided, that it was a chance to overcome their misconceptions. I find that satisfying.

You can also hope that children will grow up knowing better because they are increasingly living in a world where people with disabilities are visible, active, and part of their lives in meaningful ways.

Disability pride

You have an important contribution to make to this society. You are in a position to teach that focusing exclusively on narrow standards of physical beauty, youth, and conventional athleticism is a problem for all of us. By continuing to demonstrate that you are not looking to be cared for, but to be treated as a whole, self-determining person with the right to make your own decisions and have a full life, society gets the chance to develop values that respect everyone.

> *My own philosophy is that there is one thing you show the outside world: pride. On the other hand, living with limitations is sort of a drag. That's the reality. But you don't go shouting that to everyone in the world or it just encourages all their stupid thinking.*

Carol Gill expresses her view:

> *I think our Western world in many ways is in a moral crisis. Some of the values of the disability world can really help the greater world in sorting out this moral dilemma—to look at what's important and develop a whole new slate around what it means to be human. I think we have an important lesson to teach the world because we have to deal with our own acid test of what's human. I'm an idealist, too. I'm hoping we will win out and be heard.*

CHAPTER 6

Wheelchair Selection

Selecting a wheelchair is a major decision. All the choices you have to make can seem overwhelming if you are getting wheels for the first time. You might anticipate that you will recover from your injury or illness, so you wonder why you should even bother to get a wheelchair at all. But the right wheelchair is a liberator, not a prison. When you choose the right chair, your quality of life increases dramatically. Even people with severe disabilities can have a considerable degree of independence and activity with the right wheels. For those who no longer need it at some point, having had the right chair will mean better health and greater strength.

Wheelchair design has advanced tremendously in just the last decade. No longer limited to the aluminum folding chairs you might be accustomed to seeing in hospitals or airports, there is now a huge array of designs and options for both manual and power wheelchairs. Wheelchairs are highly adjustable—or custom built—available in various sizes, with features to make driving them easier, safer, and more dignified.

Modern chairs are also better-looking; even power chairs have become less bulky and obtrusive. There has been much effort to reduce the visual emphasis on the disability and to bring more attention to the person.

This chapter discusses the issues involved in selecting a wheelchair, including funding, researching products from various manufacturers, working with professionals who will advise you, and the many features and options of manual and power wheelchairs.

Funding your chair

Wheelchairs are expensive. A typical manual chair can cost about $2,000. A fully equipped power chair can reach prices in the range of $30,000, though they generally will be closer to $10,000.

Because you need the best chair and it costs a lot, you have little choice but to rely on outside payers. Your chair might be paid for by a small or large insurance company, managed care such as a health maintenance organization (HMO) or planned provider organization (PPO), a government agency such as Vocational Rehabilitation or the Veterans Administration (VA), or a government plan like Medicare from the federal government or Medicaid from state government.

Whether private or public, funders are all conscious of their budgets and have a lot of motivation to limit their costs. In the recent environment of political pressure to control healthcare costs, it is becoming increasingly difficult to get approval for your ideal wheels, though this depends on exactly who is paying.

Advocate for yourself

You need to be serious about being your own advocate when buying a wheelchair. Read your policies and contracts. Don't be afraid to ask questions or to make phone calls to find out what you need to know. Insurance companies and government agencies are bound under certain laws to give you information.

Don't assume your insurance policy won't cover something you need. It's worth the effort to check your policy or discuss your situation with your insurance contact person. For example, insurers might well be willing to cover the cost of a new chair assuming you have a justifiable medical need.

> I spent more years in my heavy E & J hospital-style wheelchair than I needed to, as it turned out. I was assuming, mistakenly, that my private insurance through my job would not pay for a new wheelchair. Even though people were telling me that I should get out of my old "tank" in favor of a new lightweight chair, I never did the research. I figured when the day arrived when I would have to replace my old wheels, I would have to pay for it myself.

> Finally I made the call and discovered that my policy did indeed cover the cost of a wheelchair at least once in the life of the policy. They would pay 80 percent, and I could easily handle the difference. So I made the appointment with my rehab doctor who approved a consultation with the occupational therapist, who referred me to the local dealer, and I had my first Quickie wheelchair.

There is no reason you can't question a policy that you consider inappropriate or unfair. The worst your funder can do is say no. But if you can make a good case, you just might be able to convince an insurer to reconsider. Dr. Michael Boninger, Executive Director of the Center for Assistive Technology at the University of Pittsburgh, specifies chairs for people. He advises, "If your policy only allows you a $200 wheelchair, then challenge it. If you fight hard enough, you might get the insurer to make an exception."

Funding agencies and organizations generally do not think proactively. They tend to resist paying for something now, even if it will prevent problems—and save money—later. For example, an insurer might not want to pay for a contoured back to help control the trunk of a rider's body. Contoured backs can reach prices of up to $800, but their use can prevent the need for more expensive equipment or corrective surgery later on.

Jody Greenhalgh, O.T.R., is an occupational therapist with UCSF/Stanford Rehabilitation Services in Stanford, California. She is closely involved in specifying wheelchairs for people. More than once, she has encountered someone with pressure-sore problems who has had expensive surgery. She finds that often these problems could have been avoided if the person had been provided with a better wheelchair and positioning system in the first place:

> We see patients who have severe skin ulcers. They've been on bed rest for months. A specialized wheelchair is medically recommended but denied by the insurer. The patient then requires a $50,000 surgery, after which he returns to the inadequate wheelchair. This causes the surgery to fail and pressure sores recur. The patient has to go back on long-term bed rest and repeat hospitalization.

> The insurance companies seem to be short-sighted, preferring to spend money on surgical intervention rather than paying for the right cushion and specialized wheelchair—which would ultimately save dollars and help the patient return to a productive and independent life.

You might need to enlist the help of your physician, occupational or physical therapist, or other medical professional. The initial wheelchair prescription typically includes a "certificate of medical necessity," which is signed by the physician. If your funder denies the chair specified on your prescription, ask for help from your medical team. Your doctor or therapist can write to your funder, explaining in detail why that particular chair is medically necessary for you. Greenhalgh is an experienced advocate:

> I will write a lengthier justification if a wheelchair prescription is denied. Sometimes I pull up old cases to use as examples and say, "Look, we saved money by doing this." If I persevere it really does pay off, but the process can extend for months. It means I have to spend a lot of time on the phone and paperwork rather than treating patients.

It is increasingly common for insurance companies and funding agencies to assign your file to a case manager. The case manager should be your advocate, putting your medical interests first above all. He may or may not be a nurse or otherwise medically experienced. Your case manager will talk with doctors and therapists, confirm the policies and limits of your coverage, shop for the best prices (which is part of what makes case managers appealing to the insurer), and even contact social workers to seek out additional sources of funding or equipment if the policy does not cover you.

Sometimes case managers are on staff, or the insurer might have a contract with an outside provider of these services. If there is not a case manager assigned to you, ask for one. You do not have a legal right to a case manager, but it's likely your request will be granted, especially if you are pleasantly persistent. If possible, try to get a case manager with specific background in rehabilitation equipment and your specific disability.

Following are additional suggestions for how to overcome a denial of funding:

- Submit an official appeal. Your funding contact person should be able to provide you with the appropriate procedure.

- If coverage is employer-provided, enlist the help of your employer's benefits department.

- Write to the state insurance commissioner.

- Contact an appropriate advocacy group.

- Appeal to your congressional representatives.

- Take your case public. Local television or newspaper reporters might be interested in reporting about a funder who is denying coverage for clearly needed equipment. Funders don't like negative publicity, so they might be persuaded to do the right thing. Even if you still don't get funding, the report could flush out other forms of help such as a generous donor or someone with a used chair that meets your needs.

Another way you can help yourself is to research a wide variety of manufacturers. For instance, smaller producers are very aware of the need to increase business by making their products a more attractive option to funding sources, so they try to offer good solutions at lower costs. If you can find a less expensive solution to your needs by doing this kind of research, it might reduce complications in dealing with your funding source and make it easier for you to get approval.

If you are unable to deal with funding problems, perhaps a family member, friend, case manager, or social worker would be willing to invest the effort to overcome resistance you might encounter from payers. Many local Independent Living Centers offer advice or active assistance with funding issues.

Alternative funding

If your funding source is refusing to pay for a particular chair or feature, you must decide how long you will fight the good fight. At some point it might make sense to take what they give you and enhance it on your own.

The following are some possible sources of funding or finding a chair if you have to "do-it-yourself."

- Your church or other community group might be able to contribute to a purchase or stage a fundraiser on your behalf.

- Many local agencies provide used wheelchairs for people who are not getting proper funding support.

- Your local Independent Living Center might have surplus chairs or parts, or know of someone looking to donate a chair or sell a used one.

- Med-Sell is a newsletter that lists used equipment and accessories. (See the Appendix for contact information.)

- Some major banks offer special loan programs. For example, San Francisco-based Bank of America offers a longer-term loan with no down payment required if you use it for medical equipment. Check with major banks in your area to see if they have a similar program.

In all of these cases, of course, you must get proper guidance in identifying what is appropriate for you, including proper cushioning, and have the chair adjusted to your needs.

Large versus small manufacturers

Like other manufacturers, wheelchair producers come in many varieties. There are large corporate wheelchair manufacturers, small specialized producers, and innovative new companies hoping to make a name for themselves. Naturally, you will want to find out what various companies offer before deciding which manufacturer produces the optimal chair for you. Your therapist and the dealer with whom you work will have a lot of information about the major producers, and hopefully between the two of them, they will also have a well-rounded knowledge of smaller producers. No one can know it all, however, so it is in your best interest to do some investigating on your own.

Advantages of major manufacturers

Large manufacturers employ more people and operate on bigger budgets. Greater resources mean major wheelchair manufacturers can invest more in research and development than their smaller competitors. They can afford to build many prototypes and can take a little longer to develop new designs since these large firms have a steadier stream of revenue from existing products.

Following are additional advantages offered by large wheelchair manufacturers:

- They have comprehensive lines of wheelchair products, with plenty of options and accessories.

- They can afford to spend time and money on aesthetics.

- They have been in the business long enough to have a lot of experience behind them.

- They will have refined their manufacturing and design over those years and will probably be around for the foreseeable future.

- They are reputable and generally make good chairs, assuming you select the right model, properly configured.

- Your dealer will have more experience maintaining and repairing chairs from larger manufacturers.

Find out what small manufacturers offer

There are dozens of small companies out there making wheelchairs. Since they don't have the marketing budgets of the big firms, you might not hear about them. It is very difficult for dealers to represent every option in the world, so it is a challenge for the smaller makers to reach you, to let you know if they are the best solution. However, if you decide a small-producer's chair is the right one for you, your dealer should be perfectly willing to call the manufacturer and ask them to sell you one.

Many of the smaller suppliers have no desire to knock down a Goliath. They fill niches, meeting the needs of smaller populations. Many small producers customize each chair, building it exactly to order. The emphasis on making better, innovative products or specialized ones—is a recurrent theme among small manufacturers, as is offering more personalized service. Jeff Ewing of Falcon Rehabilitation in Commerce City, Colorado, explains his company's view:

> We're not in this business as much for the money as to help people out. Of course, like any business, you need enough money to keep it going. But we're not that concerned with producing mass numbers of these chairs. We'd rather focus on a small group and help them out to the best of our abilities.

There is a lot to be learned by exploring the smaller wheelchair producers. Asking them to send you product literature is worth the few moments it takes.

Following are the most important benefits offered by small companies, including those that are newer to the industry:

- They are generally passionate about their work, concerned with quality, and interested in helping people.

- You are likely to get more personal attention.

- You might find a chair that more specifically meets your needs, even one that can be more aggressively customized for you.

- Since smaller producers don't have huge production schedules, they may be able to deliver your chair faster than a large company.

- You might be able to find a better price.

One issue you will want to consider before deciding to purchase from a small producer is how important the look of your chair is to you. Wheelchairs designed by the smaller companies often tend to look like they were designed by an engineer, whose concerns are wholly functional and whose training does not include aesthetics. Engineers are interested in the operation of the chair and the ease of manufacturing it. This is not universally true of small producers, but is more the rule than the exception. (Two small companies notable for the aesthetic aspects of their products are Paraglide and New Hall's Wheels.)

The selection process

Not only can choosing a wheelchair be difficult emotionally, it can be confusing and exasperating. The professionals who are advising you will talk with you about many issues and options. They will ask you a lot of questions. They may give you catalogs for a variety of chairs that have all kinds of features to choose from. It will likely seem overwhelming. You might think, "Just sell me a wheelchair!"

The best advice is to relax and take heart. First of all, your therapist, the supplier, and the facts of your condition and lifestyle will very quickly narrow the choices down to a much more manageable number. This is a process that takes time, and it is extremely important not to rush it. You'll have much to learn and many questions to consider. If you find the right people to work with, they will help you identify the chair that will make it possible for you to have the fullest possible life your disability allows.

Who will help you choose your chair?

The prescription for your chair will be written by a physician. You will want to make sure that she is either a rehabilitation specialist (physiatrist) or that she refers you to an occupational or physical therapist who will help ensure that you get the right chair.

Occupational therapist Jody Greenhalgh finds that some people end up with the wrong chair because they relied on their primary physician to specify it:

> The primary physician writes a simplistic prescription, and the insurer pays for inadequate equipment. Once that happens, it is very difficult to convince an insurer to pay for a more appropriate wheelchair system.

Physiatrists and rehab therapists understand the medical and physiological issues that affect your wheelchair choices. Some therapists have chosen to make a specialty of consulting on wheelchair selection.

A therapist's knowledge of anatomy and biodynamics is extremely valuable. Your therapist will study your exact disability, and do muscle and range testing. He will determine whether you have the physical ability to push a manual chair or whether you should drive a power chair. He will identify how to establish a stable posture which will allow you access to your optimal strength as you push, or study your ability to operate the various types of power chair controls. He will test your eye-hand coordination and cognitive skills. He will measure your weight and height, your knee-to-footrest distance, seat depth, back height, and all of the other specific dimensions needed to configure your highly customized set of wheels.

Your therapist is the expert on the specific requirements your physical/medical condition demands from a wheelchair. But keeping up with everything that is available in the wheelchair market is more than most therapists can manage. They can't know it all, so they rely on the wheelchair suppliers who will actually order and sell your wheels.

Your therapist will likely know the best wheelchair dealers to work with, but if you have to find one on your own, the time you spend locating one with knowledge and experience will be well worth it. It's best not to purchase your chair from a general medical supply store, one that sells all sorts of medical equipment. Such a business is not likely to have the kind of expertise you need.

A knowledgeable DME salesperson can make a tremendous difference in ensuring that you get the right wheels. You'll want someone who has a lot of experience seeing many people with different needs, and who has specialized in rehab equipment. A competent salesperson often has more information from users about what worked and what didn't than the therapist does.

Bob Hall of New Hall's Wheels in Cambridge, Massachusetts, a smaller producer and himself a chair rider, cautions against relying on a dealer who may not be as knowledgeable as one would hope:

> *Wheelchair dimensions are often over-prescribed because of lack of knowledge of the dealer. Back heights, in particular, are often too tall and limit movement in the chair. Chairs are often too wide. You can say that you need to make room inside the chair for your winter coat, but if you*

can't get through the door it isn't doing you much good. The product actu-
ally ends up being more disabling, whereas the right chair can raise your
self-esteem.

If possible, find a salesperson who has experience with insurance and funding. He can help you avoid choosing a product the insurer simply won't pay
for, and help you choose appropriate equipment that will be approved.

You may not always have a choice about the dealer with whom you will
work. Your funding source might require that you use a particular supplier
in order to save money, and such a supplier might not be well informed
about the most appropriate product for you. If you believe you need additional consultation in order to get the best chair, assert yourself with your
insurance carrier or agency so that you can work with a local source that is
better qualified to consult with you.

The consultation

A typical consultation will take place at your therapist's office and will
include you, your therapist, and a salesperson from your local wheelchair
shop. Your therapist will have a list of requirements derived from her work
with you. You will have information about your home and workplace, your
lifestyle and level of activity, and of course, your personal preferences. The
salesperson will contribute knowledge about various manufacturers and the
products they offer, including necessary accessories, such as cushions, and
optional features.

As a team, you will discuss the various factors that will determine the specific features and dimensions of your chair. The therapist and salesperson
will guide you through this process, but it is a good idea for you to have
some knowledge about the many details that must be taken into consideration. For example, seat height is related to the ground clearance required by
footrests. Seat depth is partially dependent on the kind of seat back you
choose. As various features are discussed throughout this chapter, these
kinds of interrelationships will be pointed out.

You should be given the chance to try out a close configuration of the chair
you will eventually purchase. The supplier should have chairs on hand that
can be adjusted fairly closely to your needs, and may even allow you to take
it out and live with it for a few days. Some manufacturers will actually ship a
chair to the supplier specifically for you to try out.

One rider describes his experience with the selection process:

> *I spent two days with a team in making my decision. The team included a physical therapist and an occupational therapist. The physical therapist spent time assessing my strengths and weaknesses. We then decided on seating requirements before addressing the actual chair selection. We spent a lot of time discussing my lifestyle and exactly how and where the chair was to be used.*
>
> *Once the medical needs were identified and physical measurements were taken, the last thing was to determine the exact model of chair. We were able to narrow it down to five, which I was able to try out for a few hours each. The trial included maneuvering in a simulation of the work area I use and then spending an hour or so outside on a variety of terrain. We also tried them in my van to see how they fit and the method of transfer I would need to use to get in the driver's seat.*
>
> *Luckily, I knew enough to demand this sort of evaluation and knew where to go to get competent professional help.*

Ordering your chair

From your initial consultation to the actual ordering of your chair typically takes two to three months. This includes taking time to try out one or more models. A more complex chair may take longer. If you encounter resistance from your insurer, that could also add time to the process.

Once you have decided on the model of chair that is best for you, the dealer—using information from you and your therapist—will fill out a specification sheet with the exact details for every aspect of your chair. Ask to see a copy of this list. If you have questions or concerns about anything, ask. Make sure it is complete and correct; if something is inadvertently omitted (such as clothing guards) or wrong (such as color), you'll end up with a chair that isn't what you wanted. Even if the problem can be fixed, you'll probably have to pay for it. Your therapist will sign off on this list, and it will then go to your physician, who will write a prescription for it.

The prescription and specification list will be sent to your insurance company or funding agency for approval. Once approved, the dealer will order your chair from the manufacturer. If your chair is not covered by insurance and you are paying for it yourself, a down payment of 50 percent at the time the order is placed is typical.

Your dealer should give you an accurate delivery date so you can plan accordingly.

Your role

No matter how skilled and knowledgeable your therapist and salesperson are, you are the expert on *you*. Since you are the person who will have to live with your wheelchair, it is in your best interest to take an active role in its selection, to learn as much as you can, and to take your time before making the final choice.

Do some research

Chances are you know other chair users, possibly from your rehab experience, support groups, participation in athletics, or your local Independent Living Center. Chair users tend to be very opinionated about their choices. Remember that every person is different. You can learn much from what others say, but what works best for them might not work for you.

> *My experience with purchasing the best chair for me came primarily from my own research, which included talking with other wheelchair users. I got a couple of names from the retailer, but the best information I got was from the Internet.*

Check the track record of all chairs under consideration. While major flaws are uncommon, there could be defects in the manufacture of some chairs, as with any consumer product. The U.S. Food and Drug Administration (FDA) keeps track of voluntary recalls by wheelchair manufacturers, though not all manufacturers are entirely open about such problems. You can contact the FDA for this information. Newer manufacturers should not be suspect just because they are less experienced, but there is always some risk of unforeseen problems that simply may not have appeared yet. Seek out users of a given product and speak with them about its performance and quality before selecting your wheels.

Learn as much as possible about chairs and what is available on the market. You can request product information from all companies that appear to have something you think might work for you. Wheelchair manufacturers not only have catalogs and brochures available, but they can provide a specific checklist for every model which includes all available options.

Be prepared for your consultation

Your wheelchair supplier will need to know many things about where you live and work. It is not uncommon for an occupational or physical therapist to visit you and make notes about your living space, but you will want to take an active part in making sure your chair will optimize—not limit—your mobility and comfort at home and work. Investigate your home and workplace, and then arrive at your therapist appointment or the wheelchair store equipped with answers to questions such as these:

- How wide are your doors—main entry, kitchen, bedrooms, bathrooms, etc.?

- Are there tight angles to negotiate, such as a hallway that turns sharply at the bedroom door?

- How large is the bathroom? Will it be possible to wheel your chair alongside the bathtub, or must you face it directly? Is the door smaller than the others in your house? Will you be able to close the door once inside with your wheelchair?

- What is the knee clearance of tables and desks?

- How high are cabinets and shelves that you might need to reach?

- Is the terrain around your home paved? If not, what kind of surface is it? Is it level?

- What are the surfaces where you will do most of your wheeling? Carpet, tile, concrete, packed soil?

You must also consider the vehicles you use:

- If you drive, do you have a car or a van? Two or four doors?

- What is the size of the trunk in the family car?

- What kind of public transportation might you use?

Failure to consider any one of these points can mean having to live with a constant irritant or insurmountable obstacle and facing the stress of unnecessary restriction of your mobility every day—just because you got the wrong chair. You might even be risking your safety if, for instance, you are forced to make a long transfer to the bath or shower because you chose those fixed footrests which prevent you from getting close enough.

Getting the right chair can also save you from having to make potentially expensive home modifications:

> It was many years before we could make my home wheelchair accessible. If I had known that there were power wheelchairs out there that could raise a seated person 6 to 8 inches or that had a turning radius of 19.5 inches, my life would have been so much more comfortable. And it wouldn't have cost quite so much for the home modifications.

You will also want to share important information about your lifestyle and the kinds of activities you plan to participate in. If you like to be on the go— visiting friends, attending entertainment and sporting events, taking classes—or travel a lot either for pleasure or business, you might need a different chair than if you prefer a more quiet life and enjoy being home most of the time. Information about your preferences is critical. Along with the previous lists, make one that includes:

- Hobbies and activities for which your chair will be a consideration.

- Relevant information about any "homes away from home." If you like to hang out at your best friend's place, you want to make sure you can fit through those doors, too.

- The importance of the appearance of your chair to you. Do you see yourself in something sporty? Eye-catching? Or do looks not matter much to you?

- Your usual level of physical activity, including exercise.

Your lifestyle and personal preferences for comfort are important. Without your input, your team might not fully understand your needs. The more information about yourself that you can give to the therapist and salesperson, the better they can help you identify the chair that will work best for you.

> Although my rehab folks were wonderful, my first two chairs did not suit my lifestyle. There were places I might have been able to go, people I might have been able to see, and events I could have participated in if I had had the right chair from the beginning.

Keep an open mind

Despite the variety of wheelchairs on the market and the many options available, you may not be able to find every feature and detail you would ideally like in one chair. As with other purchases, such as a car or home, some compromises and trade-offs are usually necessary. As you work your way through the selection process, try to think about the big picture and how you will use your chair over time. Establish priorities, learn from the experience of others, and value the advice of experts.

For example, it is common for people to be drawn to the appearance of a chair, but it is dangerous to be overly influenced by the look of a chair to the possible exclusion of other, more important issues. That really cool-looking rigid-frame chair might not fit into the trunk of your family car.

Doe Cayting of Wheelchairs of Berkeley, California, has seen people become too attached to the appearance of the chair, in lieu of other features more important to their mobility:

> You have to think about whether aesthetics is the most important thing for you, because the right chair is always a question of compromise. There isn't an exact right or wrong. But if you want something that looks a certain way, and I know it is not appropriate, it is my responsibility as a supplier to say no.

Fortunately, there are lots of good-looking chairs that fit many needs. Compared to the institutional-style chair that everyone had to use until the 1980s, whatever you choose will be better-looking and more to your liking than in "the old days."

Have your new chair properly adjusted

When your chair arrives at the dealer from the factory, you will need to have the store adjust it specifically to your needs. Plan on taking the time to have them fine-tune it for you and don't hesitate to ask them to continue to make changes until it is right. Dr. Boninger, of the University of Pittsburgh, finds that factory settings are not particularly optimal overall. For example, he makes this observation about manual chairs:

> The factory tends to put the wheels far back for stability, but this can force excessive range of motion as you reach back and limit the amount of stroke you can make on the wheel.

Axle position is only one of the many details of chair configuration that have a significant impact on the efficient, comfortable, and safe use of your chair. Remember that a wheelchair is really a complex web of interrelationships.

Changing the axle position or caster height affects seat and back angles, and the relationship of your arms to the wheels. Placement of a joystick affects overall posture. And so on.

Some riders learn—by observing and asking questions of a qualified technician—how to expertly adjust their own chairs, but you should not attempt to adjust your chair until you are confident in your knowledge and are certain that you have the right tools to protect the chair from scratches or stripping the heads of screws or bolts. More than one wheelchair salesperson can tell a story of a customer who called complaining that their chair was wrong or damaged, only to discover that they had made inappropriate adjustments or used the wrong tools.

The basic choice: manual or power

The first decision to be made when choosing your wheelchair is whether it will be a manual or power chair. Often this decision is obvious, or becomes clear after your therapist tests your strength, balance, dexterity, and other abilities. In some cases, though, the choice is not so simple and, in fact, it sometimes takes both kinds of chairs to reach the optimal solution.

Two chairs are actually a good idea for everyone—manual and power chair riders alike will want to have a backup manual chair for use in case their main chair is out of commission for a few days. A backup chair doesn't have to be as complete or as customized as one you purchase for daily use. If you aren't able to get your own backup chair, find out if your dealer has loaners available for those times when your chair needs servicing.

Advantages of manual wheelchairs

Manual chairs have a number of advantages over power chairs, and most people prefer to use a manual chair if at all possible. Consider the following list of "pros," but also be honest with yourself about your strength and energy—you'll need plenty of both to operate a manual chair.

- Manual chairs are lightweight and getting lighter all the time thanks to modern metal alloys and composite materials. Lightweight chairs require less strength and energy to push than their predecessors.

- Manual chairs have unlimited range, not being tied to the charge capacity of a battery.

- Manual chairs cost less to purchase than power chairs. Maintenance costs are also lower thanks to fewer working parts and not needing to replace depleted batteries.

- Manual chairs are more discreet than power chairs, being less bulky and, with no motor noise, quieter—assuming the manual chair is well maintained.

- Manual chairs are easier to maneuver for slight rotations or small movements, although the newer controls for power chairs are excellent.

- Manual chairs travel more easily than power chairs, whether on an airplane or stowed in the backseat or trunk of a car. Depending on options, a manual chair can be stored more easily when broken down to its component parts. Swingaway footrests can be removed, as can the wheels by means of the now-common quick-release axles.

- Manual chairs can extend mobility. For those with the strength and agility to master the art of the "wheelie," many curbs and single steps no longer represent an obstacle in a manual chair, as you can safely "jump" a curb or step either going up or down.

Advantages of power wheelchairs

Some riders are finding that they do better in a power chair as they age. Chronic shoulder pain from overuse or weakness from an illness might make it necessary. Some of the reasons you might opt for a power chair follow.

- A power chair conserves your energy, allowing you to go whatever distance necessary without exhausting yourself for work or pleasure activities.

- A power chair allows you to handle uphill slopes that would be an unnecessary overexertion or perhaps beyond your ability to climb with a manual chair.

- A power chair frees you from the need for assistance when going a considerable distance or on a steep surface.

- A power chair leaves one arm free to stabilize an object you might carry in your lap—such as a bag of groceries or books—while operating a joystick control.

- A power chair can include powered tilt or recline features, which aid in pressure-sore prevention, respiration, and comfort for quadriplegic riders.

Weigh your options

Choosing a power chair can be a tough decision. There are mobility restrictions that come along with use of a power chair. Power chairs are limited by battery life, are too heavy to be carried up a stairway, and don't jump curbs easily, if at all. They make more noise and are less able to make fine maneuvers. Pushing a manual chair keeps the upper body in shape, to a degree, so using a power chair can be an invitation to losing strength.

Some people resist choosing a power chair because it makes them feel "too disabled." But it's important to ask yourself how much of your daily energy you are willing to invest in pushing a manual chair. If you have marginal upper body strength, you can exhaust yourself just getting where you're going. Perhaps you are attending a college that is on a sloping site or live in a hilly town. Consider whether you prefer to trade having more energy in the day against your public image as a power chair rider. Lack of energy from pushing a manual chair around might even make a difference in your ability to hold a job.

Finally, think about how the effort needed to operate a manual chair will affect your health in the long run. Many manual chair riders with twenty or so years of pushing behind them find that their shoulders begin to give out. You are better off using a manual chair if you can, but not at the expense of your long-term health.

Using a combination of manual and power chairs

Many low level quadriplegic people have sufficient arm strength to push a chair, perhaps aided by handrims with knobs which are easier to grasp than rims alone. Some of these riders use a manual chair at all times, while others switch between manual and power chairs, depending on distance, surface, whether they might need to be lifted up stairs, load the chair into a car, and other such criteria. You might use a power chair to go to and from work, but use a manual chair at home and at the office. A blend of the two types can be the ideal strategy for your mobility. It is an approach that does not waste your energy or overuse your body.

Some manufacturers are looking for ways to offer the best of both worlds, with products that allow a power chair to be temporarily modified for manual use or a manual chair to become temporarily powered. Yet another solution is a three- or four-wheeled scooter. Scooters are considerably less expensive than power chairs, but can give a manual chair user additional mobility for traveling longer distances or climbing steep slopes.

Manual chair decisions

Although manual and power wheelchairs have many similar features, each has some features that the other doesn't have or that need to be considered in light of how the chair will be powered. If you will be riding in a manual chair, there are a number of decisions that will affect how easily you will be able to maneuver your wheels.

Rigid-frame chairs

It used to be that most manual wheelchairs folded. An engineer will tell you that when you push a folding wheelchair, some energy is lost in the flexibility of the frame. Not all of the work of your push translates into forward motion. The loss of energy in a flexible frame led chair designers to come up with the rigid-frame chair. Freed of the mechanism for folding, a rigid chair has fewer parts and is therefore much lighter. With fewer moving components, the frame has more strength. More of the energy of your push translates into motion. The rigid chair design also allows for the angle of the seat frame to be adjustable, impossible with a folding chair. The cross-frame design of the folding chair is not needed with a rigid chair, streamlining the rigid chair's appearance. The rigid-frame design has come to be a de facto standard for those who want to reduce the visual emphasis on their disability. Figure 6-1 shows a typical rigid chair.

Rigid-frame chairs are so responsive that just minor movements of your body can be enough to adjust direction—a technique riders can use to make some of the fine adjustments necessary as they wheel. Some people find rigid chairs a little oversensitive, but many swear by them and will never go back to a folding design. According to Doe Cayting of Wheelchairs of Berkeley:

> We like rigid frames because in a folding chair 40 percent of your energy is wasted by the mechanism of the frame. Greater efficiency means you won't tire as easily, and you won't have to worry so much about overuse syndrome.

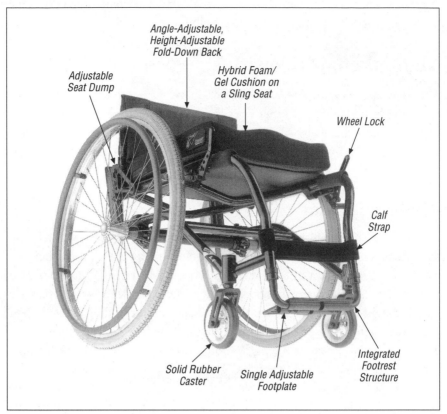

Figure 6-1. A lightweight, rigid-frame manual wheelchair

Some find a rigid chair necessary because of its more rugged construction:

> *I prefer my rigid-frame chair. I may be inconvenienced at times when I can't get close to a table, but this is rare since my chair is quite short and the ends of my toes sit directly below my knees. The durability of a rigid frame is essential, as I am quite hard on my equipment and it must endure Ottawa winters. It has few moving parts to loosen, collect dirt, and break. The chair requires less maintenance.*

However, rigid chairs can be bulky for transporting in a car and do not neatly fold up when they need to be out of the way.

> *Even though I tried a rigid-frame chair, and sure, it was easier to wheel and looked better, I found it much harder to put in my two-door car. It wouldn't fit in the trunk either.*

You will want to consider what kind of terrain you will be traveling over. Rigid frames are best for hard, reasonably level surfaces. On uneven terrain, a rigid chair will give you a harder ride and might have one or more wheels lift off the ground, preventing you from being able to wheel. This loss of control can be dangerous.

Folding-frame chairs

There are a few important reasons why some riders still prefer folding chairs. Folding chairs are likely to fit in most vehicles. On uneven surfaces, all four wheels of a folding chair are better able to remain in contact with the surface because of its flexible frame. The flexible frame also absorbs small bumps and vibrations in your ride. Figure 6-2 shows a typical folding chair.

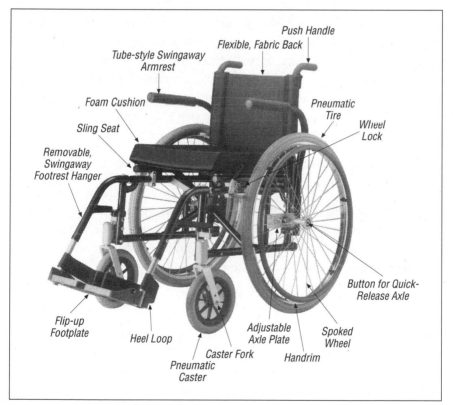

Figure 6-2. A lightweight, folding manual wheelchair

Some riders prefer a folding chair as their best overall solution for a daily street chair because of its ability to fold into a more compact unit:

> I feel strongly about keeping my chair with me in theaters, and a rigid chair would block the aisles, so I would have to let them take it away during the show. I have enough upper body strength and balance to push a folding chair without tiring myself, so for these and other reasons, a folding design is still the style of choice for my needs.

But folding chairs take more energy to push than rigid chairs and lack the other attractive qualities of the rigid design.

Chair weight

The heavier your manual chair, the more energy you will use to push it. A heavier chair is also more difficult for anyone assisting you, making it harder to push you a long distance, carry you up a stairway, or store your chair when you're not in it. The majority of chairs use an aluminum alloy, which is lightweight but strong. As you make the many choices necessary to define the best chair for you, you will want to consider chair weight versus the advantages of features that will make it heavier. For example, spoked wheels are lighter than molded wheels, but require more maintenance.

An important safety issue with a light chair is that it has a longer braking distance. You'll want to remember this while getting used to your wheels.

> When I made the transition from the hospital-style aluminum chair to a modern lightweight, I discovered that I had less traction against the pavement and so had to allow for a greater distance to slow down. It only took one close call to learn that lesson!

Wheel size

Your optimal reach for pushing will be determined in part by the diameter of the wheels. Manual chairs typically use 24-inch wheels, but wheels are available as small as 20 inches and as large as 26 inches. If you must begin a push with your arms already extended because the wheels are small or you are sitting too high, you will have very little remaining force. If you begin the push with your elbows very bent and your shoulders raised because the wheels are large or you are sitting too low, you will be overstraining your arms and shoulders to get the chair to start moving.

Wheel diameter must work in conjunction with seat height. The sequence of events leading to the decision for wheel diameter goes something like this: first you must ensure proper ground clearance for your footrests based on your leg length. Then you can determine minimum seat height, and from seat height you can determine seat angle. A seat lower at the back will bring your arms closer to the wheels and rims. Only after you know how high and at what angle your seat will be can you determine your appropriate wheel size. If you want to use larger wheels, which can be easier to push, you might choose a seat height that is greater than the minimum.

Placement and angle of wheels

Two important decisions for chair stability and optimal wheeling efficiency are where the wheel axle will be in relation to the back of the chair, and the amount of angle, or camber, on the wheels.

With most modern manual chairs, you can adjust the axle position forward or back in relation to the back of the chair. This is the point of pivot, where your weight is applied to the chair. When the wheel is moved forward on the axle, more of the chair weight is behind the axle, so it will tip more easily, lifting the front casters off the ground. At the least you want to be able to slightly lift the casters with a bit of extra push to soften your ride over bumps in the sidewalk, for instance. At most, you might use the technique of doing wheelies to go up and down curbs. The axle position will control how efficiently you can perform these maneuvers without putting yourself at risk of falling backward in your chair. When you get a new chair, you might begin with a more stable rearward position, and then move the axle forward as you gain more experience driving.

Correct wheel position is also determined by your weight and how your weight is proportioned. For example, taller people have longer legs and so have more body weight forward in the chair. More weight forward in the chair allows for a more forward wheel position without risk of falling. If you wear heavy shoes or boots, you might take that into account by moving the wheels forward. Amputees have much less forward body weight, so must use a rearward wheel position. They might even require a chair frame that allows the axle to be placed behind the vertical line of the chair back.

If the wheels are too far back, they can be hard to reach for pushing, forcing you to pull your arms farther back. Forward tipping also becomes a risk factor. When the wheels are farther back, your chair will want to roll toward the street on sidewalks, which are always sloped toward the street for water drainage. You will have to push harder on the downhill wheel to compensate for gravity pulling the front end sideways.

Another decision is the amount of camber you want on your wheels. Camber is the angle of the wheels toward your body as they rise from the floor (see Figure 6-3). Some rigid-frame chairs are available in various fixed camber angles where the axle housing is welded in place at the given angle. Most chairs use an adjustable plate that holds the axle and allows the camber to be changed.

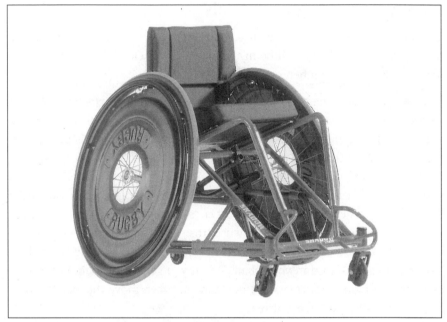

Figure 6-3. A specialized sport chair with cambered wheels

The greater the camber, the wider the wheelbase and therefore the greater the lateral stability of the chair as you turn corners or lean over. However, more camber than is necessary to give you the stability you need will add width at the floor, making it more difficult to pass through narrow spaces.

A different kind of wheel angle—one which you want to avoid—is "toe-in" or "toe-out." If your wheels were to roll independently of the chair, they would either roll toward (toe-in) or away (toe-out) from each other. Some wheel or caster adjustments can cause your wheels to be angled in one of these ways, making the chair harder to drive, and possibly applying force on the frame and axles that can cause damage in the long term. Adding camber to your wheels is especially a time when you should look for toe-in or toe-out. Your technician needs to be sensitive to this issue.

Handrims

The size of your hand will influence what size handrim should be used with a given size of wheel to ensure that you get the most efficiency in your push. The most common diameter of handrims is 20 or 21 inches. Handrims with a smaller radius from the axle require more force to propel the chair, just as a smaller gear on a bicycle makes it harder to pedal.

You will typically brake using the handrims. Standard handrims are made of aluminum with an anodized, gray coating which is smooth enough not to burn your hands from friction as you brake, but not so slick that you can't slow yourself effectively with minimum grip force. Other options include plastic, foam, or powder coatings. These coatings increase the "grip-ability" of the handrim, but are more easily damaged. Plastic handrims can be very hot when braking and might seriously burn hands that lack sensation.

Standard handrims require a strong grip, but there are other designs that allow for less gripping ability. Low level quadriplegic riders who use a manual chair can elect to use special handrims with added knobs which compensate for the wheeler's limited grip capacity.

Manual chair riders with only one arm can get a chair designed with a dual handrim on one wheel, allowing either or both wheels to be controlled with one hand.

Wheel locks

Wheel locks, also called hand brakes, are used to prevent a manual chair from accidentally rolling when you want it to remain stationary. Some chair riders have eschewed the use of brakes altogether, to the absolute horror of their therapists who subscribe to the belief that a wheelchair must be locked whenever you make a transfer to or from the chair. The instability of not having brakes can be dangerous.

> *The only people I have seen not use brakes are those that have very low level injuries and/or have some leg function. They can balance themselves well enough to transfer in and out of an unlocked chair. This doesn't work for me. The one (and only!) time I forgot to lock my brakes*

prior to a transfer I almost ended up on the ground, with the chair shooting off in the other direction!

There are other situations in which you'll be glad you have wheel locks. Just the act of reaching for an object on a table is enough to send sufficient force through your body to your wheels to cause the chair to shift, especially in a hypersensitive fixed-frame chair. If you are working at a desk, leaning forward on your arms will cause an unbraked chair to roll backward. Your wheels also give you the chance to discover that many floors are not level. It doesn't take much slope for you to roll downhill when you are in a well-maintained manual chair.

> *I am mystified by how often I see people with no brakes, being so deeply in the habit of locking my chair whenever I am not in motion. This is not because I am so thoroughly brainwashed by my therapists from twenty-five years ago, but because I prefer the stability of a fixed seat that will not shift as I use my body.*

Use of a hand brake also aids back support. Since you don't have to worry about the chair moving, you can rest your weight against the chair back with confidence.

Power chair decisions

If you will be driving a power wheelchair, you need to get the right kind of drive system for you and the right control system. You need to think about speed—and about stopping. You need to decide which type and size of battery you want to use. Finally, you want to consider safety issues. Figures 6-4 and 6-5 show the various features found on power chairs and contrast some of the design differences.

Front-, rear-, or mid-wheel drive?

Power wheelchairs commonly have the drive wheels placed either at the front or the back of the chair. Mid-wheel drive is a relatively new alternative. Each type of wheel drive entails a different style of operating your chair and takes a little while to adapt to the feel of it. If the type of drive is right for you, your skill and comfort using it will become increasingly refined, despite any early awkwardness you might experience.

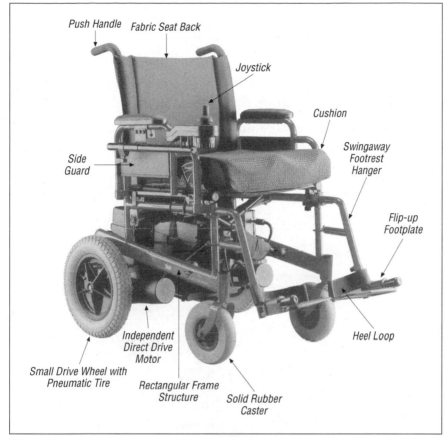

Figure 6-4. A rear-wheel drive, foldable power wheelchair

With a front-wheel drive system, you have the sensation of pulling the chair behind you. This sense of pulling means that in order to operate a front-wheel drive chair, you need greater sensitivity to the chair's movement and control. Front-wheel drive chairs are very agile—capable of making full rotations in a smaller area of space. But because front-wheel drive takes a little more skill to operate, ability and training issues must be taken into account. People with cognitive difficulties might not be able to safely use front-wheel drive.

One advantage of having the larger drive wheels in front is that you may be able to traverse a change in surface more easily—going over a curb, for example. The larger wheels make contact with the curb first, pulling the smaller casters along behind.

I live in a rural area where accessibility was initially the major issue. A chair with front-wheel drive would have better suited the terrain that I had to navigate.

If you need a tilt system, you will want to consider whether a front-wheel drive chair will be stable. The tilt system may cause the front wheels to come off the ground, making the chair difficult to operate.

When you operate a chair with rear-wheel drive, you feel as though you are being pushed forward. There is a greater sense of control over the chair, but rear-wheel drive doesn't afford as much agility.

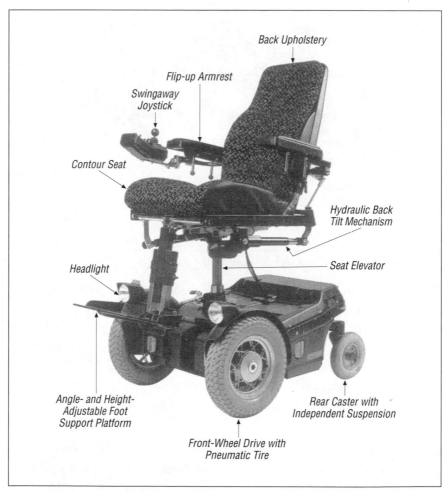

Figure 6-5. A front-wheel drive, elevating/reclining power wheelchair

Tipping is also a concern with rear-wheel drive. You may need to use anti-tippers with a rear-wheel drive chair, since it's possible for the casters in front to be lifted off the surface by the power and weight of the drive wheels in back when you accelerate the chair. (Anti-tippers are optional small wheels which attach to the chair frame at the rear and float a few inches above the ground. If the chair begins to tip backward, the anti-tippers touch down and stabilize the chair.)

If the rear-wheel drive mechanism extends out of the rear of the chair and is low to the ground, you might have the opposite problem—not being able to tip back enough. This could limit your ability to climb over an obstacle or negotiate a ramp or curb cut.

A more recent alternative is the mid-wheel drive. The mid-wheel drive design uses six wheels altogether: casters in the rear, the two drive wheels, and two more caster-size wheels in the front which are not in continual contact with the ground, but are there to help prevent forward tipping. These front casters are usually spring-loaded and adjustable.

The main advantage of mid-wheel drive is its tight turning radius. A mid-wheel drive chair can almost turn in place, making it helpful for people who must navigate small spaces at home or be able to turn around inside a van.

Mid-wheel drive helps to improve traction because more body weight is over the drive wheels, but there will always be some degree of forward tipping. Sudden stops or going down ramps are more likely to bring the front wheels in contact with the ground. Mid-wheel drives should only be used by people with good upper body balance.

Mid-wheel drive chairs do best on firm surfaces. To use them on rough terrain, the front wheels need to be raised and then more rocking occurs.

Whichever placement of wheel drive you select, there will be a range of wheel sizes to choose from. The advantage of larger wheels is that they will enable you to drive more easily over changes in grade, possibly even small curbs. The disadvantage is that larger wheels add width to your chair. Use of independent suspension—which allows each wheel to shift upward with a change in surface—can make up for the loss of maneuverability in a chair with smaller wheels.

Control systems

Power chair controls come in a number of designs and allow varying degrees of customization and programming.

Most power chair riders drive using a joystick control mounted on the armrest. The joystick should be positioned so that it can be comfortably reached by your dominant hand while you are sitting in a good upright posture with your shoulders relaxed. Improper location of the joystick can mean that you have to compromise your posture in order to put your body in the right orientation to the control. If it is not accurately positioned, using the joystick can strain the hand and arm. If you need to sit close to a desk, you will need a joystick control that is able to swing away to the side. Not all joysticks are designed to do this.

For those unable to use a joystick, several other kinds of controls are available:

- Breath controls (sometimes called sip-and-puff) respond to an in or out breath, as if you were sucking on or blowing into a straw.

- Chin controls use a small rubber cup placed just below the chin. A chin control works essentially the same way as a joystick.

- Head controls employ head movements to the back and side, with nothing obstructing the face.

The settings of your control are crucial, and you will need to work with a competent technician who understands your activities and needs. If you set too slow a deceleration rate, for example, but don't have sufficient dexterity or skill level, you might find yourself running into your furniture a lot because the chair keeps rolling once you have let go of the joystick.

How fast?

Safety should be the most important consideration when determining maximum speed. What will happen if you are going fast and a dog or a child suddenly steps out in front of you? A sudden stop might throw you out of your chair if you do not have sufficient upper body balance or are riding without the use of restraints. You might also lose your grasp of the controller in such a situation. Both maximum speed and stopping distance (deceleration) can be programmed in modern controllers, and you would be well advised to err on the side of your own safety—as well as that of anyone who might accidentally get in your way.

A safe and comfortable maximum speed depends on where you are, particularly whether you're inside or outside.

For use indoors, a maximum speed of five miles per hour is a recommended standard. When you are inside, moving in smaller spaces, a slow speed can feel fast. Traveling the short distance from your desk at work to the restroom, or from your living room to your kitchen, seems to go quickly even though you may actually be moving slowly.

A speed that is comfortable inside feels slow once you are out on the sidewalk. Outside, you usually travel farther, and you are more conscious of how long it takes to reach your destination. Traveling from your home to the corner grocery store four blocks away can seem like an eternity using the same speed you were using inside your home.

Yet outside you might be with another person who walks. Walking speed always seems slow to a wheelchair rider, yet you don't want to make your companions run to keep up with you. Average walking speed is three miles per hour, whereas a moderate running pace is eight miles per hour, numbers you can take into account when choosing your chair. Some chairs are capable of traveling as fast as eight miles per hour.

User definition of speed is now typical of power chairs and scooters. A common feature of modern power controls is a switch that lets you alternate between two programs so you can have a maximum indoor speed and a higher maximum outdoor speed. Another approach is a knob that allows you to adjust maximum speed.

Cushions

Although your wheelchair and cushion are separate purchases, which chair you choose is significantly affected by the type of cushion you will use. Chair and cushion are a team, each influencing the other. The proper combination of chair and cushion will enable you to sit in a neutral and stable posture and operate the chair safely.

Cushions come in various depths and sizes which need to be accommodated by the size of your wheelchair frame. The length of footrests, the height of the chair back, the position of armrests, and other features are influenced by how high or low you will be sitting on a cushion. Clearly, you need to decide which cushion is best for you before you can make a final decision about which chair is best, certainly before you specify the exact dimensions of your chair.

Cushion function

One important task of the wheelchair cushion is the prevention of pressure sores. Since, when we sit, only one third of the body's surface is supporting all of its weight, blood flow is restricted. In the presence of muscle atrophy—which is experienced in particular by many people with spinal cord injuries—circulation is limited further by the loss of muscle which once served as a sort of natural cushion. An additional risk of sitting is shear force, as we tend to slide forward on the cushion, causing stress across the surface of the skin. Resulting pressure sores (decubitus ulcers) can be very serious, leading to hospitalization, surgery, and—though rare—even death. The right cushion is a primary tool for maintaining the health of your skin.

The other crucial task for a cushion is postural stability. Even if you are able to walk or are an amputee with sufficient built-in cushioning, the right cushion helps to support your spine. If you already have some asymmetry in your body, you need to be supported in a way that will not increase any spinal deformity. For manual chair users, greater stability in your chair also means you can push the wheels with more confidence and strength.

It can't be repeated often enough—posture is key. Bob Hall of New Hall's Wheels puts it well:

> The wrong seating system leads to poor posture which leads to physical problems which leads to becoming more sedentary which leads to a negative emotional and personal experience. It's a dangerous chain of events.

Foam cushions

Foam technology has come a long way. No longer just the soft, airy stuff of the past, foam now comes in a range of densities and with varying degrees of "memory," holding its shape as you sit, contributing to your stability. The new foams can adapt to any shape and still provide even support, spreading pressure across the sitting surface. Different foams are often used in combination, layered for their various properties of softness, even support, and memory.

Foam is relatively inexpensive, and it is easy to cut. A therapist can experiment with shapes free of financial risk. If you have an area of skin that is broken down or on the verge, pressure can easily be reduced by cutting out a portion of the cushion. (You should not do this on your own, though, because only a doctor or therapist can identify the changes in your cushion that will help relieve pressure while still maintaining appropriate support.)

On the downside, foam wears out faster than other materials and loses its shape, but because of its lower price, this might not concern you. If you choose a foam cushion, be sure to replace it when its time is up. Old foam that is compressed can allow pressure points to form that can lead to a sore.

If you choose a gel or air flotation cushion for daily use, it is a good idea to have a backup foam cushion since gel and air flotation cushions can leak.

Gel cushions

Gel cushion designs attempt, in effect, to replace the consistency and support of atrophied muscle tissue. Highly engineered gel fluids are placed in pouches and usually attached to a foam base, so that the cushion conforms to the pressures placed on it. As a result, gel cushions provide excellent pressure distribution and are very comfortable. Many gel products also offer supplemental inserts to stabilize your legs. Your knees might tend to fall together (adduction) or apart (abduction), so such an accessory can help keep your legs straight which also aids your overall posture.

Unfortunately, gel cushions are much heavier than other types, which can cancel out some of the benefits of your lightweight wheelchair.

If you bounce up and down curbs, or commonly experience similar impact in your chair, a gel cushion might not be ideal. When you sit in a gel cushion, there is no further "cushiness" to absorb impact, a concept known as impact loading. Other cushion types are better able to absorb impact.

Another drawback to gel cushions is the possibility of them "bottoming-out" as the gel is pushed aside by your weight. You can help prevent this distribution problem by kneading your gel cushion once a day, keeping the fluids loose and spread evenly. Look for a design that divides the gel portion into several sections so that all of the gel cannot push to the sides.

There is also the chance of the gel leaking. While cushions arrive with patching kits, patches are ineffective when the breach is at a seam, which is often the case. A leak might be very minor, or it could be an extremely messy affair.

Air or dry floatation cushions

Air floatation cushions support the body entirely on air. A typical example is the Roho cushion, designed with a group of small, interconnected rubber balloons arranged in rows. Pressure is balanced by air shifting out to surrounding balloons, spreading pressure evenly against your skin. The whole system is closed so air floatation cushions can't bottom out the way gel cushions can.

If you have a pressure sore, you can tie off individual balloons to reduce contact under that area, allowing you to spend more time sitting as the sore heals. Air cushions are relatively lightweight and are waterproof, allowing for double duty in the bathtub or on a boat.

Air cushions can be less stable for those who move around a lot in their chair, but recent designs offer either low profile or quadrant options that minimize this problem. The balloons used in air cushions can be punctured, of course, and leaks do occur, although a fairly heavy duty rubber is used. But patching them is easier than with the gel design. The hard part is submerging the cushion under water to find the leak (look for escaping air bubbles).

The biggest drawback to air cushions is that they require more maintenance. It is necessary to check the pressure frequently, especially if you have pressure sores.

Urethane honeycomb cushions

Thermoplastic urethane honeycomb cushions are the most recent development in the world of cushions. Because there are many individual cells—like a beehive—these cushions are able to distribute weight evenly, but there is no risk of leaking gel or of an air bladder being punctured. The many open spaces in the beehive structure of the cushion allow air to travel more effectively. This design helps to protect against skin breakdown because your skin is kept cooler and moisture is prevented from collecting.

Urethane honeycomb cushions are very light, absorb shock, and a low profile cushion can provide significant support. These cushions can even be thrown into your washing machine and dryer, making them attractive for people with incontinence problems where the cushion will be soiled from time to time despite best efforts at bowel and bladder management.

There is not much of a track record for urethane honeycomb cushions because of their recent development, but there appears to be good prospects for this type of cushion to evolve and become more widely used.

Alternating pressure

The latest territory being explored in cushion design is the use of an air pump to create alternating pressure, of particular interest to those with more severe disabilities who are unable to perform their own weight shifts to relieve pressure.

Sitting for extensive periods of time without pressure relief causes the muscle and fatty tissues to separate, putting the delicate skin layer in closer contact with the bone. This creates even more pressure on the skin. Lack of air circulation increases the temperature between you and the cushion. Moisture collects and is trapped against the skin. All of this further increases the risk of a sore.

One alternating pressure solution is the ErgoDynamic Seating System from ErgoAir in New Hampshire. This system pumps air into and out of alternating portions of the cushion. The product is contoured for pelvic stability, with a pre-ischial cross-bar design that prevents forward slipping—and therefore shear—on the cushion. Special vent holes serve to allow the flow of air and moisture. In a five-minute cycle, compartments are inflated and deflated to shift support alternately between the ischial (sit) bones and the hips. Both areas get regular periods of complete pressure relief. The manufacturer likens it to a massage while you sit, with the resulting promotion of blood flow. In some cases, the makers suggest, a pressure sore can even heal while you sit. This cushion system can be plugged into some power chair batteries or charged in a cigarette lighter in your car.

Alternating pressure products are of course heavier—given their use of batteries and air pumps—and, like air floatation cushions, prone to puncture. However, the technology for these innovative systems is likely to evolve further in the future, as new materials and batteries are developed.

Seats and backs

Although we usually think of a seat as a single unit—such as a couch or recliner—seats, backs, cushions, and armrests are distinct when you are choosing your wheelchair. Seats, backs, and cushions have a number of interrelationships, so to some degree, you will need to think about them all at the same time. For instance, how high you will sit on the chair will be determined by the seat-to-floor height of the seat pan plus the thickness of the cushion.

Seat/chair width

Your chair should be as narrow as possible for your body size without creating contact points that can cause pressure sores.

A seat that is too wide limits mobility. A quarter of an inch in the width of the chair can make the difference between being able to get down an aisle in a store or past a couch at the home of a friend. You don't want to squeeze yourself into the seat—if you wear a heavy coat in the winter, or typically work in a business suit with a jacket, the width of the seat should take this into account—but you also don't need the wasted space or mobility limitations of a chair that is too wide. A wider chair is also heavier, given the extra metal in the frame.

A seat that is too wide will promote poor posture. If you have extra space, you are more likely to slump to one side or the other. You might think that because you would have more room to shift your position, extra seat width would be helpful in the prevention of pressure sores, but this is not a good strategy for skin management. You don't want to protect your skin by risking damage to your spine with twisted sitting postures. Rather, your skin management program should consist of proper cushioning and diet, as well as push-ups while you are in the chair. Put a high priority on good postural habits.

A wider chair also means that the wheels will be wider apart, making it necessary for a manual chair wheeler to reach farther, extending arms out to the side. Wheeling with arms extended is a less efficient way to wheel and will be more fatiguing. If the chair has armrests, they might further interfere with the process of wheeling if the chair is too wide for you, or rub against your arms as you wheel.

A wider chair does provide better lateral stability, which will help prevent a manual chair from tipping over sideways, but frankly, unless you are reckless or wheel on rough terrain, tipping sideways isn't likely. Stability can be similarly achieved by proper adjustment of the axles and plates that are typical on most chairs today. The wheels can be moved out and camber added for stability without having to incur the disadvantages and risks of a wider frame.

If weight management is difficult for you, you will want to take the possibility of weight gain into consideration when determining the seat width. You don't want to find yourself ultimately squeezed into a chair purchased when you were lighter. Your risk of pressure sores—particularly at your hip bones—will increase considerably. If you become heavier and truly need a new chair, you might have to fight with your funding source for approval, or be forced to dip into your own savings or credit limit to buy new wheels. But do you want to purchase a wider chair on the assumption that you will gain weight? Is that risking a self-fulfilling prophesy, inviting weight gain? The best solution is to reach a stable weight, whatever is normal for you, and then specify a chair that will remain appropriate to your needs while you practice the best weight control habits you can.

Seat depth

It is critical to get the depth of the seat pan right when you specify the dimensions of your chair. The seat pan should be deep enough so that the seat is in contact with as much of the bottom of your thighs as possible.

When the seat pan is too shallow, your upper legs extend beyond the front edge and more pressure is placed on your ischial "sitting" bones. This additional pressure increases the risk of skin breakdown. You are also giving up greater stability. The chair can't "carry" you if it can't make full contact with your body. Without full seat support, your body might be prevented from being in its neutral position, risking spinal curvature or muscle and tendon strain. A too-shallow seat pan also means that your feet will not rest properly in the footrests.

On the other hand, when the seat pan is too deep, you will be unable to sit properly against the chair back. You will be kept from sliding back fully in the seat, stopped behind the knees. When the seat is too deep, the only way to make contact with the back of the chair is to rotate the pelvis backward and round the spine. In other words, you will have to slump. Slumping is potentially dangerous for the spine as it can cause degeneration. This posture also makes it difficult for you to wheel efficiently in a manual chair.

A seat pan that is too deep can interfere with the position of your legs if you use calf supports with your footrests. Calf supports keep the legs in a more forward position. The seat pan might need to be shallower to compensate.

A deeper seat means a heavier chair due to the added metal in the frame. When more of the chair is ahead of the axle, you will feel as though you are pushing even more weight. If you require extra depth in the seat pan, you will need to adjust the forward position of the main wheel axles so the chair is not too front-heavy, particularly if you rely on doing wheelies in your wheeling style.

> I am very tall and recently purchased a chair that is two inches deeper than my past wheels so I could have more contact with my legs along the seat. It has worked very well, and it was not a problem to adjust the chair for wheelies and for ease of wheeling, although it did feel slightly heavier at first. Now I can't tell the difference, partly because I have nothing to compare to anymore, and I probably gained a little strength to compensate for the additional weight just by using the chair.

A crucial element that must be taken into consideration before you can determine the appropriate depth of the seat pan is the type of seat back you will use. A fabric-upholstered back requires you to sit a little farther back in the chair, and tends to loosen with time unless it is equipped with adjustable tension straps. A rigid back will not change much over time, but some are quite thick and cause you to sit more forward on the seat.

Seat height

The minimum height you can sit off the ground will be determined by physical factors. The main considerations are the length of your legs and the clearance needed for footrests. Whether you'll choose to sit higher than the minimum—and how much higher—will depend on environment, such as the height of standard tables or other surfaces, and on personal preferences.

The seat-to-floor height of a manual chair will be part of the frame dimensions ordered from the factory. It can also be controlled by where the axle plates are installed relative to the supports that carry the seat sling—the lower the axle plates, the higher the seat. On a modular power chair, the seat structure is installed on top of a drive unit and so does not depend as much on the wheel position. Instead, seat height is determined by the structure that holds the seat, which might be adjustable or available from the manufacturer in a choice of heights.

The minimum seat height for your wheelchair is determined by how much space your footrests need to clear the floor. How high you sit and how long your legs are determine where your feet will end up. In calculating minimum footrest clearance, you need to account for bumps in sidewalks, table leg supports, or any other kinds of changes in the surface you might encounter to determine how high your footrests should be from the ground. Two inches of clearance from the ground for footrests is recommended, but depending on where you will be riding, you might need more.

Whether you want your seat to be higher than the minimum height depends on a number of factors. The higher you sit, the better you can reach your cabinets in the kitchen, shelves in stores, or a bookshelf at work. Your visibility will also be a little better. Be sure, though, that your knees will be able to fit under tables and desks. On the other hand, it might be important for you to be closer to the floor, perhaps for your work. You might need to be at the same level as the surfaces you transfer to, such as your car seat or your bed. If you are a manual chair rider, you want to consider how far you will have to reach to push your wheels. Remember to add the thickness of your cushion to determine how high you will actually sit in your chair.

If you sit too low, you might strain your neck in conversation with people who are standing next to you. Some people feel that, when they sit low, they are less charismatic or appear inferior to those around them. They feel "looked down upon." However, seat height preference is an individual matter. Some folks are just happier at a higher—or lower—level. Make sure you take time to consider all the practical, psychological, and personal aspects that will be affected by the height of your chair.

Seat angle

Your chair seat does not necessarily need to be parallel to the ground. Seats can slope down toward the back. The angle of the seat compared to the ground is sometimes called "seat dump" or "squeeze." (For an example of extreme seat dump, see Figure 6-3, earlier in the chapter.)

Having some degree of seat dump means that more of your weight presses against the chair back, making you feel more stable in your seat. People with higher level spinal disabilities gain security and safety with the use of seat dump. Manual riders are able to exert more push with less effort through their arms and shoulders.

Many chairs are designed so you can adjust seat dump. Raising the rear axles to a higher position has the effect of lowering the rear of the chair and so increases the seat dump. It might also be possible to raise the caster height, achieving the same effect.

There are trade-offs for the advantages of seat dump, however, including health risks such as an increased possibility of scoliosis, and practical matters such as making transfers more difficult. Consult carefully with your therapist and dealer about the best seat angle for your needs.

Back support

Until recently, cloth or vinyl sling backs which necessarily had to fold with the chair were the only choice. Flat backs provided no lumbar support, lateral trunk stability, or accommodation of people with more advanced orthopedic/neurologic needs.

Aware of the need for better postural support, chair and cushion designers directed their efforts to making other options available. A back that must fold with the chair is much less an issue now. Rigid-frame chairs use a back that pivots down against the seat, rather than closing sideways. Power chairs designed in modules are not made to fold, so the back can now be designed with more shape, support, and upholstered comfort.

One current back design that can still close with a folding chair enhances the traditional cloth back by adding a series of horizontal looped straps down the outside of the chair back (see Figure 6-6). The straps are tension-adjustable so that each strap can be individually tightened or loosened according to the need for support at a particular point in your back.

A more recent development in the attempt to provide lumbar support for sling back wheelchairs is the PaxBac from Invacare/Pin-Dot. The PaxBac is positioned at your lumbar curve and typically provides more support than a tension back. It is made of molded foam and is designed so that support is applied on either side of the spine. (This allows the shape of the PaxBac to be narrow in the middle so that it can fold with the wheelchair.) You control the amount of back support with a strap system which attaches to the upright canes of the chair.

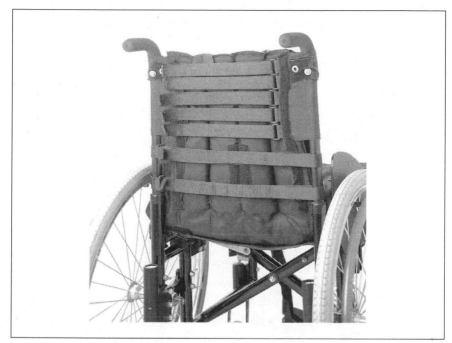

Figure 6-6. A chair back with tension-adjustable straps

Another approach to back support is a rigid back with deep upholstery. These products typically allow you to adjust lumbar support. To install this kind of chair back, the standard cloth back is removed entirely, support clips are added to the vertical canes of the chair, and the new back is hung on these clips. For a folding chair, this back must be lifted off before the chair can be folded.

If you will be pushing a manual chair, you'll want to weigh the benefits of greater back support against the additional weight of a more supportive back. Keep in mind that with extra back support you will be able to maintain more firm contact with the back of the chair as you push, enabling you to exert more force on the wheels.

If your strength and balance are more limited, your need for other back support features increases. For instance, if you have limited side-to-side stability, you can choose a back cushion that wraps around you, curving to your sides to help support you laterally. If your balance is precarious or you tend to slip easily from neutral posture, you might require additional lateral support accessories or a hip and/or chest seat belt.

There is also a psychological component to having supports. Karl Ylonen of Care Corporation in Vancouver, Washington, points out:

> A lot of people have a fear of falling sideways or forward. The more snug you get them in their chair, the more comfortable and secure they will feel.

For people whose bodies are not symmetrical, the chair back might need to be customized by a rehabilitation engineer who works closely with your therapist and wheelchair supplier. This more advanced approach can involve making molds of your body to make a highly specialized support system specifically for your needs.

Back height

You need sufficient support for your lower and upper back. Your balance may be limited by being unable to use your legs. If you are paralyzed as high as your abdomen and trunk, you are not able to use those muscles to stabilize your upper body. Too low a back might leave you unnecessarily fatigued from having to balance yourself rather than allowing the chair back to carry you.

At the same time, lower chair backs have become popular, partly as an image issue because they lessen the presence of the wheelchair. A lower back also allows you to rotate more freely, with your shoulders unobstructed. While this is an advantage for those with sufficient balance, it can encourage you in the habit of twisting your body and extending your arms to reach, rather than turning your chair. Over time, such a habit will strain your back, shoulders, and neck.

Many current wheelchair designs allow the vertical support rails of the back of the chair to be set at various heights so that back height can be customized. The upholstery has the ability to adapt to the support heights, with any extra material folding back underneath or running along the seat pan beneath the cushion. It is then held in place with Velcro.

When you order your chair, you will usually specify a back height which is then adjustable within a range of a few inches.

Footrests

One of the risks of using a wheelchair—particularly for power chair users—is to have your foot fall off a footrest, or be improperly supported to begin with, and then be injured by getting caught on an object or literally run over by the chair itself. In order to achieve good support for your feet while maximizing mobility, you'll want to take care to choose the right footrests—including hanger angle, type of footplate, and type of supports—for you.

Fixed or swingaway?

There are essentially two types of footrests—fixed and swingaway.

Fixed footrests are increasingly common, spurred by the growth and popularity of rigid-frame wheelchairs. They are integrated into the frame of the chair, held in place by telescoping tubes which slide into the frame to be adjusted for your leg length.

A fixed footrest typically has a single metal plate which holds both feet, rather than a separate plate for each foot. The single footplate attaches either between two tubes which extend from the frame or is clamped onto a tube which is part of the frame itself. The single footplate is therefore a design that can add to the structural rigidity of the chair. And since it involves fewer moving parts, there is less maintenance risk. For an example of a fixed footrest, see Figure 6-1, earlier in the chapter.

Swingaway footrests are the historical norm and remain an option for some folding wheelchairs. Individual footplates are attached to the bottom of hangers—metal tubes which attach onto the frame structure. A spring release allows the hanger/footrest mechanism to be held in place, but easily released to swing the whole unit aside or remove it completely. The ability to remove your footrests can help when sitting at a table with a large base, getting into a very small elevator, approaching a bathtub, or putting your chair into an automobile trunk. For an example of swingaway footrests, see Figure 6-2, earlier in the chapter. The footplates of swingaway footrests usually flip up to help you transfer to or from the chair. Flip-up plates are mandatory for folding chairs, or the chair would be prevented from closing. (If someone else folds your chair, be sure they know the footplates have to be lifted first, to avoid damage to your chair.) Some folding chairs offer the option of a full-width plate which can also flip up as a single unit to allow the chair to fold. The single plate offers added structural stability as well as more freedom for the positions of your feet.

As you wheel, your feet are kept from sliding off the footplates by heel loops—strips of sturdy material attached and looped across the rear of the footrests. Instead of heel loops, some chairs—usually rigid-frame chairs with single footplates—use a support strap that passes across the frame behind the calves, keeping your feet in place by preventing your legs from sliding backward. Some people find their feet are less stable with a calf-support strap, particularly if they have a tight hanger angle. Feet can more easily slide off the footplate, although tipping the footplate at more of an angle can help.

Angle and position of footrests

The angle of your footrest determines where your feet will be in relation to your knees. A tight angle will put feet under the knees. Some footrests even angle backward, so that feet are farther back than knees. A wider angle, of course, will bring feet forward so they are in front of the knees. Which angle is best for you depends on a variety of factors, including leg length, physical limitations, and personal preference. In addition to the angle of the footrest, you might also want to consider footrest designs that keep your feet closer together. Finally, consider the best angle for your feet as they rest on the footplate.

Recent designs have brought the angle of the footrests closer to the body, putting the legs into more of a perpendicular position. Table legs become less of an obstacle, removing the need for flip-up footplates for some people. A tighter footrest angle means a shorter "wheelbase" from rear to toe, and so allows you to turn around in smaller spaces. You need sufficient range of motion to bend at the knees and ankles to use these closer footrest angles.

Some people like to be able to see their toes so they can tell where their feet are. If you are conscious of your posture and concerned about your feet being even and flat on the plates, you might want to choose a more forward angle. Those with longer legs might need a more forward angle in order to bring the feet up away from the ground. This option might be more convenient for them than choosing a taller seat height, which can raise the knees too high to clear desks or tables.

For people with flexion contracture, where the knee will not open to a ninety degree angle, the feet need to be supported underneath the leg. Some chair producers have an optional footrest that can be adjusted back underneath the chair. This is generally available only for manual chairs, since batteries and motors usually take up this space on power chairs.

The angle of the footplate itself can be either fixed or adjustable, raising or lowering your toes relative to your heels. The more forward the angle of the hanger, the more upward an angle the plate needs to be at to accommodate the natural posture of your feet. Most manufacturers offer an adjustable footplate as an option. This is especially useful for people whose feet are different, who go through changes with contractures in the legs, or who have progressive conditions that affect foot angle.

Tires

Tires influence the comfort of your ride and the amount of maintenance your chair will need. Some riders also consider the choice of tires an important aesthetic consideration. Generally, wheelchair tires are made of a gray rubber designed not to leave scuff marks on floors. Your choices range from pneumatic—air-filled—tires to solid rubber tires, with tires that attempt to offer the best of both in between. As you decide which type of tire will serve you best, keep in mind that larger tires will add width to your chair.

Pneumatic tires have inflatable tubes in them like bicycle tires, so they offer a more cushioned ride and are better able to squeeze their way over obstacles. Like bicycle tires, they can be punctured by a tack or piece of glass picked up on the street. The risk of punctures is greater for power chair tires because the extra weight of the chair against the pavement can help a sharp object pierce the rubber. Obviously, getting a flat tire means you might find yourself stranded away from home or going back for a repair riding on the deflated tire. Riding on a flat tire can cause damage to the rim of the wheel. Flats can be minimized by using heavy-duty, thorn-resistant tubes or Kevlar tires. (Kevlar is a material used for bulletproof vests.)

Pneumatic tires need replacement more often, since the depth of the rubber before reaching the fiber lining is thinner than a solid tire. The rubber wears down from normal use, particularly the more shallow treads of most manual chair tires. Knobby tires with a deeper tread are also available. They will last longer and provide better traction on unpaved surfaces, but are harder on the hands of manual chair riders.

Thin-profile pneumatic tires—used on manual chairs—have less surface area in contact with the pavement, so there is less friction when turning. This makes the chair more agile, critical for sport use, and preferred by some riders for daily use. Others find the thin-profile tires less comfortable in their hands.

Solid rubber tires make for a rougher ride. You will feel each bump of the pavement, but your tires will never go flat. You might value the security of knowing you will not get a flat, like this power chair user:

> I found when I had air tires on my chair I would get flats an average of two or three times a month. It happened at very inopportune times, like when I was alone or on vacation. Switching to solid tires has been a godsend. Now I don't have to avoid that broken glass. I can go right through it.

Many power chairs have solid tires with a deeper tread that lasts longer while providing better traction. Solid rubber tires tend to be slightly heavier than other options, since they contain more rubber.

A recent variation that is a compromise between pneumatic and solid rubber tires uses a rubber insert. The insert is placed inside a tire as an alternative to an inflatable tube. The tire doesn't need to be pumped up with air, so obviously can't go flat. Manual chair riders will find that the resulting apparent tire pressure is softer, and that the chair won't roll as easily. The wheels will also lose momentum faster which means having to push more often. However, some power chair users swear by rubber inserts.

Yet another variation is the foam-filled tire, a special design that has better rollability and a softer ride, but cannot go flat.

Casters

Casters are the smaller wheels at the front (usually) of your wheelchair that allow the chair to turn—and keep it from tipping over on two wheels. Casters rotate on their forks as you change direction in your chair. They can be large or small, soft or hard. The kind of casters you choose has a lot of impact on your comfort and mobility. You will want to weigh the advantages of small casters against those of large casters.

Small casters allow tighter footrest angles, thus their popularity on rigid-frame chairs. Small casters are less likely to get in a position that prevents them from rotating when you turn. Greater agility has made small casters very popular, but since they are hard—typically made of solid plastic or rubber—they make for a bumpier ride. Some small caster wheels are the same type as those used on rollerblades or skateboards. You will feel every crack in the sidewalk, and you will need to lift the casters by doing a mini-wheelie with an extra push in order to clear thresholds at doorways. The smallest types of casters can even be stopped by very small obstacles, like a stone on a sidewalk. They might get caught in a sewer or ventilation grate on the street. These kinds of sudden stops, as you know, can mean being thrown out of your chair.

Pneumatic casters are larger, at least six inches in diameter. They will provide a very soft ride. Any air-filled tire is at risk of puncture, but it is also true that a flat caster will not strand you the way a flat main tire will. The chair itself will also last longer with larger, soft casters, as the vibration from harder tires causes more wear and tear on the frame.

Large casters can handle obstacles and rough terrain more easily. Picture a hard caster approaching a three-inch curb, and you can sense that it would require more force to roll over the curb than a softer, larger tire. The Terra-Trek all-terrain chair from Kuschall has very large, pneumatic front casters, partnered with heavy-duty knobby main tires.

Before choosing a large caster, you'll want to consider your ideal footrest angle. When larger, pneumatic casters are used, your heels must be moved forward with a greater footrest angle to clear the rotation of the casters, extending your overall length, "wheel to toe," if you will.

Larger casters can also obstruct your movement suddenly if you are close to a wall or some other raised surface. As the caster begins to rotate, it becomes blocked by the wall, stopping your movement. You won't be trapped; you'll simply have to maneuver so that you get the caster free of the obstacle. Some people find this stressful, but many users learn to avoid these situations.

A compromise between the two extremes of caster options is the four-inch solid rubber caster. It cannot be punctured and is not stopped by small obstacles, but it does still transmit more vibration through the chair.

Suspension systems

Cars have shock absorbers to soften the ride, so why not wheelchairs? This thought is occurring to an increasing number of chair designers. Outdoor terrain and vibrations from wheeling on sidewalks with all of their bumps and potholes have an impact on the tissues of the body. It is not good for us to be shaken up every day, so a soft ride is protective for people who encounter lots of vibration when they wheel. If you have back discomfort that is aggravated by the bounce of your wheelchair, adding a suspension system can reduce the impact enough to spare you some back pain.

As we've already discussed, one concern about rigid-frame chairs is that they are less able to keep all four wheels in contact with surfaces that are not level, such as an outdoor trail or a city sidewalk with bumps and dips. This instability can mean a temporary loss of control which potentially could be disastrous. Independent suspension designs enable rigid-frame chairs to have better contact with the ground.

Smaller power chair producers have also shown a lot of interest in suspension.

Specialized chair systems

In addition to the variety of options for a basic chair, there are additional features available if your physical condition requires more support, alternative methods for pressure relief, or the ability to shift to a more horizontal position. Two of these features are tilt and recline—mechanized systems which allow either the whole chair or just the chair back to recline. Other specialized features include lateral supports, which give you additional cushioning to hold your body steady, and head supports.

Your doctor or therapist will no doubt recommend such features if:

- Your upper body balance and stability are seriously limited
- Your disability involves structural deformities, spinal curvature, or muscle contracture
- You are at risk of fainting or dysreflexia
- You do not have the strength to shift your position on your own

Make sure you have expert assistance when choosing a tilt or recline system, lateral supports, and head support. It's important to make sure you have the optimal system for your needs and that the specific models you choose are compatible with the rest of your chair.

Armrests

Power chairs almost always have armrests, but some manual chair riders feel that armrests get in their way. It's true that armrests can interfere with wheeling when you want to get your body into the push by leaning forward, and people with shorter arms in particular might find that armrests interfere with a comfortable relationship to the wheels. Armrests can also get in the way of reaching to the side or to the floor, or prevent you from being able to get close enough to a table at work or in a restaurant. In addition, armrests add weight to the chair—a significant amount in some cases.

But before you decide against armrests for your manual chair, consider the following benefits of having them:

- Armrests can help prevent spinal problems. When you put the weight of your arms on armrests, you relieve some of the load on your spine.

- Armrests may be important for transfers into and out of the chair.

- Armrests are helpful for shifting your weight in the chair, a crucial habit for the prevention of pressure sores.

- If you have limited upper body balance, your safety may depend on having the added stability armrests provide.

Generally, armrests are removable, so nothing says that you have to use them all the time. Many chair users purchase armrests and then use them only when it is appropriate for them. As always, the choice depends on your individual needs and activities.

> My habit is to get dressed while sitting in my chair, and I rely on armrests to lift myself high enough to pull up my pants. More recently I've been spending more time at the computer and find that armrests offer some relief to my neck and shoulders. Otherwise, I leave them off.

There are several types of armrests. The typical armrest is wide enough to support the arm, padded, and covered with vinyl upholstery. This type of armrest can be in the desk style—which has a shorter upholstered section allowing you to pull closer to desks and tables—or full-length, which might be important to support a lap tray if you use one.

Some armrests lock down and can be used as a grip to carry a folded chair or used by people who might carry you on a stairway. If the armrests on your chair are not fixed, be certain to let someone helping you know this before they attempt to lift your chair—especially if you are in it. Locking arms also ensure that the armrests will still be with the chair when you reclaim it after an airline trip.

High level quadriplegic riders can choose sculpted armrests, possibly with straps, to keep their arms in place. Some riders may have enough dexterity to operate a joystick control on a power chair, even though their arms are generally weak. Sculpted armrests can aid them in keeping their arms in place while driving the chair. Sculpted armrests might also include supports for the hands and fingers to keep them from curling into contracture.

Many modern manual chairs have tube-design, swingaway armrests that can easily rotate away from the chair. The horizontal portion is covered with a soft, water-resistant material. These armrests tend not to be comfortable for resting your arms, because they are round and not very wide. Tube-design armrests are more appropriate for doing push-ups and correcting yourself if you feel off balance.

There are also flip-up armrests, a good solution for those who need/want armrests only part of the time, but who don't want the bother of taking them off and putting them back on.

Whatever type of armrests you choose, it is important to adjust them to the correct height. Armrests that are too high will lead you to elevate your shoulders, which can cause tight muscles and pain in the neck and shoulders. If armrests are too low, you will be encouraged to slump to the side to make contact, increasing the risk of developing spinal curvature.

Clothing guards

Clothing guards—also called sideguards—protect clothes from being soiled by or getting caught in the wheels of the chair. They are optional, but if you will be riding your chair outside very much, clothing guards are a practical choice. You can select armrests with built-in clothing guards. Those who do not use armrests, or who prefer the tubular type which include no side panel, can use separate sideguards. Clothing guards can be made of fabric, plastic, or metal.

The advantages of using cloth sideguards are that they are lightweight and can be easily loosened when you need to move them out of the way, during transfers, for instance. The disadvantages are that the flexibility of cloth sideguards makes them tend to bend outward from general use. When this happens, your clothing will not be completely contained.

Since plastic sideguards do not get crushed down as the cloth ones do, they are more effective in holding in your clothing. The main disadvantage of plastic sideguards is that they require extra care during transfers. You can injure your skin by hitting the hard edge, potentially causing a sore. You might also break the sideguard. Finally, plastic guards can be an obstruction if you sometimes sit cross-legged in your wheelchair.

CHAPTER 7

Home Access

Access means more than installing grab bars and ramps. For a person with a disability it means being independent in his or her home and being able to participate fully in the family. Subtle details can affect the quality of life for a person with a disability, such as a door threshold that is a bit too high or carpeting that is a bit too plush.

This chapter looks at what you can do to make your home environment accessible and your daily life fuller and more convenient. We begin with a look at overall design: the needs we all want met in our homes. Next, we turn to things to keep in mind when planning adaptations: appearance, using professionals, public and private space, your strength and stamina, the size and features of the wheelchair, dimensions required for various activities, and creative solutions to expensive problems. We next look at modifying building features—ramps, doors, windows—and utilities—heating/cooling, electrical power, and telephone.

Then we examine changes that can be made to individual rooms, focusing on the bathroom, kitchen, and bedroom. We close the chapter with brief looks at finding a new home or apartment and training the people you live with to be aware of your needs—for example, training them to not leave shoes in a place that blocks your path.

Fundamental needs in the home

A home should be flexible enough to handle everyone's needs, without people finding themselves trapped by obstacles or unnecessarily dependent. *Building for a Lifetime*, by Margaret Wylde, Adrian Baron-Robbins, and Sam Clark, documents the results of research conducted at the Institute for Technology Development under a grant from the National Institute for Disability Rehabilitation and Research. It details the concept of the Lifespan home, which not only accommodates people with disabilities, but considers the needs of all family members at all stages of life and health, including children and elderly people.

The authors describe four fundamental needs that homes provide:[1]

- **Privacy.** A space of your own and a chance to be left alone.
- **Belonging.** The ability to share spaces with friends and family, to be able to join in preparing meals and social activities.
- **Control.** The ability to go where you want and do what you want.
- **Safety and security.** The ability to open doors and escape in an emergency.

In the Lifespan model, you evaluate your home, keeping in mind these four aspects and looking for the highest possible quality of life for everyone, rather than simply thinking in terms of getting in the front door and using a bathroom.

Each person finds his or her own priorities. This woman moved into an accessible apartment in New York City:

> *My apartment was built for a wheelchair user. The kitchen has a roll-under sink. The bathroom door is very wide and opens out. The bathroom is very large with a huge turning radius. The switches are lower and the outlets are higher, but that doesn't mean as much to me as being able to use the bathroom and wash the dishes. My balance is really good so I don't rely so much on grab bars.*

You might resist making home modifications. The process can amplify negative emotions about your disability or give it more solid form. Particularly if you have a progressive condition like multiple sclerosis or ALS, planning for a future of additional disability can be upsetting. Louis Tenenbaum is a carpenter and building contractor in Maryland who specializes in access modifications. He describes his work with a client:

> *She fought me all along the way, because she thought that making changes was giving in to her disability. But in the end, every one of the changes has increased her independence.*

Universal Design

A new philosophy known as Universal Design aims to increase independence for everyone in the home, while keeping the home attractive. When efforts began to remove architectural obstacles, terms like barrier-free or handicapped-accessible design were widely used. These are terms that tend to stigmatize a building, implying it has been somehow compromised or institutionalized. Increasingly architects and product suppliers are developing alternatives that fit seamlessly into the overall design, with respect for aesthetics.

The late Ron Mace was an architect with a private practice and director of the Center for Universal Design at North Carolina State University. He had polio as a child. Mace saw that making the world accessible benefits everyone. He saw that the existing terms did not promote integration and in fact generated resentment.

> Universal Design says, why not change our thinking and design for everyone all of the time? Let's not call it "design for people with disabilities." Let's call it "good design."

Proponents of this philosophy speak of a home that can "age in place." As you and your family members get older and encounter any of the variety of physical changes humans encounter, your home can remain friendly and usable, or at least easier to adapt.

Most people eventually experience a disability of some sort, even if only for a matter of weeks using a wheelchair or crutches. A broken leg or temporary disease could mean being physically limited for months or years. An entrance without steps and an accessible bathroom are suddenly useful at such times. The demographics of the United States are shifting dramatically toward an older population. As you age, you will value features of Universal Design in a home. You might be able to stay in your home longer, despite an illness that might otherwise mean moving to a residential care setting.

More and more, people with disabilities are out in the world, making friends, raising families. These people will be buying homes and deserve a selection in the marketplace. It makes good business sense for builders to incorporate Universal Design principles.

Here I have a big down payment and a pre-approved mortgage, but because I use a wheelchair I have much, much less to choose from than anybody else. It is extremely frustrating, because the place where I will live is the key to the quality of life I want to make for myself. This severely restricted market for accessible homes is keeping me from my dreams, and I don't appreciate the idea that I should have to compromise. You'd think that they would want my money.

Universal Design also makes monetary sense. The cost of later modifications is usually much higher than doing it right in the first place. The price of lever handles, door closers, grab bars, sinks, accessible showers and tubs, and shelving modifications in the kitchen will continue to fall as the demand increases.

Money is a very real issue when you are faced with modifying your home. You might not be able to afford all of the work it would take to achieve full access. Tenenbaum notes that you often have to make tough choices:

I worked with a woman recently where we decided that her best solution was to build an additional room on the first floor, but [the design also] meant she wouldn't be able to go upstairs to yell at her kids about throwing their clothes on the floor. It's very hard, because we're being controlled by budget. Universal access is a goal, but we often have to compromise our goals because of other constraints.

Universal Design also suggests building for adaptability, an approach referred to as "handicapped-adaptable." With some foresight and simple measures during construction, future accessibility needs can more easily be met. For instance, make sure that walls in bathrooms are reinforced in advance for grab bar installation. Ron Mace explained:

With adaptable design, they don't have to put the grab bars in. You can just put them in where someone needs them. Or in the kitchen, the builder puts the base cabinet under the sink, but makes it removable. He just doesn't bolt it down. You take a couple of screws out and put it in storage.

Building codes sometimes offer builders an alternative. They can make a certain percentage of units accessible, or they can make more units adaptable. Variations in a city depend on local policies and the choices made by housing developers.

Private homes and accessibility codes

At this time, there is no requirement for private, single-family homes to be made accessible. The building industry has resisted such provisions, fearing it will impose excessive expense on them.

Current building methods do not lend themselves to easy accessibility. For example, the typical style of home-building puts the main floor up at least several inches to prevent water from flowing in from the ground level, in theory at least. Homes are also raised to allow a "crawl space" for air to circulate under the home, again to remove moisture, or to make room for windows to allow light into a basement space.

When you consider accessibility codes in terms of how legislation would apply to private homes, the issue gets trickier. On one hand, some people hesitate to force accessibility on private homes:

> People should be allowed to build the home they want. Maybe I, in my wheelchair, can't deal with a sunken living room, but that should not prevent someone from having one, if that is what they want. We have no business telling people how to build their homes.

> This is coming from a wheelchair user who hates visiting people in homes that are uncomfortable or difficult for me. But I would never tell someone that they must build their house to suit me.

On the other hand, millions of people with disabilities have to live someplace, and in the present environment have very little to choose from. You could be forced to leave a neighborhood you prefer, or have to spend extra money for adaptations, just because there are no requirements for basic features of access.

> But why not require that all new private homes be required to meet minimum standards of accessibility, rather than just public or apartment buildings? We don't accept that someone can just decide, "Oh, I don't feel like having my new house meet all of those expensive fire-safety and structural integrity requirements." The public interest is said to be best served by ensuring a minimum standard of safety for both the first residents and any future residents. Is it unreasonable to expect this of basic accessibility?

Access questions extend beyond your own home. Your life takes you to the homes of relatives and friends. People throw parties. Someone you love might need help because they are not well. The "visitability" of other homes is a significant factor in the quality of your life.

> When I visit a home where I need a lift up the steps or have to control my liquid intake for lack of a bathroom I can use, my hosts are very apologetic. Consistently, people wish that they could provide a setting that works for me. Some will go out of their way, as a dear cousin of mine recently did by building a portable ramp for the garage entry.

> Visitability is always important. When I go to visit my great-aunt and uncle in Illinois they always put up a ramp at one door and hook up the hand-held shower.

To date, two American cities—Atlanta, Georgia and Austin, Texas—have established a visitability ordinance.

You will decide how much you hope or expect others to accommodate you. Friends and relatives also struggle with money issues, and if they live in multi-story homes there will be only so much they can do. They will need your help to understand your needs. Perhaps you can even offer some guidance on specific measures they can take, do a little research into products, and share a creative process with them to optimize your access as much as possible.

Will it look like a hospital?

Many people fear that making their home accessible will make it look institutional and damage future resale value. Ramps, grab bars, lowered switches and raised outlets, or kitchen counters that leave space for leg room all raise the specter of not being able to sell the home when the time comes.

It is a fallacy that an accessible home must become unattractive to potential buyers. Remember, when you think in terms of Universal Design you are making your home safe, comfortable, and convenient for everyone. Because the design quality of products—from grab bars to kitchen and storage systems—has improved, your home can remain attractive and not look like a hospital.

Building contractor Louis Tenenbaum puts it simply:

> *Beauty really is in the eye of the beholder. One person's institutional is another person's attractive. Personally, I think what's ugly is breaking a hip because the environment was unsafe.*

Adapting what's there

Most people with disabilities will be faced with adapting an existing home or apartment. Adaptation for access is not what architects and builders are thinking about when they design and construct housing.

The degree of adaptation you can make depends on:

* What you can afford

* What control you have over your home—owned or rented

* The existing design features of your home and/or property

Adaptation might not be that big a deal if you are fortunate to live in a home that doesn't need a lot of changes.

> *I was fairly lucky that when I was disabled both my parents' houses needed only minor modifications to be made accessible (bars, hand-held shower, wider bathroom door). Both houses were one story with no more than one step to get in.*

Start with measures that cost nothing, such as moving furniture around to make space and teaching your family to not leave items where they impede your path. You might move to another bedroom in the home, rearrange kitchen cabinets, or remove the door to the bathroom in the master bedroom. It might even be necessary to accept not having access to certain parts of your home without assistance.

Next, there are measures which don't cost much money. Wooden ramps can be built easily; portable, folding metal ramps are available at reasonable cost. Doorknobs can be converted with inexpensive lever handles, and door hinges can be changed to a hinge type that pivots the door aside so the door's thickness no longer blocks your way. Grippers, reachers, and various other tools help to extend your reach and use what strength you have.

Remote control systems allow you to turn almost anything on or off in the home, as well as open doors or answer the telephone.

More expensive is the construction cost associated with major work such as widening doors, pouring a concrete ramp and grading the land outside, replacing a bathtub with a roll-in shower, or adding a new room to the house. You might also consider taking down a wall that is not load-bearing—perhaps between the dining room and den—to open up space for ease of movement. Depending on your income and where you live, tax credits might be available for some of these expenses. Some banks extend long-term loans with minimal down payments for disability-related construction.

Take care not to use up all your resources on one adaptation. If you use all your money to build an accessible addition, you won't have funds left for changes in other parts of the house. The result could be that you are isolated in your shiny new wing of the home, unable to freely interact with the rest of the household.

If you are doing substantial work or buying significant new items such as major appliances, this is a chance to improve your home with quality construction and well-made products which will last, with a minimum of maintenance. Adapting a home for access can be a chance to increase the convenience of your home for everyone, and improve its long-term value.

Considerations during planning

Save yourself later headaches or regrets by taking enough time in the planning stage. You will avoid surprises, speed the construction process, have a more satisfying working relationship with the contractor or worker, and save money.

Using professionals

Doing construction in the home is quite stressful. The stereotype—often true—is that things take longer, cost more, and disrupt your life in ways you never imagined. Many people find themselves in conflict with the contractor or their spouse, arguing over scheduling, costs, or quality.

It is easy to underestimate what construction will cost, even if the task seems simple. Contractor Louis Tenenbaum observes:

We volunteer with a program at the local Independent Living Center where we help with consulting and evaluation. They had the impression that they could do a lot for $2,000 per house. That's just not true. $2,000 doesn't go very far.

Working with the right professional is a way to get good advice on the reality of the work—the costs and the actual tasks. Many builders are still not experienced with accessible design, beyond simple tasks like adding grab bars or using wider doors. However, there are contractors who make a specialty of accessible construction. It is worth some effort to find the most experienced people. You would be well advised to interview a number of builders, find out about their experience, invite them to evaluate your home, and ask for references.

Some architects have also emphasized access in their practice, either for doing modifications, new buildings, or both. While it might cost more to pay an architect's fee, architects understand how to maintain the quality of your home's appearance and overall function. Architects will also have worked with local contractors, so can advise you on who does quality, reliable work. Ron Mace noted:

It happens all the time that people build something ugly instead of something that is well integrated and looks good. They make terrible, brutal home modifications, sometimes at great expense, because they don't know what they can do.

Adapting a home is a multi-disciplinary process involving many players. Therapists have a contribution to make, because they understand how the physiology of your disability affects your interactions with the home. Louis Tenenbaum says:

Occupational therapists tell me that I should learn about the various medical conditions. I say, "Yeah, but you have to learn something about construction."

The process also includes you. Observe the details of how you function in your present home. Note what is stressful, fatiguing, inconvenient, or awkward. Make notes to have with you when you start to discuss changes. No professional can automatically know about your specific needs and preferences. If you can clearly describe your needs from your everyday experience, you will get the most from their services.

Defining the problems

Start by defining the problems. Take time to evaluate your home, consider how your disability needs to be accommodated, do research and reading, and invite in people with experience. Check with your local Independent Living Center, many of which offer evaluation services or even programs to help perform or finance changes. Tenenbaum finds that people often come to him with preconceived notions about what to do:

> *I find the most important thing is to avoid discussing solutions until we identify problems. For instance, the problem is "How do I get into my house?" not "How do I get in my front door or in my garage?" Or even "How do I build a ramp?"*

Considering private and public space

Maintaining the separation between private and public space is important to your quality of life. The bedroom is a private space, while the entry foyer and den are public. A bathroom is a private space, but even so there can be the bathroom with your private toiletries and adaptive equipment, and the bathroom that guests would use.

Some families whose homes have all bedrooms upstairs find themselves changing a downstairs room into a bedroom for a person who can't go up the stairs. Tri-level homes also pose problems of this sort. There may be only one level where you have access to a bathroom or the ability to freely come and go from the home.

Putting a bedroom on a lower level can violate the separation between public and private space. The normal flow of family life is disrupted by the loss of family space downstairs or by the movement of activities upstairs in which you can no longer join. Guests coming in may see a bed or medical equipment, perhaps in what used to be the living room. This kind of exposure can be uncomfortable for the whole family—especially the person with the disability.

If a formerly public space must be made private, try to relocate the public space somewhere that is still accessible. One family in a tri-level home made a bedroom of the ground floor living room, because it had the easiest access. The father—the chair user—opted to accept being assisted up a ramp around the side of the house to get to the new living room on the next level.

Too much privacy can mean isolation for the person with the disability. Even if the solution is to build a totally accessible addition to the house, keep in mind the need for everyone to share in the community of the family.

Product selection

Choose the best products you can, even if they are more expensive at first. Well-designed products will last longer, be easier to operate and simpler to maintain, and often be better looking. Well-designed products don't tax your strength; their operation is self-evident; they provide you with auditory and visual cues that they are operating correctly.

Consider all features when choosing products. A door handle might be easy to turn, but have a key lock which demands fine dexterity or pinching strength. A flat stove surface might make it easy to slide pots onto and off the heating element; it should also indicate by some color that it is on to prevent accidental burns.

Strength and stamina

Keep both strength and stamina in mind as you consider adaptations you make in your home. Strength is how much force you can exert briefly. Stamina is your ability to continue performing an activity. For example, opening a door or making the bed by lifting the mattress are strength tasks. Making a door spring less tense or choosing a lighter mattress can preserve strength. Washing the dishes or doing container gardening are stamina activities. Locating a kitchen or gardening task so that you can sit comfortably affects how long you can work.

Wheelchair width

If you are selecting a new wheelchair, you should know the narrowest door or passageway that you will need to get through. A narrower chair doesn't necessarily mean narrower seat. Frame design and wheel type also have an effect on overall width.

Your chair can be adjusted to optimize your access. The more camber you use—adding angle to the wheels to increase your base—the wider you are. If necessary, you can adjust your wheels to be absolutely vertical, making your chair as narrow as possible. If you have adjustable axles, you might also gain some clearance by bringing your wheels closer to your body. Obviously, your stability in the chair is a high priority, but the fraction of an inch you might gain could make the difference between getting someplace or not.

Dimensions

There are published standards which detail exact dimensions—often expressed as a range—for wheelchair clearance and accommodation. In reality, the ideal measurements depend on your specific needs. Just because a home does not technically conform to accessibility codes does not mean there will necessarily be obstacles for you. You might not need every recommended access measure, so might as well save your money.

For instance, a circular area five feet in diameter is typically recommended as the space necessary to fully turn around in your wheelchair. You might actually need more or less space. You might need more if you need to elevate your footrests and have a ventilator on a tray behind your chair, or less if you are using a high performance, lightweight, rigid frame manual chair where your feet are under your knees. Front- and mid-wheel drive power chairs can turn in smaller spaces than rear-wheel drive chairs.

Consider whether you even need to turn around. Going backward out of a small room like the bathroom might not be a large problem. On the other hand, having to wheel backward often, over a greater distance, could lead to stress in your neck and shoulders from having to crane around to see where you are going.

> *I once lived in an apartment with a small bathroom. I couldn't turn around, but I could close the door once I was inside, and get to the toilet, the tub, and the sink. Because I am flexible enough to reach behind to open and close the door, and because I can wheel backward accurately, it was fine, although not ideal. Everything else about the place was just right, so I decided to accept it.*

By all means, acquire the published standards; they have much to offer. But consider them a guide, not law. Do your best to think in terms of principles—being able to move, reach what you need, be independent, and use your energy efficiently.

Being creative

To modify your home, you don't always have to call a professional contractor, pay top dollar for new products out of catalogs, or even restrict yourself to products that are designed solely for access. Keep your thinking—and your eyes—open to solutions in unexpected places. You might have a friend who just loves tinkering and solving problems. Give him a call. Those skills can come in very handy.

Your building contractor can use the same creative approach, as did a builder in Canada for this person with a spinal cord injury:

> While I was in the local Auxiliary Hospital, waiting for our home to be constructed, we phoned a company to see what it would cost to have a door opener installed. They wanted $2,000 plus traveling to come about 75 miles to install one. My contractor said, "That's ridiculous." He bought a garage door opener for $270, mounted it sideways above the patio doors with a rod and a chain so it pulled the doors open or closed instead of pushing them. Then he hooked the on/off switch to doorbell buttons inside and out, and I could go in and out whenever I wanted. It worked like a charm, and altogether it only cost $450.

Creative contracting solutions should be done with care. Automated equipment needs to be properly installed. Anyone adapting equipment needs to understand how it will withstand the stresses placed upon it, and ensure that the structure holding it can support it. For example, a standard garage door opener is a fairly heavy item not designed to operate on its side. Improperly executed, a low-cost approach can lead to injury, as this woman with a mobility disability notes:

> It is usually cheaper in any situation to rig up something that was intended for another purpose. But when you call a supplier you are pretty much asking them about the installation of equipment specifically made for that purpose. A supplier has their reputation and liability to think of. If they jerry-rigged something and the door somehow closed on you or hurt you in some way—well, they would be the ones in trouble. If a door opener made for that purpose malfunctions, then you can go back to the manufacturer for satisfaction. If you are using something made for another purpose, the manufacturer is going to say, "Too bad."

Many creative ideas don't involve expensive or heavy equipment, only simple solutions. This contractor found a simple solution to the problem of keeping a door open while someone helped the chair rider up a ramp:

> *One easy modification that comes to mind is a chain with a hook on a post at the edge of a porch where I built a ramp. It connected to an eye that I attached to the storm door. This allowed the gentlemen caregiver to hook the door open when he was pushing his wife in her wheelchair, so that he did not have to hold the door with his knee or something. Though it is a small thing, it did make things easier for him. The low tech way— that's what I love.*

Typical building features

A number of building features impact the ease of access to your home. Doors, flooring, windows, electricity, and other features need to be considered for the ways in which they obstruct your independence or can be better designed.

Entrance

Getting in the door is the first order of business. Ideally you would prefer to go in the front door like everyone else, rather than being relegated to the back door, and have more than one entry. The primary entrance is ideally close to the car, and allows you to bring things into and out of the home as easily as possible. In an apartment complex this might mean convenient access to an elevator from a parking garage.

A paved, reasonably level, smooth surface is best for approaches to doors, patios, decks, gardens, and parking areas. Widths of five feet are considered ideal. Consider whether the entrance should be protected with an overhang. Chair riders often need a little extra time to get a door open, so will be exposed to the weather. An overhang also suggests the need for additional lighting, so you can find your keys, see the pavement when approaching the door, and see the doorknob well enough to operate it. A small shelf next to the door gives you a place to put down a bag of groceries while unlocking the door.

If you can afford more extensive changes to a private home, you might regrade the driveway to bring it up to the level of the house. This way, you take advantage of the car to get up the slope, so you won't have to push or drive your wheelchair uphill.

Ramps

A ramp is a common and generally affordable solution. Some people might simply lay down a piece of wood so a chair rider can be hauled up it in his chair, but that might not achieve independent—or safe—access.

The usual slope recommended for ramps is 1:12, which means that for every one inch of rise there are twelve inches of horizontal run. This angle can be too steep for some chair riders, as well as for some people who walk, or in winter or rainy conditions. A gentler slope of 1:20 is likely to be usable by most people. Figure 7-1 shows the difference between a 1:12 and a 1:20 slope.

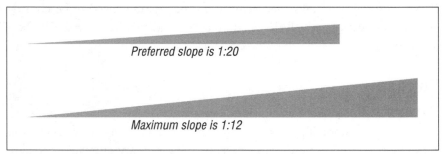

Figure 7-1. Preferred and maximum ramp slopes

The angle you choose also depends on space. The less the angle of slope, the more distance the ramp will run. If there isn't much room, more slope might be the only approach. Some riders do have the strength to climb slopes even greater than 1:12. But no matter how strong you are, when you have a bag of groceries in your lap, you can't climb as easily since you can't involve your upper body as well. And, of course, there is a point at which too much slope will be likely to cause the wheelchair to tip back altogether.

The ramp does not have to run in a continuous rise, but can "switch back," making a turn and coming back in the opposite direction. Or you can use a dog-leg design that makes one ninety-degree turn—an approach that can be used to run part of an exterior ramp along the side of the house, minimizing its visual impact. Such designs need a level landing at the turn. All ramps must have a level landing of five feet for every thirty inches of rise.

Tenenbaum emphasizes the need for a landing before a doorway:

> *The main thing is to have a landing at the top. Make sure you have room to be out of the way of the door when it swings open. People sometimes mistakenly run the slope right up to the door, with no curb or handrail.*

Ramps of concrete and asphalt are ideal surfaces that require little maintenance, but for rises of more than one foot, these materials will usually not be practical. Too much concrete or asphalt can crack under its own weight. Wood or metal grating is used for ramp surfaces. If using metal grating, be certain that openings are not large enough to catch a crutch tip or a shoe heel. Take drainage into account so the surface will stay dry and free of puddles.

Handrails are an important safety element of a ramp, just as for a stairway, and are usually advisable even with a gentle slope. Provide handrails on both sides. Some chair riders prefer to pull themselves up the ramp by grabbing the handrails, which is sometimes easier than pushing the wheels. Rails should not be more than one and a half inches in diameter so that they can be gripped reliably. A round shape is best. Handrails should not be too close to the wall—one and a half inches is recommended. Handrails should extend one foot beyond the bottom and top of the ramp so it is possible to have support as you approach the rise and until you reach secure, level ground. For exterior ramps, provide for nighttime lighting.

A ramp has a strong visual impact. Take into account the design of your home, and use compatible materials, colors, and patterns. You want to avoid communicating, "A disabled person lives here and we had to make our home ugly because of it." Rather, you want the design to communicate, "Our home is a place that welcomes everybody." Landscaping can better integrate the ramp into the design of the home.

A poorly designed and aggressively installed ramp can indeed affect the value of your home. Ron Mace observed:

> *The ramp is the cheapest thing you can do, but it has the disadvantage of being very obvious. It devalues the home in the view of realtors. They usually discount the house, because they feel that in order to put it on the market, you're going to have to spend more money to take the ramp off. It's something that nobody else will want.*

You don't want to build a ramp in a way that will feed into these attitudes. Regrading is desirable, if possible, or you could install the ramp in a way that it is easily removed but still structurally sound. Alternatively, perhaps the ramp could go inside a garage; this can be the most convenient place if you will be driving and typically enter the home through the garage door. Putting the ramp in a garage also protects the ramp—and the person using it—from weather.

Temporary and portable ramps

Temporary ramps are often acquired or built. In some public settings, a removable ramp might just get left in place rather than building something more permanent. Inspect such a temporary ramp for stability.

> I fell out of my wheelchair on a ramp at a funeral home. The ramp was removable and when my front wheels hit it the whole ramp moved. I fell and the electric wheelchair came down on top of me. I broke my elbow and scraped my knees.

Portable ramps in various lengths are available for sale. Some are individual tracks that you set a proper distance apart to accommodate wheel position. This design makes them lighter overall and easier to transport, but either track can shift independently out of position. Other types are full width, some of which fold up to reduce their bulk for transporting. Check what weight these ramps can handle. If you are a large person in a power chair equipped with a recline system and a ventilator, you might find yourself having an experience similar to this man with his new, portable metal ramp:

> We made it into the house all right, but on the way out the left ramp collapsed, nearly tipping me and my chair over, and almost ruining my wife's and my attendant's backs. When I phoned the dealer, the first thing they said was, "Were you in the wheelchair when the ramp collapsed?" I said, "Yes, I was." They replied, "I'm afraid your warranty is void then. If you look in the owner's manual you'll see that they are not recommended for use while the wheelchair is occupied." I looked and sure enough that's what it says.

Interior ramps

Ramping inside the house is more problematic, since not as much space is available. There is a tendency to keep the ramp from taking up too much precious floor space by making it shorter and steeper. But the steeper the ramp, the more likely you are to lose control going down, get stuck on your footrests at the bottom, or not have the strength to push yourself up it. If you are in peak condition, you might have no trouble, but as you age—or when you become ill or tired—such a ramp could become more of an obstacle and risk. In general, building next to a wall is advised because it allows you to put a handrail on at least one side of the ramp.

The Ramp Project

In 1991, the Minnesota Center of Independent Living (MCIL) developed the Ramp Project, which has helped people build quality, appropriate exterior ramps for very low cost. Their program is based on the use of volunteers who pitch in to help construct and move ramps. MCIL reports that many ramps have been reused in different locations thanks to their modular approach, which was reviewed and modified by a professional engineer.

The plans for these ramps—with specific structural details—are available from MCIL for a modest price. They offer a booklet that includes planning guidelines, and also discusses issues such as permit approval and how to order materials. MCIL has developed a modular ramp system that requires no footings. That means it is not necessary to dig down into the earth to set posts in stone or concrete below the frost line—the usual construction approach. Their design is stable and does not have problems with shifting.

MCIL conducts a rental program that allows people to pay off the cost of materials and then keep the ramp for as long as they need it. They have even managed to arrange for insurance to cover volunteers during construction.

Lifts

Lifts can be used as a way to get to an outside entry or up interior stairs. They have some disadvantages, but can be a solution when nothing else works.

Many homes have a front porch with perhaps four or five steps, a driveway next to the house, and small front yard. There just is not space for a ramp. A mechanical lift would be the solution. Ron Mace said:

> I recommend lifts when there isn't enough land or room to put up a ramp. Besides, ramps in icy locations are not much good half the year. In winter settings, even if there's space, it can make sense to do a lift anyway.

A lift can cost as much, if not more, than constructing a ramp. Being mechanical, it can break down. A lift is not attractive. Although landscaping can conceal the lift, and you can locate it in the least conspicuous place you can manage, lifts are bulky, and it is more difficult to integrate one into the appearance of your home. An exception is the Everhard lift, which is enclosed in a concrete pit underground.

It is important to take care of a lift: keep it lubricated, observe weight limits, and have the dealer make regularly scheduled maintenance checks. Lifts need more maintenance in winter environments.

For interior stairs, a vertical platform lift could be a solution for a short run of four or five steps, but not for a full flight of stairs. Installation of a full elevator is a much more elaborate and expensive undertaking, but is an option if you have the resources and space. Elevators do not have to look commercial or institutional. For instance, the elevator door could be designed so it looks like a normal, interior door.

Most stairway lifts consist of an individual seat. Depending on the stairway, a lift could also be a platform that could accommodate a wheelchair. But most full stairways are not wide enough to accommodate a platform lift. Platforms also have a harder time with curves and turning a corner at a landing.

The seat lift can be a good solution, but you need to have good balance and the ability to make transfers in order to be stable and safe using it. Most seat lifts include a footrest platform, and the seat flips up out of the way for people who walk the stairs. All come equipped with a seat belt. Seat lifts usually include an obstacle detection system that will stop the motor if it encounters resistance. These lifts can follow a curved path or turn corners at landings, although this option makes them more expensive. A second, inexpensive wheelchair could be kept upstairs, since you would spend less time using it and it would not have to hold up to rigorous daily use, but perhaps be used only for the bathroom and bedroom.

Doors

Doors are the most likely bottleneck to free movement through the home. A number of conditions could make a door an obstacle. A doorway should:

- Have sufficient maneuvering space at the approach
- Be wide enough for a wheelchair to pass easily
- Have hardware that can be easily gripped or turned
- Require little force to open
- Have a low threshold

A door without one of these qualities could rob you of independence, and threaten your safety if you need to use the door in an emergency.

When you are thinking of how to modify your home for maximum access, think of the functions of a door. Doors provide safety, privacy, acoustic control, climate control, and aesthetics. The function of safety should not be compromised. However, you can weigh other priorities. Any door that does not provide these functions might not be needed at all. If a door only gets closed when you sweep behind it, why not remove it altogether?

Door width

A door must be wide enough for you to fit through. Wider doorways also protect the door frame from damage and allow you to carry an occasional wide package on your lap. Bathroom doors are typically the most narrow in the house. Bedroom doors can be narrow or oriented to the hallway in such a way that you can't wheel straight through. While making the door frame wider is not always an option, there are other possibilities to give you more clearance, such as using a different kind of hinge that takes the door out of the way or using a pocket door.

Wider doors do not add to the cost of a new building. There are many benefits, according to Mace:

> When you use wider doors, there's nothing different about them. They're just doors. Buy a wider door and you're putting in less wall. The wall actually costs more than the door. It's a direct tradeoff that doesn't cost anything. It doesn't look any different from any other door. I've never heard anybody complain about the look of a wider door. It's a lot easier on

moving day. It increases circulation and air flow, and increases views into the room. Deaf people get better sight lines.

Door types

Many people report that sliding glass doors are the easiest to operate, but they sometimes have difficulty getting over the metal channels at floor level. Sliding doors are best installed in a recess in the floor to make the surface flush, assuming that water infiltration would not be a problem. Sloped thresholds—or "mini-ramps"—can also be installed to help wheels over the frame. Some sliding door designs use lower-profile channels.

A pocket door slides into and out of the cavity of the wall, so it takes up no space from the door frame. The door rides on easily gliding tracks that require little exertion to operate the door. When the door is open and fully tucked into the wall, there is usually a small hook on its edge, which you grab with your fingertip to pull the door in order to close it. This can be a dexterity problem for some people. A D-pull handle solves this, but then will limit the ability of the pocket door to fully recess into the wall. If enough clear space is not left to pass through the doorway, you can cut a notch in the wall to recess the D-pull so that the door can open all the way (see Figure 7-2).

Installing a pocket door in a wall is a significant construction task, and some people complain of difficulty with maintenance. If properly built, the door should glide easily and stay on the track. A less costly and simpler approach is to install a surface-mounted pocket door. Such a door can be attractively installed on the outside of the wall, with proper trim and hardware, and without the problem of having to cut a notch for a D-pull. The only drawback is the loss of some wall space (see Figure 7-3).

Closets typically use double-leaf or folding doors. These door types don't impose themselves as far into the room when they are opened. Two smaller doors can provide better access to a closet space. Folding doors are often inexpensive and not of high quality. They tend to jam, fall off their tracks, or require more dexterity to operate.

Door hardware

Door hardware has a large effect on independence. A door with difficult-to-use hardware is also more likely to be damaged as it becomes necessary to

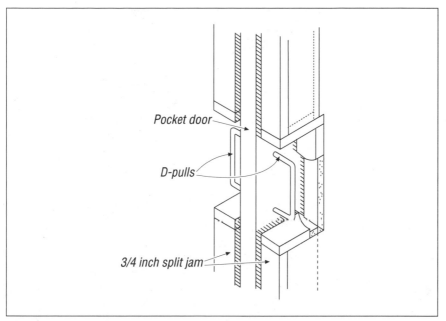

Figure 7-2. Detail of recessed D-pull on pocket door

push, kick, or use the wheelchair itself to get through it. Lever handles and D-pulls are the easiest to use. A hook latch or handle with a thumb latch require dexterity and strength.

Lever handles should be used on both sides of entry doors. Contractors or installers might think that a person with a disability will only open the door from the inside, but be assisted when coming from the outside, which of course, may not be true. A second door pull, placed closer to the hinges, can help you close a door you've passed through. The latch can be too far to reach once you are through, so the additional D-pull allows you to close the door without strain.

Lock hardware also can be inaccessible. Many people are unable to put a key in a lock, grasp it with their fingers, and twist it to turn the lock. Some people tend to install many locks for an increased sense of security, but locks can serve to imprison and endanger someone who has difficulty operating them.

Keyless locks are now commonly available; a keypad is used to enter a code with gentle pressure from a fingertip. Generally, you set the code, so you can change it occasionally for security reasons. You also can never lose your

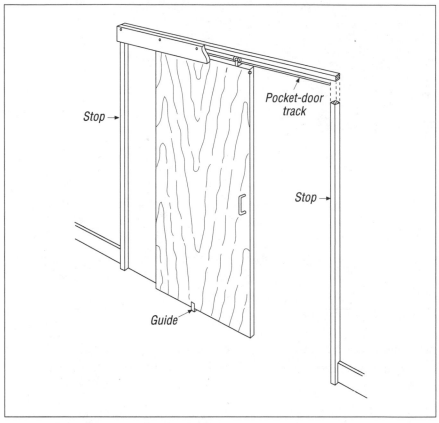

Figure 7-3. A surface-mounted pocket door

keys—though you can forget the code. Make sure the control is installed at a reachable height. Some of these products come as an integrated system that includes a doorbell, mailing slots, or intercom.

Often a small bathroom is rendered inaccessible simply because the door swings into the room. The door can't be closed because there is not room to wheel far enough into the room to clear the door. This can be solved by reversing the swing of the door. You can remove the door and put the hinges on the other side of the frame so that the door swings out instead.

The thickness of a standard-hung door occupies one or two inches of the space of the door frame when it is opened. There is a replacement hinge available which pivots so that the thickness of the door is effectively removed from the passageway when it is opened. These hinges are easily installed and inexpensive. Figure 7-4 shows how this type of hinge works.

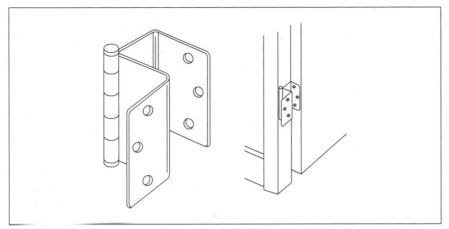

Figure 7-4. An offset door hinge

You may be able to remove a bathroom door altogether. If privacy is an issue after removing a door, hanging a curtain in the doorway can often solve the problem.

> *I removed a bathroom door in one place where I lived. It was never a problem because the bathroom was accessed through the bedroom, so I could simply close the bedroom door for privacy. In another apartment where I lived, I simply never closed the bathroom door because the room itself was too small for the door to close while I was inside. If I had guests I simply told them to stay in the living room, and I turned up the music!*

Another common obstacle is a screen or storm door at the front door of a house. Having two exterior doors can be solved with automatic door closers or by enclosing the doorway area with a porch. Then you can deal with each door separately.

How easy is it to open the exterior door? Most doors in a home do not have a closer, which applies some spring resistance to the door when you open it. Apartment buildings, however, will likely have closers on the door to the apartment, and certainly on the door at the street entrance. The spring tension needs to be adjusted so it is not difficult for you to open and then pass through comfortably. There might be conflict with building management who want to keep the spring tension tighter at the street for security reasons. But it is management's responsibility to properly maintain the door to close securely without requiring greater spring tension to slam it closed.

Floors

Flooring surface has a big effect on how easily and comfortably you are able to use a manual chair at home. Since many quadriplegic, elderly, or weak users switch to a manual chair while at home, floor surface has significant impact for many people.

Most floors in a home are carpeted. A thick pile carpet on a soft undermat is very difficult to wheel on and will fatigue you quickly. It is more difficult to wheel in a straight line on thick carpeting, which forces you to constantly make adjustments with each wheel as you go. You will not coast very far either. Since you tend to repeatedly travel the same paths in your home, a thicker surface will develop visible tracks.

> *Eventually, tracks start to show in the carpet because I usually follow regular paths at home. They sort of disappear when you vacuum, but eventually they get pretty set in. It's just part of the wheelchair experience, I guess. They used to have a thicker pile carpet in the hallway of my apartment building, and friends who didn't come over very often used the tracks to help find my door!*

Carpets with tight weaves provide better rollability. A pad underneath the carpet is not usually necessary, but if required comes in thinner profiles. Some people have installed industrial grade carpeting, designed for public environments like offices.

Many homes use large rugs over a wood floor. Rugs are unfriendly to wheelchairs and can get twisted up in the front casters. A rug can be secured with velcro. If you are placing it over carpeting, only the half with the hooks is needed, attached to the underside of the rug. Velcro strips in various widths with a sticky backing are available in rolls from office supply stores.

Hard floors are very easy to roll on. For wood floors, make sure no nails or screws are coming up from the surface that could threaten a tire. Look for wood splinters that could puncture a tire or get caught in the wheel—and then in your hand. Stone or ceramic tile can be very bouncy to wheel on. Deep spaces between tiles are usually the source of a bumpy ride, though the tiles themselves can be made with an uneven surface. The spaces between should not be too wide, and the grout which fills these spaces should be close to the top level of the tile for a smooth wheeling surface.

Floors need to be level. It doesn't take much slope for you to begin to roll downhill. Frankly, it is hard for builders to get all floors perfectly level, and a building inevitably settles a bit over time. If an existing house has noticeably sloping floors, however, check for problems with the foundation. If you are going to use a very heavy power chair, that is all the more reason to ensure the structural integrity of your building. If you are building something new, you should strongly emphasize this point with the building contractor.

Your wheels will carry some amount of grime on them, especially if you have deep treads or wheel on dirt or wet surfaces. You might want to use large floor mats at entrances, create a mud room for cleaning off your chair, or even have a different chair for use in the house. Keep a towel handy by the door to wipe your wheels clean. You can also keep a towel in the car in case you visit someone's home with dirty or wet wheels.

Windows

Quality of life is related to having natural light come into the home. Windows also help maintain contact with the outside world. You can look out to see what might have caused a sound or see who is asking for entry into your home. Using operable windows for ventilation is an efficient way to manage temperature, and is the best way to get fresh air throughout the home and circulate impurities out of the air.

What if you are adapting an existing home? Even if adding or changing windows is beyond your budget, you can orient furniture—particularly the bed—so that there are views to the outside. You can add landscaping to make the view more appealing or trim branches to let in more light.

There are different types of windows.

- Casement windows open toward the outside by turning a crank. The hinge is usually on one end of the window, but is sometimes found in the middle. Casements are easier to open than other types, and are more likely to open enough for an emergency escape. Handles can be found for the crank that are large and easier to grasp for ease of opening and closing.

- Vertical sliding sash windows are common in homes. Opening them usually requires two hands and considerable upper-body strength and balance. They are often too heavy for a person with a disability to lift. The latch is usually at the top of the lower sash, often out of reach in the sitting position, but there are products which locate the latch at the sill.

- Horizontal sliding sash windows cannot unexpectedly close due to gravity and are easy to open. They usually are designed with a lip which runs the entire vertical edge of the moving window, offering variety in where to push or pull. They come with different kinds of latches, some of which are spring-loaded, placed high, and require pinch force—a difficult-to-use design. A simple latch placed at the bottom which is easily lifted and stays in place is best and commonly found. Only one half of the total window width can be open; this might not leave sufficient room for escape in an emergency.

As with doors, remote window openers are available for many of these types of windows, depending on the brand and design. Cranks for either sash window type particularly lend themselves to being motorized.

Walls

Do not place rough textures on areas of wall that you are likely to touch, such as plastered surfaces that are laid on with a decorative texture or some wallpapers such as grasscloth. These surfaces are often rough enough to injure your hand if you slide it across the surface or need the wall for sudden support.

When turning a corner in a manual wheelchair, it is much easier to make the turn by placing your hand on a wall, rather than grasping one wheel while you push the other. The same is sometimes true for going through doors: placing a hand on the wall as you pull the door open can make it easier. Unfortunately, that means that each time you will leave a little bit of oil and dirt from your skin on the wall. This eventually starts to show as a dark area. Choose wall coverings that are easily cleaned and that don't show dirt as well.

When a circulation path passes close to a wall, it is more likely to be bumped or scraped by a wheelchair, no matter how skilled the rider. Wainscotting with wood or with vinyl or plastic covers protects the underlying wall surface and can be attractive.

Furniture

Just because you are a wheelchair user doesn't mean that you will always stay in the chair. Many chair riders are able to easily transfer to furniture—and want to. It can be a real relief to get out of the chair.

Be conscious of the surface you choose to sit on. Just because it is soft doesn't mean that it will provide appropriate support for the prevention of pressure sores. The foam in some upholstery is soft enough to compress almost all the way, resulting in focused pressure on your skin. You might supplement a chair or couch in the home with a foam pad, a piece of lamb's wool, or the cushion from your wheelchair.

Knee clearance at tables will be a key issue. A central support for the table is more likely to be in the way of your feet when you sit on the side of the table. Many dining room tables include a skirt around the edge that might be low enough to keep your knees from going under the table. Tables sometimes come with extra leaves to extend the end of the table. The extra leaves hang out over the edge, and often allow that extra inch or two of clearance for your knees or feet. This explains why chair users so often find themselves sitting at the head of the table as a dinner guest.

> I had my table put up on blocks so I could roll under it. Same thing with the table for my computer. I hired someone to make the changes for me, and it was a very simple solution.

Stacking tables and folding chairs, such as director's chairs, can be kept aside for clearance and then used for company. Coffee tables which go in front of a couch are an obstruction, both to travel within the room and to your ability to transfer to the couch.

> I have friends with two couches and a large table in between. If there are other guests while I'm there, I simply cannot get into the rest of the house. No room left to pass.

Lighting

When you are considering lighting, think about being able to reach and operate switches and being able to change bulbs. Typically, room light switches are located just inside the door. The placement of a switch might be too high or require a degree of dexterity beyond your ability. When you are unable to reach a switch, a noise-actuated switch can be installed that responds to a clap or a loud vocal sound. Unfortunately, these switches sometimes respond to sounds when you don't want them to, turning a light on as you sleep or leaving you in the dark prematurely. A more costly approach is to literally move the light switch down, cutting a new hole, and filling the old one.

Of the many types of light switches, rockers and push buttons take the least dexterity, involving no gripping or pinching. Thumb wheels, rotary knobs, and slide bars are generally more difficult. Figure 7-5 shows various types of controls and the difficulty of operating them.

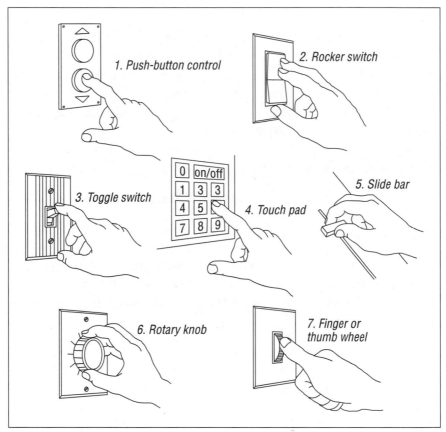

Figure 7-5. Electronic controls, from easiest (1) to most difficult (7).

A remote control unit is a reliable solution for people with limited hand dexterity. These systems usually involve no electrical rewiring; there is a small unit that you plug into the power line, and then program the remote control to recognize it.

The design of a fixture might prevent you from changing a light bulb. Many lights require that you pinch a small set screw to remove a hood or globe in order to access the bulb. A lampshade might have been replaced too tightly by a friend or family member to be removed. Some attention to detail can make a big difference in independence. Multiple light sources, fixtures with two bulbs, and a backup desk lamp help ensure you won't get left in the dark. Ceiling fixtures can be found on retractable cables to bring it down for a bulb change; grabber arms can be handy.

Outdoor lighting is important so you can see the path and avoid any surprise obstructions. Motion detectors can turn a light on when it picks up the arrival of your vehicle or your approach from the sidewalk. Motion detectors then can turn the light off after a set period of time which presumably leaves you enough time to get inside the house. Timers can be installed and programmed to turn the exterior lights on at a given time each day.

Electrical wiring

The first question to ask is whether you have enough power. If you are charging a power wheelchair, have a bed with motorized adjustments, use a ventilator or oxygen, have a remote control system for lights and so on, these will place considerable demands on your power supply. The last thing you want to risk is overloading a circuit and shutting off a ventilator. Using plug taps, power strips, and extension cords so that you can plug more items into existing outlets than would otherwise be possible can quickly overload a circuit and present a real fire hazard.

It might be necessary to add more power to your home or reroute existing power to where it is needed. Some outlets—such as in the basement or garage—might be underused, and more valuable when routed to the bedroom, for instance. Running new wires through walls—if necessary—can be very costly and disruptive, but is the first choice for aesthetics. An easier and less expensive approach is to use cable raceways which are surface mounted. They can be placed unobtrusively or covered by moldings.

In the bathroom, incorporate ground-fault circuit interrupters into outlets in the wall. An interrupter is not a major piece of equipment, but will shut off power at the plug rather than at the main circuit if water gets in.

If you need it and can afford it, a battery backup system can be installed which will provide you with a number of hours of emergency power if the system goes out. A generator that runs on a small gasoline engine is another backup option. Call your local authority—city, township, etc.—and let them know if someone in your home is at risk if power is lost. In the event of a blackout, the local emergency plan should put a priority on protecting people whose lives might be threatened without electricity.

Some local utility companies offer special rates for people with disabilities, or have programs that allow you to spread out payments during winter months when the bill might be substantially higher. You should also ask if they have a registry or special number to call in the case of an emergency, in the event you need a high priority for having your power restored.

After you've checked that you have enough power and can protect yourself in the event of outages, you'll also want to look at other matters of safety and convenience.

Power receptacles low on the wall are often obscured behind furniture and can be difficult to reach. You can effectively raise power outlets with a power strip—several receptacles on a strip at the end of a two-foot cord. It gives you flexibility for where to position the power, and often includes electrical protection from power spikes which can injure sensitive electronic equipment. There is usually a master switch which allows you to turn off several items with one push of a button. Accessible Work Systems makes a product called the Upright Outlet which effectively elevates a power receptacle by twenty inches. When these items are used, people are less likely to pull plugs from the wall by grabbing the cord, which damages the wiring and increases fire hazard.

Heating, ventilation, and cooling

Temperature control is very important for people with certain disabilities. With multiple sclerosis, excessive heat can encourage exacerbations. People with arthritis are sensitive to temperature variations, as are older persons who generally need more heat. Some people with spinal cord injuries are unable to sweat, so need to keep cool. People on fixed incomes have difficulty spending more money on heating, ventilation, and air conditioning. Some people address the need for more heat with space heaters, which are often inefficient, expensive to run, and more likely to cause a home fire.

The placement of thermostats is important in controlling temperatures. Put the thermostat within reach for everyone and make sure it is not in direct sunlight. Zoned heating and air conditioning can be an important feature for a bedroom where a temperature-sensitive person sleeps or spends more time during the day. Some thermostat designs are more difficult to use; avoid designs that require pinch and hand strength or on which the numbers are too small to easily see.

Think through emergency procedures for utilities and make sure that shut-off valves are accessible to every family member. For example, you can install a gas shutoff valve that can be turned easily by a long lever-type of handle, without great strength or tools.

Before spending money on expensive heating and cooling equipment, take measures to control air movement and sunlight with passive energy methods:

- Be sure windows and doors are well insulated.
- Weather-strip around door and window frames.
- Make sure that doors to the outside have a good seal at the threshold.
- Spray an insulating foam into walls.
- Manage the sunlight: when you need heat, open shades and let the sun shine in; close shades when you're warm enough.
- Awnings or eves of the correct depth will block the sun in summer and let it in, in winter.

Fireplaces can remove heat. The heat of the fire travels up the chimney flue, and creates a vacuum effect that actually draws warm air out of the house and out the top. Be sure not to leave the flue vent open when you need to keep heat in the house.

Telephones

The ability to communicate over distances is key for people with limited mobility. The phone can be the link to your social world, maintaining relationships through calls with friends and family. A phone line for an Internet connection can be a link to a wider community, as in the case of this man with Friedrich's ataxia:

> The Internet has enhanced my life a great deal. I'm an amateur writer, and the World Wide Web has been a great research tool for my writing projects. I have been able to converse with some great people

about many different things. By using a computer I am more independent than I would be otherwise. The computer has been the impetus for some of the best things I feel I've ever done. I use a wheelchair, my hand/eye coordination and balance are very poor, but the computer allows me to function as a productive member of society.

It is helpful to have an additional telephone line for an Internet connection. When the computer is hooked up to the Internet, no one else can call in or out. If you have a business and a fax machine, you might find it necessary to have several phone lines.

Telephone jacks are best placed near electrical outlets, since computers, fax, and answering machines also need power. General advice is to have at least one phone jack in each room where you are likely to spend more than a few minutes at a time.

A telephone line is also a lifeline. A speaker phone with a speed-dial button might only require pressing one or two buttons, without having to pick up the handset, in order to make an emergency call. There are services that allow you to carry an alarm button which will make an automatic phone call to a healthcare facility or security agency. Some medical equipment can have similar features, in which a phone call is made if the machine experiences a shutdown that could be life-threatening. Dedicated phone lines might be needed in these cases.

Many telephone companies have disability programs to provide special equipment. For example, Pacific Bell gives people speaker phones or head-sets free of charge once you and your physician fill out the application.

Telephones are available with large, lighted buttons which are easy to press. Quadriplegics with little arm movement can freely access the telephone via puff-and-sip control systems that allow them to choose from a prepro-grammed list of numbers or dial a new one. Hands-free telephone access is possible.

Remote—or cordless—telephones are very helpful. It can take some time to get to a fixed telephone set—for instance, if you are not in your wheelchair when the phone rings—and you might miss calls. (You can let people who call you regularly know that you might need more time to answer.) A remote phone goes where you go, which is especially helpful in the bathroom. These products have improved a great deal in recent years. The sound quality is good, multiple channels are available in case you get static, and 2.4 GHz phones can have a range of 1,000 feet or more.

> Now that I have a remote phone, I never miss calls. I can take it in the bathroom or outside. I never hear someone hanging up just as I pick up the phone because it took me a little longer to get there—especially if I'm doing the dishes, because I have to dry my hands before I can touch the wheels, whereas someone who walks can dry their hands as they walk to the phone.

Intercoms

Intercom systems allow easy communication or monitoring and are especially useful for people who have very restricted mobility or who must spend a share of each day in bed or on a breathing apparatus. Intercom systems can be helpful for monitoring guests at the front door. Commercial systems are now available for the home with video capability, so you can see who is there and be able to speak with them as well.

There are two types of intercom systems. One uses its own wiring, usually threaded through the wall cavities—an approach which provides the clearest sound. Wiring is best done during new construction, but is possible to install in an existing home; surface conduits can be used.

The other type of intercom system uses carrier current. The intercom is integrated into electrical wiring, which carries the signal alongside the electricity. Components plug into outlets in order to transmit the signals. Some static is picked up from the shared wiring. These systems are generally less expensive than intercoms with their own wiring.

Home control systems

There are now elaborate home control systems that allow you to:

- Control the volume of televisions or sound systems
- Adjust lights
- Lock and unlock or open and close doors and windows
- Control heating and ventilation
- Turn on appliances of all kinds
- Use telephone systems

Some systems are designed for ease of use, with disabilities in mind. When you shop for a system, learn the details of how it operates. Operation should be clear, intuitive, and not demand much memorizing of commands. Controls should be easy to operate without fine dexterity or the need to apply much force. The controls for a home control system can be integrated into a power wheelchair. For instance, a head switch could be used to open or close a door. Voice-activation or puff-and-sip controls can be positioned at a bedside for a quadriplegic user.

The functioning of a home control system also relies on the installation of appropriate mechanisms such as automatic door closers. Each home control system may provide some of its own mechanisms for doors and windows. Appliances you already own might not be compatible with some control products.

As with intercoms, there are hard-wired versions and carrier current types of home control systems. The X-10 standard is an example of a carrier current type of system. Modules are purchased which plug into power outlets and then the appliances to be controlled. Such a system can be expanded over time, as your budget allows.

> *Everything is working fine with the X-10 protocol; I've never had a problem. It controls lights, electric devices, temperature (heating/air conditioning), built-in alarm system and medic-alert, with scenarios that you can program. For instance, when I enter the bathroom, the lights fade in by themselves and fade out after a predetermined number of minutes. You can control everything either by phone, with a remote, or by a touch-screen panel.*

Ron Mace liked the product because it met his criteria for Universal Design:

> *The X-10 product came out as a consumer product—not a disability access/adaptive technology product.*

Alarm and warning systems

A loss of mobility implies increased risk in the event of an emergency. Early warning is critical for a person with a disability.

Warning alarms include smoke, fire, and gas detectors. The alarm design should consider a variety of sensory needs. A buzzer or siren for warning might not be sufficient. Products are available with strobe lights which can waken sighted people from a deep sleep and thus also serve people with hearing disabilities.

Check alarm batteries often. Smoke and heat sensors need to be placed high up on a wall or on the ceiling, since heat rises. Provide some means for a person with a disability to turn off the alarm, even if that is with a broom handle kept nearby. Some homes and apartment complexes have systems which notify a security office or the police or fire station in the event of fire or emergency. Be sure that everyone in the household knows the codes for setting and defeating these systems.

It is a good idea to inform building management or neighbors that someone is in the household who might need assistance in an emergency. Local police and fire departments might also keep such lists. Find out what kind of emergency assistance programs exist in your community. Put a wheelchair symbol in your bedroom window to identify yourself, and develop an escape plan with your family, neighbors, or attendant.

The bathroom

The bathroom is often the space that is the greatest challenge to make accessible. In a 1993 U.S. Census Bureau report, 4.5 million people with disabilities reported having difficulty bathing, and 2.1 million had trouble using the toilet. Millions of people are inconvenienced—even endangered— by inaccessible bathrooms. Any impediment to easy access to the bathroom can lead someone to delay their bowel or bladder program. A bathroom that is easy to use protects your health (see Figure 7-6).

An existing home might have several bathrooms. They don't all have to be accessible. Ideally, there should be an accessible bathroom on each accessible floor of the home.

Creating a larger bathroom for access does not have to rob the rest of the home of space. Ron Mace explained:

> All we need to do in bathrooms is increase the size by about a foot to get enough maneuvering space for a wheelchair. If you plan it carefully, you're only adding about five square feet, and you can get that by just taking a few inches out of adjacent rooms. You hardly notice the difference, except that the bathroom is a bit more luxurious.

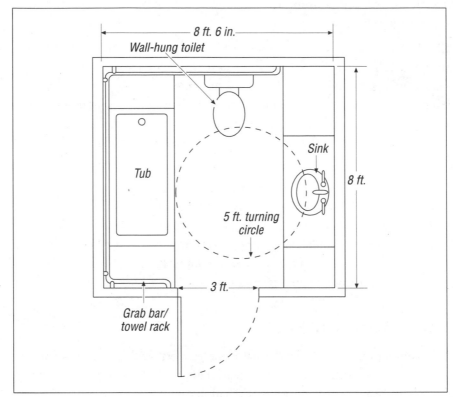

Figure 7-6. A small, wheelchair-accessible bathroom

Builders of new apartments benefit from providing access.

> *People who move into an apartment with a large bathroom don't even know it's for access. They just love it. It turns out to be a marketing plus.*

Safety

The bathroom is a site of many household accidents. The U.S. Consumer Product Safety Commission reports that more than 110,000 accidents occur in bathtubs and showers each year. Some chair users make several transfers each day from their chair to a toilet or bath. More than for any room in the house, you need to think of safety as much as simple access to the space.

For a chair user who is able to stand to use the shower or bath, a slippery surface can be extremely treacherous. Various floor materials respond differently to being wet. Some new ceramic tiles or rubber-based linoleum surfaces have better slip resistance. Keep the bathroom floor clear of small objects on which you could slip, and use cleaning products that do not leave a slippery film.

Toilets

Toilets are often installed too low for people with disabilities. This can be solved with a riser to elevate the seat, available in various heights. Some riser products lift out of the way to allow others to use the lower seat. A company called Med/West makes a power elevating toilet seat which you can set to a preferred height. You could also replace the toilet with a wall-mounted unit. A wall-mounted unit not only lets you put it at exactly the height you need, but also frees up floor space underneath which increases the turning radius available to you by allowing additional clearance for your footrests.

Chair users have their own needs and preferences for how they position themselves relative to the toilet. Some people don't get onto the toilet or only get on occasionally. Those who use catheters empty their bladder into a plastic container which is then dumped into the toilet. Others wear a leg drainage bag and need to be able to get the drainage tube into the toilet to empty the bag.

The side of the toilet or bidet needs to be placed at the right distance from the wall. If the side of the toilet is too close, you risk bumping the wall during transfers. If it is too far away, you could fall between the wall and the toilet while reaching for the tissue dispenser or a grab bar.

Toilet paper holders or items which might extend from the surface of the wall need to be placed for easy reach from the toilet. They should not be too far away or behind the plane of the shoulder, making it necessary to reach behind oneself. Many people lean forward and drop their head as they transfer from the toilet to the wheelchair; make sure nothing is in the way of your head.

There needs to be sufficient clear space in front of and next to the toilet or bidet to get your chair in the optimal position for transfer. In public, far too many so-called accessible bathroom stalls are wide enough to enter, but leave you sitting directly facing the bowl. If you are facing the bowl, you need to do a full 180-degree transfer—a treacherous feat at best. For safe transfers, it is generally necessary to be able to achieve a 90-degree angle to the toilet. Some people being assisted are best transferred from a position next to and parallel to the bowl.

Tubs and showers

Getting into a bathtub is difficult for many people with disabilities. They cannot step or lift themselves over the edge of a tub or, once in, cannot lift themselves back out. Yet they yearn for the luxury of a good long soak, after having to typically settle for showers or, worse, sponge baths in bed.

One design which lets you down into the tub is a sort of balloon which is "inflated" with water. The balloon lowers you down into the bath when you release the water from inside it. You refill it from the tub tap to raise yourself back up. Some people also use sling lifts in the bathroom to make transfers onto a shower chair or down into the tub. A portable lift can do double duty in the bedroom and bathroom.

Sitting on the floor of a tub is a problem for people with posterior muscle atrophy. There are a few tubs designed with a foam base under a heavy, vinyl-like covering. Some people have found success with the proper density of foam which provides support but does not float. An air floatation cushion could be used if it can be partially filled with water to keep it from being buoyant, which would make you unstable in the tub.

A tub becomes usable as a shower with a shower chair or tub seat. Some designs allow you to get into the chair outside of the tub, and then pivot or slide into place. A hand-held shower head gives you or your personal assistant the ability to hold the shower head to rinse easily.

Anti-scald controls are now commonly available. They control water pressure, which can affect water temperature when it fluctuates.

Shower and tub controls are typically placed in the center of the wall over the spigot, which can be difficult to reach from a chair when you are outside the tub. Controls would ideally be located closer to the outside wall and lower down for easy access. Many people who prefer to sit in the tub would benefit from having controls on the side wall where they can be reached from inside the tub. In either case, a single, lever control is easiest, compared to knobs or handles that require a strong grip. Make certain that the contractor understands the reason for the location of controls, because they—and building inspectors—are accustomed to seeing controls in the center and could unwittingly override this valuable access detail.

A range of bath and shower units are being developed for the convenience and comfort of those with disabilities. For example, the Freedom Bath is a bathtub with a side wall that raises and lowers, and includes a seat formed inside the tub (see Figure 7-7). You can transfer onto the seat at normal height, raise the wall, and fill it with water for your bath. After emptying the bath water when you are done, bring the wall back down for an easy transfer out. There is no need to deal with the dramatic change in level to get to the bottom of a bathtub, but you can still be immersed for a good soak. It is the size of a normal bathtub.

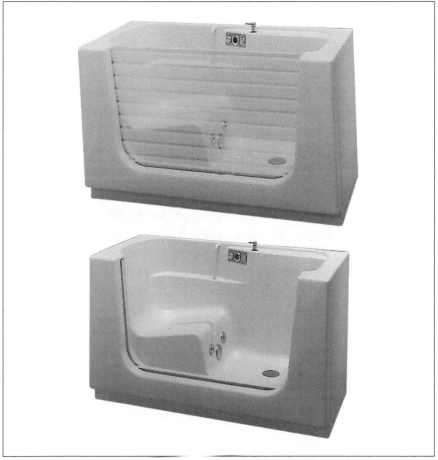

Figure 7-7. A side-entrance bathtub

Some stall showers have a molded seat built in; others use a fold-down platform which lifts out of the way for use by people who stand. You might need to add a cushion to such a platform, in which case you need to be careful it would not slip and that you are very stable. Prefabricated shower units are designed to roll into, accommodating rolling shower chairs designed for the purpose. Prefab units have only a small lip at the edge, rather than the three-inch or larger lip that are common to most stall showers. These units can be used in new construction or replace an existing bathtub.

A more advanced solution is to build a wet room—a space, sometimes just the open corner of a large bathroom, that is tiled with a drain on the floor. Faucets, shower heads, and handholds are installed on the walls, also tiled. You wheel into the area in a rolling shower chair to wash.

Grab bars in the bathroom

Grab bars are essential, particularly around the shower, toilet, and bidet. A grab bar needs to be attached to a solid structure in the wall, typically horizontal reinforcement between vertical studs that can be drilled into. Builders are now encouraged to provide support structure in bathroom walls for the eventual addition of grab bars, but it is not yet a standard construction measure. When sufficient structure is not already present, it is sometimes necessary to break into the wall to add the structural backing.

> *I moved into a newly built apartment complex that used the handi-capped-adaptable approach. In my smaller, second bathroom they couldn't put a grab bar in the bathtub because they hadn't reinforced the wall. There was nothing to attach it to, so they just put the grab bar verti-cally at the front of the tub. It's totally useless and just a waste of money.*

Sometimes a brace can be added across studs on the surface of the wall which can then carry a grab bar. But a brace near the bath or shower becomes a trap for water which will eventually cause damage. Another approach is to sheathe the wall with 3/4 inch plywood, which creates a strong structural base for grab bars. The plywood sheathing is more costly than adding one or more studs, but allows installation of support at any location you choose. Grab bars need to be able to carry as much as 300 pounds. A towel rack is not a grab bar. It is not able to carry your body weight.

A mobile home might have some walls which are only made of particle board, fiberglass, or sheet metal. These materials are incapable of supporting a grab bar, but it might be possible to add reinforcement behind these surfaces. There are grab bars available that clip on to the side of a bathtub or toilet, and don't require structural support from a wall. Be very certain they are firmly installed, check the attachments regularly to keep them tight, and then test carefully in advance by applying force in several directions before relying on them for support.

While there are standards which advise specific grab bar heights, optimal height and position for grab bars depend on your exact capabilities and size. A grab bar that is standard height might be too high for some people because of their height or because the muscles they would need to use are weak or unavailable.

Some people benefit from supports immediately next to the toilet, functioning as armrests. For others, these can be obstructions during transfer from a wheelchair. Some products are hinged from the wall, so can be raised out of the way during a transfer, and brought down for safety and stability while using the toilet.

In *Building for a Lifetime*, the authors suggest thinking in terms of handholds—places in the room where people might require support as they bend or lean in the course of their business. Handholds can include a shelf, countertop, or a ledge around the bathtub. This kind of thinking might mean you reinforce the support of the sink, for instance. The authors recommend using "a generous supply of handholds."[2]

The selection of access products for the bathroom has expanded. Major bathroom appliance manufacturers have been applying their skill to the design and appearance of accessible fixtures. Grab bars, for instance, are available in options beyond the once-standard stainless steel. They can now be found in a variety of colors and designs. An accessible bathroom is an enhancement to your home, and you should have no reservations about proceeding with such changes.

The bathroom sink

Many bathroom sinks are set in a cabinet top. The cabinet can be removed from under the sink to allow room to get close to the sink, after making certain that the cabinet is not supporting the weight of the sink. Remember to cover the water pipes under the sink with insulation to ensure that you don't burn your legs.

The best sink faucets are single lever types. Anti-scald devices are useful here. Use a spout that extends far enough out so it is easy to get your hands fully underneath the water, unobstructed by the back of the sink.

Choose a faucet with an easy-to-use control for closing the drain. The old style rubber plug with a chain is easy to use.

Regulating air temperature

There are unique temperature management issues in the bathroom. Warm water in the bath or shower generates heat and humidity. On the other hand, you tend to feel chilled when you open the shower curtain and let in the cooler air from the rest of the room or house. For people with temperature sensitivity, heat and cold can be managed with:

- A dedicated air conditioner
- An infrared heat lamp
- A wall-mounted heater
- An exhaust fan
- An operable window

Because of the amount of water in a bathroom, a space heater placed on the floor is dangerous and not recommended. In bathrooms, windows tend to be installed higher for privacy, but may be important for ventilation and temperature management. Some window controls can be extended with a chain or a pulley system to allow them to be operated from a lower position.

The kitchen

The kitchen is much more than a place to make food. It is a central gathering place and social center for the home. Access to the kitchen is crucial for participation as a full member of the household.

When looking at kitchen design, think in terms of the two-cook kitchen. Leave wider aisles, and create work spaces that allow knee clearance so the wheelchair will not obstruct circulation in the space. Then the chair user can join in, rather than become an obstacle that prevents others from working with him in the kitchen.

To be able to cook from your wheels, you need a surface low enough for cutting vegetables and other food preparation tasks. Normal height counters can still be reached easily to hold items not in use, but are usually too high for a seated person to comfortably use for cooking preparation. At the least, you can set a cutting board on your lap, possibly with a piece of thin foam underneath to level and support it.

Ideally, provide a lowered work surface. The surface should be within reach of the sink and stove so that you won't have to be moving back and forth as you work. The surface should have knee clearance and unobstructed leg room. A cabinet could be removed and a height-adjustable surface installed, controlled either by a manual hand crank or a motor. Lower surfaces also let children get more involved in the cooking process, and elderly or temporarily injured family members can sit on a stool to work in the kitchen. Space underneath this counter might also accommodate a serving cart or recycling bins.

Lowered surfaces can also be created with pull-out counters installed into the kitchen cabinets. They are hidden when not in use and greatly expand counter area for all users. They are especially valuable near the stove where foods can be cut and placed directly into pots. A pegboard with hooks or a countertop container allows you to keep commonly used utensils like a spatula or spoons within reach at all times.

You should not have to struggle to operate anything in the kitchen, or risk having something heavy, hot, or sharp fall in your lap because a sticky drawer forces awkward movement.

Kitchen sink

Ideally, it should be possible to sit straight at the sink, saving you from the need to twist continually while washing vegetables or dishes. A shallow sink can help provide both better leg room and spare you from having to reach down into a deeper sink. If you are installing a garbage disposal, it is best placed to the side and rear to preserve leg room. A garbage disposal can help keep trips to the trash can to a minimum. Pipes and plumbing underneath the sink must always be insulated to protect your legs from burns.

Height-adjustable sinks are possible thanks to flexible drain pipes which allow the sink to move. Flexible pipes can be used underneath the drain while maintaining a trap—the U-shaped form that keeps water in the hose and prevents gases from rising back up through the drain into the house.

Use a single lever handle on the sink. Use a spout that is high enough so that there is room underneath to place pots. The spout should also extend far enough forward for minimal reach and be able to rotate. People with the ability to grip can benefit further from a hand-held spout.

Appliances

In general, choose appliances that are easy to operate, with clearly readable controls that function intuitively. All appliance controls should be in the front, especially on the stove, so that you will never have to reach over a hot heating element.

With an electric stove, choose a stovetop that includes a warning light when a burner surface is turned on, to prevent accidental burns. A stove with raised heating elements presents a greater risk of a hot pot falling off the edge since it has to be lifted to be moved. Ceramic stovetops allow pots to be more easily slid safely to a counter surface at the side. A disadvantage of the smooth ceramic stovetop is that there is less capacity to catch spilled liquids, increasing the risk of burns for someone who is seated near it.

Stovetop burners should be staggered so it is not necessary to reach across one burner to access another. It should be evident which control affects which burner. An angled mirror above the cook-top is very helpful to see inside pots from a sitting position.

Oven doors generally open downward, forcing you to either lean over the door or position yourself to the side, assuming there is space next to the appliance. Either way, you are not in the best position for balance, especially to handle heavy, hot items. A wall-mounted oven with a side-hinged door allows you to be closer, but also increases the risk of a spill, unless there is counter space immediately adjacent where you can set a hot dish without having to drive the chair. A pull-out surface immediately underneath the oven is the ideal.

Microwave ovens are often installed up high, over a traditional stove. This location can be too high for some people, who need the microwave placed on a counter top or installed into cabinetry at a lower level. Microwaves come with various types of door latches, some of which require pressing a button while pulling. These are difficult for people with reduced gripping ability.

Dishwasher designs suffer from the same issue as an oven with a door that pulls down, although there is not any risk of burns. A dishwasher needs to have sufficient clearance at the side so that dishes can be put in directly after being rinsed in the sink.

In refrigerators, put the heaviest items at chest height where they are easiest to access. Side-by-side refrigerator/freezers put more freezer space within easy reach.

Kitchen cabinets

In the traditional kitchen, a great portion of cabinet space can be inaccessible. Cabinets are too high, too low, or too deep to be fully accessible by someone sitting or older household members who also have difficulty reaching or stooping. Cabinets can be made more useful by any of several measures that improve visibility, accessibility of contents, or height.

- Use shallow cabinets which keep more items within reach and within view.
- Use windowed doors to save the need to search for items by opening many cabinets.
- Remove cabinet doors altogether, particularly on lower cabinets where you have to move away from the door as you open it.
- Put the most-often used items on shelves that are easiest to reach.
- Use a grabber arm to get items on shelves that are out of reach (see Figure 7-8).
- Adjust cabinet shelves to a more convenient configuration.
- Store more items on the counter. A small stack of shelves can make good use of a countertop, or small cabinets with doors can be built in.
- Place a lazy Susan in a cabinet or on a countertop.
- Move overhead cabinets lower to bring them into easier reach.
- Install automated units that can be lowered to counter level.

Drawers bring objects within reach and view and into the light. The back half is as useful as the front, unlike a cabinet. Use roller tracks that glide easily, and do not overload the drawer with heavy items that will make it harder to slide in and out. Provide handles that don't demand fine dexterity or

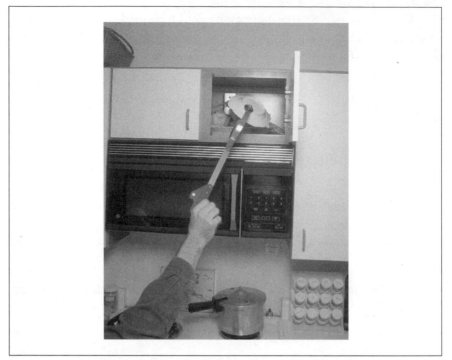

Figure 7-8. Using a grabber arm for a high cabinet

strong grip. Cloth loops added to handles can help people with no grip open drawers. Be sure there is room for the wheelchair next to the drawer.

It is not necessary to reach every shelf in every cabinet in your kitchen. Louis Tenenbaum observes:

> *My experience in the kitchen is that we use a whole lot fewer things than we have. What it's really about is spending the time to figure out what things you need to have close by. In many cases, the things you don't have close by, you use rarely. For stuff that you only use when you have company, wait until your guests arrive, and ask them to get it down.*

Kitchen electrical issues

Switches and power outlets are typically placed on walls at the back of counters. These are especially difficult to reach in corners of L-shaped or U-shaped layouts. Outlets can be relocated to the front of floor cabinets or just under the surface if there is an open space for leg room. A switch/outlet box can be placed underneath a surface where leg room has been provided, taking care to put it to the side so it does not obstruct or potentially injure your legs. There is some risk at this location of a cord getting caught by an arm or your chair, or grabbed by a curious child and of an appliance being pulled off the counter. Many kitchens have false panels, particularly underneath the sink, where a hole could be cut and wiring extended to install an outlet.

Another option is to place power underneath overhead cabinets—which also keeps them beyond the reach of children. A cable raceway can run underneath the front edge of upper cabinets, providing a series of outlets along its length.

Most kitchens benefit from lighting placed underneath upper cabinets. These lights make counter tasks easier to see, and also bring light switches within reach. Choose fixtures that will not create glare or shine directly in your eyes from the seated angle. Natural light is appealing in a kitchen, so provide shade controls that can be reached from the seated position.

Kitchen layouts

The most efficient layout for a kitchen is a U-shape, which puts more surface within reach without a user having to move. A drawback is that deeper spaces in the corners are more difficult to reach. The U-shape layout also makes it easier to provide room for you to fully turn around in your chair.

A kitchen with two longer parallel surfaces has its advantages, too. If properly arranged, you can be within reach of surfaces and facilities on either side of you and have a pull-out surface installed at a good height for cutting and food handling. The shape of the space is not the only issue in how well the kitchen will work. It is just as critical to establish good relationships between all features of the kitchen and make best use of accessories.

Figure 7-9 shows another good option for a kitchen layout.

If you need to make do in a kitchen with major appliances that are difficult to use, don't discount the value of your local appliance store. Toaster ovens, crock pots, waffle irons, griddles, rice cookers, and hot plates are lightweight, easily positioned, inexpensive, and energy efficient. You could do the majority of your cooking with these small appliances, if you needed to, until you could afford the more involved modifications to your kitchen.

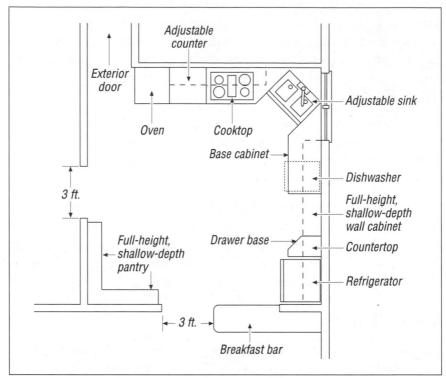

Figure 7-9. An L-shaped kitchen

Bedrooms

The ideal bedroom is spacious enough to allow full turning radius, particularly next to the bed, where people often are forced to back out of a space close to a wall. Backing up is easy for many wheelers, but awkward for others, in which case the wall or bedclothes can suffer from contact with the chair. Narrow spaces next to the bed can also make it very difficult to get to a telephone, typically kept on the bedside table.

The bedroom is a place where electrical power might be needed for adjustable beds, home control systems, medical equipment such as ventilators or oxygen machines, television, stereo, or computer systems. The trick in planning is to be able to reach all of these things. Once in bed, for instance, how do you turn off the lights? A bedside lamp with a chain switch (which might need to have a loop added to it for those who can't grip) could be the answer, though it should have a heavy base so it won't easily tip over. A more advanced solution is to put switches in the wall directly next to the bed.

Beside the bed, you might need room to have a lamp, a book to read before you go to sleep, medications, or remote control units, especially if you use an environmental control system. It could be difficult to twist far enough around to reach a bedside table which is placed back against the same wall as the headboard. A bedside stand with wheels can be rolled forward after you are in bed.

Bedroom dressers and tables often have drawers which do not slide easily or use handles which require strength and agility in the fingertips. Better designs use ball-bearing tracks so the drawer slides with little force, and handles large enough to grip with all of your fingers. Even then, adding loops can help make drawers more accessible, such as for this woman with rheumatoid arthritis who also has a vision impairment:

> *For the bedroom, we added brightly colored belts to drawer handles, so that I can loop my arm in them, to see inside. To make it more of a family thing, we put them on everyone's drawers, as this way I am not singled out and it actually made it easier for other family members to get into the drawers, too. Also, some of my blankets have loops at the top, that I can loop my arm through to pull them up or down.*

The ultimate bedroom is a master suite with an accessible bathroom and roll-in closet. These spaces could use pocket doors which are easy to open and close, and don't invade any space by swinging out.

A close relationship between bedroom and bathroom is highly desirable. Getting dressed is more effort for most chair users. A private route to and from the bathroom spares you the need to dress until you are fully prepared for the day. If you receive assistance, you are best served when the helper has easy access to the bathroom. A lift can be installed on a ceiling rail which travels from the bed directly into the bathroom. This allows you to go from your bed directly into the tub or shower.

The more time you spend in the bedroom, the more important it is to have an escape route. There might be a door to a deck or patio, but at least there should be a window large enough to get out.

It might not be possible to have access to an upstairs bedroom. Depending on your resources, you could consider installing a stair lift, converting a space downstairs, or adding a new bedroom. If you add a bedroom, ensure full access to the rest of the house. Louis Tenenbaum describes seeing a plan for a bedroom addition:

> There was no way for the father—quadriplegic from a work injury, using a power wheelchair—to make the turn through the kitchen from this new master suite.

Storage and utilities

There is now quite an industry in closet organization, with shops, catalogs, and consultants presenting products for optimal efficiency. The typical closet has a horizontal rod for hanging clothes with a shelf above it. Both can be out of reach for a wheelchair user. Hanging rods must be lowered or a height-adjustable product installed. Sometimes this allows installation of another rod higher up that can be used by a standing person.

Apart from moving rods, storage space can be gained with an array of accessories. Stacking storage boxes, drawers, and shoe bins can make the most of existing closet space, while bringing more items within reach. Placing folded clothing in drawers or shelves can be easier on the arms, sparing you the need to extend your arm forward to lift clothing on hangers off of the rod.

Every home has a space for tools, wet boots, brooms, and where laundry gets done. In an apartment these things get squeezed into a closet. If you have a utility room, consider the height of shelving, ability to access closets, and the type of washer and dryer. A small, stacking washer and dryer unit can be very hard for a wheelchair user to reach. Front-loading types are easiest to reach.

> All the washers in my apartment building laundry room were top-loading. I couldn't reach them, so I wrote the management and they put in two front-loading ones. Everybody in the building likes them a lot, so they're not always available.

Outdoor spaces

Access to the outdoors and any yard is an important consideration. Ramped sidewalks or ramps from rear patios and decks expand access to the outside for family barbecues, working in the garden, or just sitting in the sun. A sun porch added to the rear of the house or a screened-in balcony in an apartment offers greater opportunity for fresh air, protects from bugs and direct sunlight, and removes the need for a screened door at the entry, which complicates access.

Some surfaces are easier to wheel on than others. Thick grass, especially on damp ground, is difficult for wheeling, and grass can hide invisible depressions a wheel could sink into, tipping you over. If you intend to wheel on a lawn, keep the grass cut, and inspect the yard for depressions to be filled in. On unpaved surfaces, gravel and stones make an unfriendly surface, whereas crushed limestone or packed clay makes it more passable.

If you will be encountering substantial rough terrain, wider, knobby tires can help or you could use an all-terrain vehicle instead of a wheelchair. Clearance of footrests can make access difficult if footrests are too low, since there is a greater chance of the main wheels settling a bit in soft ground. Rugged wheelchairs like the Iron Horse are favored by some farmers.

Finding a home

You need to take responsibility for determining whether a home or apartment can work for you. Telling landlords or real estate agents that you require wheelchair access will usually not do the job. They could either exaggerate or minimize your needs. They don't know how you adapt nor what is hard or easy for you to do. They may think that you must have a home formally designed for wheelchair access, according to general standards and codes.

You will have better luck getting what you need with newer construction. Depending on the state you live in and whether the developer gained any exceptions to accessibility codes, a certain portion of new apartment units or townhouses in a newly constructed complex are generally required to be accessible. This might mean "handicapped adaptable," an approach in which the unit is designed to be adapted in certain ways if it needs to accommodate a wheelchair user. For instance, the management would be prepared to install lever handles on the doors and plumbing, add grab bars, or switch the stove/oven unit for one with controls on the front.

Thanks to the recent history of access codes and the ADA, the building environment is much improved. Builders tend to be more aware of the standards and of product offerings that satisfy legal requirements. But there is a difference between the codes and what really works best. If you have the chance to influence the design of a home or apartment complex before construction, you might be able to offer some guidance to a builder who is interested.

> I had a hard time finding accessible housing after I was injured. I finally met with a builder in my area who was planning a new apartment complex. Because of my contact with him, he made two apartments in the complex very wheelchair accessible (roll-in shower, etc.), and all apartments are accessible (wide doorways, level entrances). He would not have done so without my influence, not because he didn't care, but because he wasn't aware of the needs, or how easy and inexpensive it was to make the apartments accessible.

This is unfortunately more the exception that the rule, particularly if you are buying, because of business and permit approvals. A builder might not be allowed to accept money for a housing unit until it is finished. Since you can't commit to the purchase in advance, builders can't risk making special accommodations since they can't be certain you will end up actually buying it.

Developers are just beginning to witness direct demand for Universal Design in their new apartments and homes. Ron Mace described how some consumers are planning ahead:

> We had a developer come to us who said that six clients had recently said they had heard about Universal Design. They wanted the developer to build houses that would last the rest of their lives. These were families without a person with a disability. They were baby boomers who saw their own parents have to leave their homes when they got older and couldn't climb the stairs or use the bathroom anymore.

Mobile and modular homes

Some people have found a workable solution for accessibility in mobile and modular homes, which are usually limited to one floor. A mobile home is attached to a steel frame which provides structural stability. It can be placed only in a mobile home park or other site zoned for mobile homes. A modular home is more akin to conventionally built homes. However, it is largely constructed indoors in a factory, transported to the site, and then placed onto an already-constructed foundation. Modular homes can be located in most residential areas, depending on local zoning ordinances and building codes.

Mobile and modular homes are built with the outer shell providing the structure. Interior walls are generally not load-bearing. Because of their construction, there is usually more flexibility in modifying interior design. Modifying an existing unit can also be much easier since interior walls are less likely to be structural. Doors can be widened and walls moved without worrying about the ceiling falling in. A ramp added to a mobile home will usually need to be structurally freestanding, since the building is not designed to carry the additional load.

Beyond physical changes

You might need to train family members and friends about keeping a clear path for you around the house. People who walk tend to leave shoes, bags, or packages recently brought into the house in your path of circulation without realizing they are obstructing your way. You also need to train others to return chairs fully back under the table and out of your way. You often need to remind people a few times before it really sinks in. Most people will understand and adjust.

Often, other people tend to think that since a chair user spends all day in a chair you must be accustomed to it.

> When I have guests to my home, I end up staying in my wheelchair more than I otherwise would. Part of the problem is that there is a lot of competition for my favorite recliner—definitely the most comfortable spot in the house! But the other issue is that people don't understand my preference to get out of the wheelchair.

If you're not getting to move out of your chair enough, feel free to speak up and let others know your needs, saying something like, "I'd really like to get out of this chair and be more comfortable."

What else is involved in making a home usable aside from building ramps, enlarging doors, or buying the right stove? Louis Tenenbaum suggests:

> I often think that to make all this work, these homes need reasonably priced friendly maintenance contracts. I think that is going to have to be a vital component of independence living.

CHAPTER 8

Intimacy, Sex, and Babies

Whatever your situation—newly injured or living with a disability all your life, young or mature, single or in a committed relationship—sexuality is a part of your nature. You can find a way to express your sexuality in a way that is satisfying and meaningful for you and your partner.

Adjusting to a new disability has its difficulties. Some loss of sexual function occurs with many injuries and disabling conditions. However, this is a matter of adaptation. You are fully deserving of love and sensuality. Understanding the physiological impact of your disability is crucial to knowing your limits and therefore your possibilities. Unrealistic expectations are far more destructive to your sensual life than the actual physical limits.

Advances have been made that allow paralyzed men to participate in intercourse and fathering a child. Women's experience of sex—a topic largely neglected in the rehabilitation community until recently—is getting more attention, in addition to the question of having babies.

This chapter looks first at the pressures that culture and our expectations place on a narrow range of sexual activity. We then look at options for intimacy and finding partners. Next, we turn to sexual activity itself: talking it over, concerns about revealing your body, orgasm and other sexual responses, changing expectations and style, bowel and bladder issues, male erection, etc. Finally, we look at reproduction and parenting.

Sexual beings

Is sex possible for a disabled person? Absolutely.

Is childbearing possible for a disabled person? That depends.

These are big questions. It is human nature to desire intimacy and to reproduce. These needs are in no way diminished by a disability.

Sexuality does change for a person with a disability, often in dramatic ways. You will need to ask questions, experiment, and perhaps readjust some of your notions of what sexuality means. There are physical limits and adjustments you might face which can affect your sexual options.

At the Baylor College of Medicine, the Center for Research on Women with Disabilities conducted an extensive study, drawing from the responses of 475 women with disabilities and 406 able-bodied women. Margaret Nosek, Ph.D., principal investigator in the Baylor study, says about that study:

> We found that women with and without disability had the same level of sexual desire, but the women with disabilities experienced a lot of frustrations and barriers in having sexual activity at the level that they wanted. They had trouble finding partners, and so the rate of marriage and of living with a partner was much lower for women with disabilities.

Ultimately, the study is reassuring:

> What we also found is that many women with disabilities have overcome the effect of those [negative] stereotypes and have had wonderful success in developing relationships, families, and satisfying lives.[1]

Especially interesting is the finding that level of disability is unrelated to the level of sexual functioning or satisfaction. Other factors were found to be the cause of limited dating, relationship, marriage, and childbearing options.

Even for the most confident women with disabilities, it was harder for them to find partners. Nosek observes about the Baylor study:

> There were many, many women in our study who were very self-confident, had high self-esteem, had a positive body image, and yet they still experience big problems finding partners. The reasons they cited were that potential partners were afraid of their disability, couldn't handle physical limitations, or assumed the woman was not interested in sex.

This woman has been with her partner for the last twenty years:

> Many things have changed. When I was young, I defined myself as a sexual athlete of sorts. I liked playing around with everybody. I enjoyed experimenting with wild positions, etc.
>
> Well, that ain't me no more. Now, most intercourse positions are simply too painful or too fatiguing for me (including some of my former

favorites). The medications I take to keep the depression at bay also make it difficult to achieve orgasm.

I spent years feeling guilty about not being the woman I once was. It's still a struggle, but I know I have many positives on my side of the ledger to start with.

I've begun to get my gut around the notion that sex is 99 percent mental, and that the point of sex is to share love with someone.

In a study on sexual response in women with spinal cord injury conducted by Marca Sipski, M.D., and Craig Alexander, Ph.D., at the Kessler Institute for Rehabilitation in New Jersey, they found that:

When questioned about activities and preferences, there was no significant change pre-SCI and post-SCI in the types of activities, nor was there any relation to the extent of injury. Where sexual satisfaction significantly decreased after SCI, sexual desire did not diminish.[2]

The study goes on to conclude that those who had a greater number of partners pre-injury had more partners post-injury. Sexual experience and confidence have been found to correlate with successful sexual adaptation for those who acquire a disability.

There are indeed challenges, but most chair users still have many options for sensual contact available to them. You can discover that you are not only still a very sexual being, but that sex in the context of disability can offer some surprising and gratifying new experiences.

Intimacy and sexual pleasure

Intimacy really has little to do with sexual function. Caring touch is what truly satisfies—giving and receiving it. Loving and being loved is ultimately a more powerful human exchange than "raw sex." Love can be expressed in an infinite variety of ways, as simple as a touch or a kiss or cuddling together. These experiences have nothing to do with genital contact, and are clearly available to anyone.

At its best, sexual intimacy is an experience of unity, of joining, of feeling as if there is no longer any boundary between you and your partner. For couples who don't have this deep a romantic connection, sex is nonetheless an act of trust, a choice to make yourself vulnerable, and an opportunity to share the incredibly powerful experience of human sexuality. The remarkable sensations, the sense of bliss, the shift in consciousness, the quality of relief and clarity—are all life experiences possible in sexual intimacy. These qualities are no less available to people with disabilities. They simply take other forms.

Sexuality is about fun and trust and sharing pleasure with another person. Sexuality empowers you with self-worth and reduces the stresses of your daily life. It can even be healing.

Mitch Tepper is the founder of the Sexual Health Network, and is a doctoral student in human sexuality education at University of Pennsylvania. Tepper—a quadriplegic—has noticed that while there is much written about issues of erection, ejaculation, pregnancy, and disability in marriage, there is little said about sexual pleasure for people with disabilities:

> There is growing evidence that sexual knowledge and sexual self-esteem are related to the ability to experience sexual pleasure and orgasm. It seems that knowledge is power, power fuels self-esteem, and self-esteem opens the door to sexual pleasure.[3]

Culture and sexual mechanics

Modern culture places so much emphasis on the mechanics of sex that the range of sexual possibilities becomes very narrow. Advertising, media, and the easy availability of explicit materials on videotape and the Internet focus on the clinical act of intercourse. This focus places undue strain on sexual adjustment to a disability, as this woman with traumatic brain injury says:

> Results-oriented sex—he gets one big O [orgasm], I get one (or three), then we've "had sex"—is not very compatible with what my body likes right now. Too bad I've grown up in a culture that trumpets this sort of sex above all others.

Men are expected to maintain an erection and complete the sexual act in ejaculation. For women, the ability to move their hips and to control the vaginal muscles seem indispensable.

Orgasm is particularly glorified as the indispensable goal of sexual contact. Glorya Hale, in *Sourcebook for the Disabled*, says:

> Although the aim of most sexual expression may be reaching orgasm, it's clearly not necessary to have an orgasm for both partners to achieve intense sexual satisfaction.[4]

Initially, any sexual limitations at variance with "norms" as described by the culture can appear to mean a life sentence of loneliness and sensual deprivation. This need not be the case.

Cultural pressures are hard on everyone. Able-bodied persons also struggle to find true sexual identity amidst this cultural noise and the emphasis on externals—large breasts, sculpted muscles, the right car, impeccable grooming, etc. For a person with a disability the challenge to find sexual identity can seem horribly amplified. False cultural myths promoted for commercial motives can rob you of self-esteem and incorrectly lead you to believe that you have no sexual identity.

Recent disability

Immediately after an injury or the onset of a disabling disease, you are still defined by your previous identity. A sudden and dramatic change is not easily absorbed. Finding a sexual identity is part of the larger process of finding your identity as a person with a disability.

Sandra Loyer, Clinical Social Worker at the University of Michigan Medical Center, works in the Department of Physical Medicine and Rehabilitation. Loyer is part of the team that is immediately involved with spinal cord injury patients. She says:

> There are guys who come out of surgery and their first question is "Will I ever get it up?"

People also labor under their existing beliefs, as reported by women studied by the Baylor College of Medicine:

> For women disabled in adulthood, it is often a realization of their worst nightmare. The have grown up absorbing the social stereotype that women with disabilities are asexual and are a burden to their families, and they feel that this type of life has now been thrust upon them.[5]

Often, medical personnel, counselors, family, and friends find the topic of sex and disability uncomfortable. They avoid the issue and instead reinforce the notion that sex is not an option. Doctors have been known to suggest that a person with a disability forget about a sex life and move on to other things.

At one time, these attitudes were presented to the medical community as fact. One study in 1967 stated that "to those who have it, paraplegia is sexually totally disabling."[6] It was left to people with disabilities to find out for themselves what was possible, weighed down by such beliefs and the resulting lack of support and information.

In their book *Enabling Romance*, Ken Kroll and Erica Levy Klein tell of a quadriplegic who had been told by his doctor that he could not be sexual. Then he met a woman with whom he had an immediate physical attraction:

> *Much to Gary's delight, he found that, despite his being paralyzed, his relationship with Beverly awakened feelings of sexual excitement he never thought he'd experience again.*[7]

The book tells that they went on to a long-lasting marriage and satisfying sex life.

An assumption that you will not be sexual is not only foisted on people born able-bodied. A twenty-three-year-old woman with cerebral palsy recalls:

> *I think the toughest thing about sex with a disability you are born with is the assumption that you are so innocent and childish you don't think about that stuff. I didn't date in high school. I ended up being good friends with people, but none of the guys would have thought to date me. I met my first when I was 19. He's also disabled, and we had a very passionate relationship.*

There is often not time in rehab to address sexuality when other medical and rehabilitation tasks must take priority. Staff might also be lacking sufficient training in sexuality. Sexuality educator Mitch Tepper gives seminars on sexuality and disability to professionals, and observes:

> *I am surprised at how little training rehab staff have received about the unique needs of people with disabilities with regard to their sexual identity.*

The problem is more pronounced for people who acquire their disability at a young age.

> *I learned nothing about sexuality or reproduction in rehab, because I was in a children's rehab hospital and I guess the powers that be didn't think young people should know about sexuality.*

In the Baylor study, only 59 percent of women felt that they had received adequate information about how their disability affects their sexual functioning.[8]

Negative attitudes still exist, and some people in the healthcare community still carry their own personal discomforts or myths regarding sexuality and disability. Don't allow anyone to convince you that sex is no longer an option, regardless of your disability.

In *Enabling Romance*, Randi—a nurse who discovered a deep relationship with Tom, a quadriplegic, while he was a patient in rehab—describes his change after they became intimate sexually:

> *It is in this one area that I've seen Tom change from a shy boy into a confident man. These changes have carried over into other parts of our relationship and into his ability to cope with his disability and the world in general.*[9]

The question of how you will function sexually is one that takes time to answer, as your body reaches medical stability and as you begin to learn from your own experience. Time is on your side. According to Mitch Tepper:

> *Time since injury is associated with a general increase in self-esteem; however, an increase in sexual self-esteem often lags until people face the issue of their sexuality. That is the point where there is growth potential.*

Putting sex aside for a time?

You are not obligated to be sexually active, as people who practice abstinence by choice will tell you. You might be engaged in work or a community of friends and family that is satisfying, that provides you with affection and fun and affirmation. Intimacy takes many forms, and not everyone needs to be sexually active in order to feel whole.

It can also be understandable to choose to set sexuality aside when your disability demands so much of you in addressing day-to-day matters. Reasons to abstain might include the difficulty of finding a partner, fear around muscle spasticity, bowel and bladder weakness, the presence of catheters or other appliances, fear of infections, or the simple loss of the urge—more likely repressed than actually gone. You might be taking medications that suppress sexual impulses. For most people, even during times of abstinence, the desire for sensual expression remains. You may need to integrate these other issues of adaptation into your life first, moving on to sex when the time is right for you.

Some people may use their disability to avoid sexual issues they had been struggling with all their life. Disability can be a convenient excuse to simply give up the game, driven by fears that you may not even be fully aware of. However, not addressing fears or other feelings means that you might miss out on the potential for greater personal fulfillment through discovery of your sexual identity.

Past abuse, failure, or adjustment to your disability might simply feel over-whelming. A period of recovery and healing might be necessary and entirely appropriate before you can address your sexual identity. Just remember that for many people with disabilities, these issues have been surmountable.

Emotional struggles

All of us face the work of sorting through our sexual psyche. The challenge of discovering your identity as a sensual disabled person can amplify this challenge. In the *Journal of Rehabilitation*, A. Frankel notes:

> *Most people have unconscious conflicts about sex which they keep buried. A devastating injury or disease serves to unearth these conflicts.*[10]

Loss of sexual function—multiplied by the burden of inaccurate messages from caregivers, family, and the broader society—can erode your self-confidence. If you were already struggling with issues of sexuality prior to your disability, they will certainly not just disappear. They will have an impact on your overall adjustment to your disability, and so need to be addressed as directly as the physical or social needs.

Even if you accept that you will have some sexual limits, and want to relax and have as much pleasure as possible for yourself and your partner, there can be a feeling of having been left on the sidelines. You might find yourself experiencing feelings of resentment toward your partner for having what seems to be a more substantial sexual response than you experience. Despite the advice of many rehab professionals or caregivers, thinking positively is not easy, nor is it automatic. You may want to take pleasure in your partner's enjoyment and in providing your partner with sexual satisfaction, but still struggle with negative feelings. If negative feelings can't be worked out through trusting communication, the support of a counselor may be called for if you want the relationship to succeed.

Orgasm is different for everyone, defined in each individual's terms. If you have acquired a disability later in life, you should know that you can redefine orgasm. This is about a process of finding what orgasm is for you, even if it is different from what it might have been in the past. As this married C5 quadriplegic man found:

> An orgasm is really in your mind. Sure, before my accident there were sensations that felt good, but it feels just as good in my mind. [11]

Able-bodied partners may find themselves feeling guilty over the fact that they are capable of sensations which are not possible for you. Just as you may struggle with emotions unique to your sexual experience, the feelings an able-bodied partner might experience are natural and deserve to be recognized and discussed. Your emotions are not the only emotions going on. Intimate partners react to each other.

Overemphasizing intercourse

For those who were sexually active prior to their disability, the memory of sexual sensations remain, amplifying their sense of loss. They know what they are missing, so the idea of redefining their sexuality might feel like nothing more than compromise and loss. These feelings need not last as you discover what previous—and new—pleasures are now available.

People disabled prior to the loss of virginity might carry an unresolved curiosity about intercourse—feelings that might never be satisfied in their lifetime. They might envy the general able-bodied population, and imagine an able-bodied sex life to be more ideal than it actually is.

Losing the capacity for intercourse in adolescence is very difficult, coming at a time when the anticipation of a first sexual experience is extremely high. This grand sense of expectation can linger for a long time. We have missed a rite of passage. Eventually we find that our maturity is based on values and accomplishments other than genital intercourse.

For a man unable to maintain an erection, having to stop short during intercourse can be saddening and disappointing. The psyche wants to continue, but the body will not obey. A man might feel guilt for asking his partner to make a compromise, to accept with him only what is possible, when he imagines that his partner wants more than he can provide. In such moments, you don't want to be trapped in being overly attached to intercourse; you can move on to one of many other options and continue to enjoy your intimacy. In time, you'll probably work your way back to the moment you thought you had lost.

Staying stuck in what you want to happen increases the distance between you and your partner. It reinforces your association of tragedy with your disability, and costs you the pleasures that remain.

For a person with a disability, sex may become more precious precisely because of the existence of limitations. Once you have lost certain options, those that remain become more valued. If you experienced early fears that sexual activity might not be an option—or worried that sex would be complicated—the discovery of deep intimacy in a relationship becomes all the more precious. Changing the emphasis from intercourse to sensuality and caring intimacy—wherever it may lead—is key.

A 1993 study of men with spinal cord injury performed by Drs. Craig Alexander, Marca Sipski, and Thomas Findley of the Kessler Institute for Rehabilitation in New Jersey found that:

> Post-injury there was a dramatic reduction in the percentage of subjects engaging in penis-vagina intercourse. The majority of subjects preferred penis-vagina intercourse pre-injury. Post-injury, however, subjects seemed to prefer a wider variety of sexual activities with not as strong a preference for one activity. Moreover, preference for penis-vagina intercourse decreased substantially while preference increased for oral sex, kissing, and touching.[12]

Once you gain sexual experience in the context of your disability, you will find that your relationships are not defined by your disability as much as you might have imagined.

> I'm blessed with having experienced a relationship with a very wonderful and loving woman. Although we are no longer together, it is not because we failed as a couple, but that the circumstances of our lives did not allow us to make a commitment at that time. I can no longer doubt that someone can be attracted to me because of my disability.

Partners

You might already be in a committed relationship, have a partner and wonder if it's going to last, or be thinking about embarking on a search for a new partner.

Your body image

The body goes through certain changes—depending on the given disability—about which you might feel insecure or self-conscious. Muscle atrophy which results in very thin, sometimes skeletal limbs is common with spinal cord injury. Amputees have their stumps. There might be scars from surgeries, leftover effects of skin rashes, or other skin conditions. Higher level spinal disabilities can result in a distended stomach and loss in tone in the abdominal muscles. Quadriplegics have curled fingers and thin hands which they cannot use for handshaking or for certain sexual activities. Spinal fusions or the insertion of rods in the spine can impose a very upright posture that others may misinterpret as an uptight body language. You might adopt a stiff posture for fear that movement will induce muscle spasms. These physical realities all affect the signals put out to potential partners. They also influence your sense of self.

Over time, we adapt to our "new normal" because we no longer have the direct comparison of what our body looked like prior to our disability. Once again, you become accustomed to your new shape and it is just your familiar body. Your wheelchair is now a part of your body image, and is often the first thing that someone reacts to when they first meet you. Body image is an important factor in your choice of wheelchair, although it shouldn't outweigh function.

Body image is a powerful force in how the world views you as a sexual person, as this paraplegic woman in her thirties found out in the early years after a spinal cord injury:

> It wasn't easy at all to develop my sexual identity as a disabled teenager. I was fourteen, so I never got to wear hose or walk in high heels. Our culture defines so much of a female's sexuality by the appearance of her legs.

She went on to marry, have children, and discover a clear and satisfying sexual identity for herself:

> I don't have time to feel sorry for myself as a woman in a wheelchair, because I'm embracing life now.

The Baylor study reports:

> Women with disabilities who had a more positive sexual self image
> and who perceived themselves to be approachable by potential romantic
> partners also had higher levels of sexual activity.[13]

It's not hard to imagine that these things would be true for men as well. As one woman explained, "The sexiest thing to me is self-confidence." Feelings of shame and embarrassment can be overwhelming, yet again and again, people with disabilities have found that these feelings become irrelevant in the presence of a trusted, intimate partner.

Existing couples

There is a cultural assumption that an able-bodied person who stays with someone after the occurrence of a disability is either masochistic or heroic, but there are no rules. Some couples will stay together, some won't. Staying together is more about people and their values and what they mean to each other, not any social notions about being an "invalid" or a "caretaker."

> My doctor told me that I would have to forget about my girlfriend
> and move on to others. It turned out that he was right, but not especially
> because of my spinal cord injury. It was getting time to move on anyway.
> She might very well have made the transition with me if she were the
> right partner for me in the first place.

> I had a conversation on an airplane with an accomplished business-
> man who told me about a young couple who were recently married. The
> man had become a quadriplegic during the engagement, and they still got
> married. My flying partner said that many people doubted her motives or
> their chances of success. They saw a woman giving up her future. I asked
> what he saw. He answered, "Two people in love."

A sudden disability can be a strain to marriage. Some couples might have allowed sexuality to be so much the foundation of their relationship that, in the presence of a sudden disability, they don't have enough of a foundation in the other aspects of their relationship to carry them through. The issue of changes in their sexual relations can be the final straw that breaks apart a couple whose relationship was not strong to begin with.

In the Baylor study of women with disabilities, several issues with existing partners were reported:[14]

- A woman with a disability may blame herself for everything that goes wrong in a relationship.

- Her husband may take advantage of her self-blame and collude in blaming all their marital problems on the disability.

- Nearly half of women with partners responding to the study sometimes felt like a burden to their partners.

- Nearly half also felt that their relationship suffered because they were less able to contribute to housework or participate in previously enjoyed activities.

Dr. Margaret Nosek states:

> You find relationships that go beyond the physical. Many women reported they found new kinds of activities they can do with their partners. If the relationship is good, they'll find other doors that can be opened.

> Some reported cases of later onset disability where the men they were with just couldn't deal with it, and it broke up their marriage. In other cases it didn't, it made them significantly closer. Success in marriage didn't depend on when the disability happened, whether they were born with it or it happened later in life.

Some couples don't succeed. A man who broke his neck ten years into his marriage recounts its subsequent breakup. His wife had been very supportive during his rehabilitation and return home, but then they ran into severe difficulties.

> The only thing that I was so disappointed about in her was she was so fearful of making love to me again. And I wanted to please her needs, not worried about my pleasure. Maybe 5 percent curious to find out if I could do more than I was told. For fourteen months, every time I would bring up the subject she would say, "I'm not ready yet," and end of discussion!

> Then two months later, her reply would be, "I don't know if I'll ever be ready." Before I was injured, our sex life was great, we did just about everything to please each other.

> *In October, we had our eleven-year wedding anniversary. The first Friday of November, she came home later than usual and said, "I don't know how to tell you this, but I want a divorce. If you hadn't broken your neck I wouldn't be leaving."*

The statistics about couples staying together are encouraging. The rate of divorce after disability is only slightly higher than in the nondisabled population. Successful couples have achieved a bond that goes beyond simple matters of sexual function. Though important, loss of sexual options have less impact than you might think on an existing relationship that is strong. Such a couple is capable of adjusting and enjoying each other. A woman in her forties describes her relationship:

> *I married my partner because we communicate so well. Talking about sex is not easy to do, but it's critically important. At first, all discussions had to take place well away from the bedroom, because there's lots of potential for hurt feelings and misunderstanding in the heat of the moment.*
>
> *Now I treasure the intimacy that we share. I appreciate the cuddles and the sensations that aren't painful. Hand-holding and kissing have always been wonderful. I've learned to stop thinking of these as "foreplay" and enjoy them for their own delights.*

The right partner—married or not—can make an important difference in one's overall adjustment to a new disability, as this spinal cord injured paraplegic man says:

> *Fortunately, for the year prior to the accident, I was in a relationship with a strong woman. She helped me through the hard times and showed me that my sexuality—now different—could be enjoyable. She was there for me and this was very important in my recovering with a reasonable amount of sanity.*

According to Sandra Loyer, men have a greater challenge adjusting to a disabling injury to their wives. She says:

> *They're afraid they'll hurt her, that they have nothing to offer, whereas women are more naturally nurturing. Sure, there are more sensitive men these days, but it's still harder for them.*

Adjustments are possible. The following forty-year-old woman is a C5 quadriplegic who has been married for twenty-two years. She became injured by a gunshot eighteen years into her marriage.

> We had a great sex life before my injury and we still do. My disability has never turned off my husband. We had the Big Sex Discussion while I was in rehab and had our first post-injury sex there, too. I assured him that he wasn't going to "break" me or anything. One of his concerns was about doing something wicked to the catheter. So for us, aside from the physical changes, our sex life has remained the same. I have a theory why this is: We were very much in love and very close before this happened, and we still are.

Finding partners

If you're not currently in a committed relationship, how do you get started?

Finding love is tough enough for anyone these days. Single Americans complain more and more about the difficulty of finding companionship, much less a mate. Singles clubs and personal ads abound, flooded with people on the hunt for a partner. Bringing a disability into these environments is hardly an advantage.

This twenty-three-year-old man with a spinal cord injury struggles with finding a partner:

> My hormones are raging, but I have no outlet. I go out a lot with friends, but even friends who were potential lovers before are now certainly just friends. I can't seem to shake that "Wow, you are a great person" line. I know that in the long run I will end up with someone who is great, but I could really just go for a one night stand or two! I'm a pretty good-looking guy so the prospects are there, but what do I do!?

Likewise for this woman born with a disability:

> I would like to be involved again, but I know that I can't meet people sitting around the local bar, like many of my fellow college students. Frankly, I'm clueless.

Women have a greater challenge finding partners. The culture has historically promoted the idea of the male as aggressor. Women were supposed to wait for men to approach. This has changed somewhat, with women more able to make the approach, but some disabled women still find that men are less likely to approach a woman with a disability.

This woman born with spina bifida found that growing up with a disability had its challenges:

> I felt really inadequate next to my female friends. I thought they were inherently more attractive simply because they didn't use a wheelchair. I think I got around it by being more assertive. The stereotype of the woman waiting for the man to make the move didn't work for me. If I was attracted to a man, I would make the first move.[15]

According to the Baylor study, women with disabilities reported their perceptions of the obstacles to dating:[16]

* Someone who is interested in me might not ask me out because of what others might say.

* Many people do not ask me out because they assume I am unable to have sexual intercourse.

* People seem surprised that I might be interested in sexual intimacy.

* People I would like to date see me as a friend, not as a romantic partner.

Margaret Nosek elaborates on the cultural differences that women face:

> The nurturing role is the role of the woman. So if the woman is the one who needs the help, they're up a creek. There are very few male partners or male family members who are willing to make the sacrifices necessary to provide the kind of assistance needed by a woman with a severe disability. The man with a disability has many more resources than the woman. The man gets it because it is the traditional role of women.

When it comes to attracting partners, women in the study found themselves in a paradox: you can scare off potential partners by aggressive pursuit, but if you don't pursue partners, they're gone.

The good news in the search for partners is that there are more singles on the market now. People are marrying later. Women have more options for a profession and independence than society once allowed. Life expectancy is much longer as medical advances preserve our health; making a commitment when you are still young can mean being together for quite a long time, so what's the rush? With later marriages and the increased divorce rate, there are a lot of unattached folks out there looking for love.

You certainly won't meet anyone by sitting at home. You can meet people through volunteer activities, political groups, clubs of all sorts, classes at the local college or community center, or professional organizations and trade shows. Independent Living Centers sponsor activities, including social and educational events. Although the percentage of success is not high, you might meet someone through personal ads. It's worthwhile to say hello to someone interesting at the grocery store or movie theater. You never know.

It is not unusual for couples to meet in hospitals or clinics. Therapists, nurses, volunteers, and other staff get a unique chance to know the person beyond the disability. Friendships form, and sometimes romance results. These can be equal and sincere meetings of people for whom the opportunity to see each other regularly allowed intimacy to develop. Mitch Tepper notes:

> These people are professionals with less fear of disability, so some are capable of forming authentic relationships.

At the same time, these relationships have no guarantee of success. Says Tepper:

> Some people also need to control or take care of someone. That might be why they're in the health profession in the first place.

There are dating resources specifically for persons with disabilities (see the Appendix). Resources might connect you to someone for a letter writing relationship, possibly on the Internet, or you might meet someone in your area to spend time with.

You will face some extra challenges as a result of having a disability. In *Enabling Romance*, a 36-year-old disabled man used a personal ad to seek a partner. He was open about his disability and received no response, and then:

> As an experiment I placed an ad in a magazine without mentioning I was disabled. I received three responses. I was so thrilled! But then, when I replied to their letters and explained that I was in a wheelchair, I never heard from any of them again.[17]

This is really the only approach—be honest. It can help to first discuss other areas of interest, but don't wait too long to identify your disability. If the other person is unable to accept you, it is best to move on with no regrets, possibly having made a friend in the process.

Women can have a more difficult time finding a male partner. There is more social pressure on women to fit the supermodel image; men tend to be more attached to the public image of having a beautiful woman on their arm. Margaret Nosek doesn't think that media images make people with disabilities aspire to fit those images so much as they lead others not to consider a person with a disability as a potential partner:

> I think that the media have a more damaging effect on the general public than women with disabilities. I think it's very similar for men and women.

Trading signals

Humans give out certain cues to attract a mate: a deeply ingrained, evolutionary system of physical signals. In *The Anatomy of Love*, Dr. Helen Fisher writes that:

> Men tend to pitch and roll their shoulders, stretch, stand tall, and shift from foot to foot in a swaying motion. Some women have a characteristic walk when courting; they arch their backs, thrust out their bosoms, sway their hips, and strut.[18]

These signals are hard to give while sitting down, so the disabled person is at some disadvantage. They must exaggerate their body language and use other signs to transmit the message of interest to someone they might see at a party, a museum, a restaurant, and so on. According to Fisher, the ensuing stages include getting close enough to begin a simple conversation, achieving those first subtle touches of a forearm or shoulder, and getting into a body synchrony, where two people begin to mirror each other's movements and posture. You will need to find other ways to overcome your physical limits. For instance, eye contact is very powerful and gets the message across just fine.

The impact of your sitting in a wheelchair is undeniably powerful, and you might find yourself drawn to circumvent its effect like this quadriplegic woman in her early twenties:

> I will get out of the chair just to break the contact to make it easier for other people to approach me.[19]

In some cases, the message that a wheelchair sends—that the person in it has a physical limitation—can be welcome. A man who uses a chair because of his difficulty walking finds that his awkward gait has been an obstacle to meeting potential partners:

> *I never get the girl if she sees me walking. But if we meet where we're sitting and she gets to know me first then she realizes I'm a nice guy and it doesn't matter to her if I walk weird.*

If you doubt someone showing signals of attraction could be interested in someone in a wheelchair, you might miss important cues. Be open to signals, while taking care not to mistake friendly signs for more than they are. Go gently, and allow things to take their course. Respond subtly, and if a relationship is meant to proceed, it will.

Who are you "limited" to?

Some people believe that they must find someone to "match" them physically. University of Michigan social worker Sandra Loyer incredulously remembers a young spinal-injured male who asked her:

> *Because I'm like this does it mean the only girlfriend I can have has to be like this too?*

Other people assume that a disabled partner will need an able-bodied partner to provide care. Relationships based on dependence may not be satisfying. Sex researcher Mitch Tepper warns:

> *Be wary of relationships based solely on dependence because they have a tendency not to succeed or be enjoyable in the long run. Seek interdependence. You must have things to offer the relationship, too.*

You aren't limited to disabled partners nor are you limited to able-bodied partners. The goal is to be with the right partner. There are many examples of successful relationships between a person with a disability and an able-bodied partner. There is a pattern emerging from the various writings and studies on relationships and disability. When people let their personalities shine, take care of their health, assume interest rather than rejection, and are able to communicate openly and honestly, they are attractive human beings, disability or not.

Able-bodied partners

There are many more able-bodied persons out there than disabled persons. The odds alone seem to suggest that a person with a disability needs to take their search for love into the wider world. Yet many able-bodied persons who meet a disabled person will doubt that you have sexual inclinations at all. Don't let that stop you. You might get the chance to set them straight!

Some potential able-bodied partners might have unresolved issues about disability that they could impose on you, such as insisting that you use braces rather than a wheelchair or remain under the covers in bed because they are uncomfortable with seeing your body.

Disabled men might consider it good news that many women are nurturing and open-minded. However, according to Loyer, there are also women with less than ideal motivations:

> *There are women out there who find guys in wheelchairs very appealing. They might not be healthy reasons, for example, they may feel they "have them where they want them," or they are looking for men who won't mistreat them the way other men might have. It can also fulfill the need to be needed.*

There is nothing wrong with finding a nurturing person—male or female, straight or gay—but you need to know that you are recognized for who you are, not that you are only seen as "safe."

There are reasonable concerns someone could have about involvement with a person with a disability. Given the same situation, you might ask the same questions. "Will he be dependent on me, now or later in life?" "Are there emotional traumas too complex for me to deal with?" "Will it limit my freedom to do things I enjoy that she can't, like walk on the beach? How important is that to me?" "Will there be resistance from my family and friends?"

Mitch Tepper has an approach he calls "inoculation against rejection":

> *The answers aren't always based on you, but on their own previous experience with relationships and with people with disabilities. It might be more frightening because they're just unaware.*

To build a solid relationship with an able-bodied person, these reasonable questions need to be addressed. Tackling these questions is not just for the other person's benefit; you want to know what you're getting into and whether your commitment to the relationship is based on reality.

An able-bodied woman in her thirties, asked if she imagined a disabled partner would be necessarily dependent on her, says:

> *No, not if the person was independently minded (and my impression is that most handicapped people fight very hard against the image of dependency). My concern would be that they would be limited in certain activities I would want to share with a partner (like hiking, for example). I would also think that it would require a certain basic patience that I'm not sure I have. I like to move fast, and I might have a problem slowing down my pace to match that of a disabled partner. But we're talking about a hypothetical partner here so it's hard to say.*

She has reasonable questions, knows her needs and desires, but realizes that she can't know until faced with the actual situation. It is exactly this opening that creates the opportunity for two people who are interested and attracted to explore how their relationship might work out. She might be surprised to find that there are plenty of hiking possibilities they can share, and that she might have to keep up with her disabled partner! Perhaps she might even find that hiking becomes less important in exchange for a loyal and loving partner who enhances her life in many other ways.

Finding a comfort level around how much help an able-bodied partner will provide in day-to-day life is an important question you will face. Given the greater degree of accessibility in the world today, and the availability of adaptive devices and technologies, couples can have less to work out than they might think.

Often, a disabled person will imagine more reluctance on the part of an able-bodied partner than the partner actually feels. This able-bodied single woman in her forties says:

> *I can imagine disabilities that would be an impediment, and others that would not. I suspect the difference would come into play at the point of attraction, not at the point of "choice to be sexual," though. For instance, I had no problem imagining myself in Jane Fonda's place with Jon Voight (in the film Coming Home). Once attracted to him (hell, he's Jon Voight!), I imagine no insurmountable problems.*

Nondisabled partners usually find out that their concerns are unfounded. This woman in her early forties is in a relationship with a paraplegic man, and says:

From the beginning I was attracted to him, both physically and emo-
tionally. Somehow I just knew that his disability would not be an issue.
For one thing, he didn't call attention to it. As we became involved, I
learned certain details like how I can help with the wheelchair at the car
and not get in the way! But he helps me as much as I help him. It's not an
issue. His "limitations" are not a burden, since we are so close, have such
a good friendship, and are such wonderful lovers.

Ask yourself whether you might be trying to reinforce your self-image as a complete person through an involvement with a nondisabled person. It is not unusual to want to reduce your association with the identity of disability in this way. This doesn't mean that your motives are therefore suspect or tainted. A certain satisfaction can come in strengthening our connection to the broader world through a healthy relationship with an able-bodied part- ner. It is simply important to be aware of the degree to which you might be motivated by this issue, and whether it may be distracting you from focus- ing on the characteristics that constitute a healthy relationship—love, trust, commitment, and shared values.

Disabled couples

A couple where both partners are disabled is a mixed blessing. It might be easier in some ways to find a partner who also has a disability, whether through disability-specializing dating services, involvement in the local dis- ability scene or Independent Living Center, or getting to know someone on the Internet. You might imagine that another person with a disability will be more of a kindred spirit, or that you won't have to take time trying to explain the way your disability affects your life.

Two disabled persons, understanding that each may have feared not being able to satisfy a sexual partner, might make for a uniquely powerful intimate alliance. They can be more sensitive to the necessary changes of a differently defined sexual style, free of performance pressure and focused on the simple enjoyment of touching, kissing, and the many sensual options which remain.

There are many disabled couples in successful relationships. But in public, a disabled couple are not seen in intimate terms, as this married couple found:

People usually assume that you're together for something other than
a relationship. We've had people ask us if we were brother and sister.[20]

But just as an able-bodied partner might be cautious, this can be just as true for another person with a disability. After all, they have their own stuff to deal with. Why would they want to take on more? If you share the fact of having a disability, it can be a means of camaraderie and increased intimacy, or it can be a double burden.

It goes both ways for Cindy McCoy, writing in *New Mobility* magazine. Now in her forties, she has had multiple sclerosis since the age of twenty-one. McCoy is now in her third marriage, this time to a man with cerebral palsy. She writes:

> *If the compassion and camaraderie between us are deeper and more satisfying due to the shared challenge of coping with disability, then perhaps that balances the times when double disability equals double distress.*[21]

Relationships are always relationships, no matter who is involved. They can succeed or fail. It always comes back to one question. Do you love each other? And then a few others. Do you communicate well? Do you have complimentary skills which you can combine to create a home and manage your day-to-day affairs? Can you build a shared social community, and be confident in the individual friendships each of you should have? Are you willing to work on yourself at the same time that you are committed to working on your partnership? No matter how many disabilities there are in a relationship, those are the answers that matter.

Prostitutes and surrogate partners

Since it is can be difficult to find a partner, being with a professional might solve the need for sensual experience. Some have explored the use of prostitutes or sex workers, such as this twenty-six-year old paraplegic quoted in *Enabling Romance*:

> *Despite my paralysis, I wanted and needed sex, and prostitutes seemed like the easy way out. I was a virgin, yet I had this driving need to find out what sex was all about. I started going to this very kind and sincere call girl who taught me a lot about sex and about my own physical capabilities as a man.*[22]

The book relates that he ultimately found a steady lover.

Mitch Tepper notes that there are risks in interacting with a prostitute. At the worst, it is possible to acquire a sexually transmitted disease such as HIV from a person who has that much sexual contact with many different people. There have also been cases of a sex worker luring people into situations where they can be robbed. A prostitute is also unlikely to understand the emotional aspects of your disability experience. They might be insensitive about issues such as ability to attain or maintain an erection, scars, scoliosis, or spasms. As Tepper describes:

> I know of a situation where a mother bought a $300 call girl for her disabled son. He thought she was beautiful, and she was studying to be a nurse. He had a great experience. That is going to be more the exception than the rule. Not all sex workers will fit that description.

Some have pursued more formalized experiences using professional surrogate partners in association with sex therapists. Tepper explains:

> It's a three-way relationship. The sex therapist assigns you a sex surrogate who helps you develop your sexual and relationship skills. They also teach you about dating, anatomy, giving and receiving pleasure. The relationship is about building your comfort level with a partner. Usually there is sex with the surrogate, but it could be toward the end of the series of meetings. A typical example would be an older person who has never had sex, and feels too much pressure to succeed on their own. Their nervousness prevents them from being able to establish a sexual relationship, so the surrogate helps them over it.

These possibilities are mentioned here only as options that some disabled people have explored, with varying degrees of success.

Going it alone

Masturbation can play an important role in your discovery of a new sexual identity as a person with a disability. It might be easier than starting with a partner, no matter how recent or long-term your disability might be. The emotional demands of being with a partner at this time can be overwhelming. This is not to say that the right partner couldn't share the process of exploring your sexuality with you in an atmosphere of deep and giving acceptance. However, don't overlook self-stimulation as an option which can help you find your sexual identity and ultimately find a partner, if that is your desire.

Cultural taboo might influence your thinking about masturbation. There can be subconscious messages telling you it is a shameful thing to do. Masturbation is normal and healthy.

Ejaculation or orgasm is not the only acceptable criterion for being sensual with yourself. Masturbation does not need to be fixed in those terms. Touching yourself, fantasizing, using vibrators, magazines, videos, or the Internet to enjoy stimulating erotic material—any of these can be a means of expressing yourself sexually. Self-loving can bring up satisfying experiences you have had in the past and be a break from sexual loneliness—an experience hardly limited to those with a disability.

The sexual experience

If you have a partner, the first sexual experience can be something you'll want to prepare for.

Getting started with someone new

Having met a new partner, it will be necessary to explain your unique sexual style. At first, this can be a daunting task. Explaining about catheters, bowels, levels of sensation, and other details is not very sexy. But by demonstrating your willingness to be open and honest you will set the tone of mutual intimacy needed in a healthy sexual relationship. If you show you are unafraid, you will help your partner relax into the process with you.

A new partner might not be comfortable asking what is possible, so it will fall to you to raise the issue. This is the chance to demonstrate that you want to be with this person, that you are attracted to and excited by him or her. Once you know the feeling is mutual, then you are in for a wonderful experience, and your partner is likely to be open and accepting about understanding your needs.

> *One time I had become romantic with a woman, and we had enjoyed some very satisfying kissing on several occasions. The opportunity arrived for her to stay the night, and I did not explain that I had limited penile sensation and did not ejaculate. I just wanted to have what I imagined to be a normal experience without having to explain things. Inevitably, we reached a point where her expectations were not met. She felt she was perhaps not attractive enough, and suddenly there was an emotional*

obstacle which we never overcame. I learned clearly that the pre-sex talk is crucial for a satisfying and mutual experience.

You may need your partner to assist with clinical tasks such as changing a catheter or helping in the bathroom. This can have a negative effect on creating a romantic mood, but it can also be a shared process that enhances intimacy, even as an opening to sexual intimacy. Once these duties are addressed, a couple can enter into the space of closeness and passion just as any other couple must—with patience, gentleness, and doing those simple things that begin the process of arousal.

The style with new partners is to relax into mutual discovery, to discuss and learn about each other's needs, to find every possible touch and contact that is pleasurable, and to separate from the various cultural pressures which create skewed expectations. Getting started with honest discussion and exploration puts the focus where it belongs: on people loving each other, and expressing it through touch, trust, and sincere giving.

Pretty damn sexy.

First revelation

Revealing your body intimately—despite the fact that you may be very accustomed to being naked with a physician or a personal care assistant—is a very vulnerable encounter. It can be a poignant test of trust with a person you choose as a sexual partner. As put by a young quadriplegic woman:

When I'm in a new relationship with someone I'm just not sure about, it's still a threatening thing [to reveal my body].

First exposure deserves to be handled with care. But success with well-chosen intimate partners who will show you acceptance will expose the invalidity of your fears. Your partner is able to make the same adjustment as you are to your "new normal," though you may need to allow him/her time.

Bodily appearance, while meaningful, does not play as large a role as you might suspect. Besides, while in the act of intimacy, lying next to or on top of each other, we are not seeing much of the body anyway. We are reveling in touch and intimacy.

Be in good health

Your general level of health has a direct impact on your sexuality.

If your body is pressured with physical and emotional demands, you are less able to enjoy your sexuality. Depression and stress have specific physiological effects through hormones and enzymes that are released in response. They can impact your immune system, reduce your capacity to relax and be open to sensations, and draw your attention away from your partner.

Eat a good diet, balanced with a range of foods that are whole and free of chemicals. Control the amounts of sugar, alcohol, tobacco, and caffeine in your diet, all of which deplete the quality of your blood and circulation, promote fatigue, and lessen sexual response.

Control your weight. If you are overweight, you will have to work harder if you use a manual wheelchair and will increase the risk of pressure sores. If you are fatigued and wearing dressings on a sore, this will limit your feelings of being attractive as well as limit possible positions.

Use of drugs—prescription or otherwise—can impact sexuality. Speak with your doctor about the impact of any prescription medications you take. If you see different doctors, make sure each of them knows what the other has prescribed. Some drugs—particularly spasticity control, pain management, or tranquilizing medications—can directly interfere with sexual arousal, ejaculation for men, or menstruation for women.

Always learn the detailed effects on the body of any medicine or substance you elect to use. For example, some disabled partners have an interest in the drug MDMA, also known as Ecstasy, to heighten their sensual responses. While it may have this effect, it also impedes sexual function. MDMA contains an amphetamine, and the aftermath can include prolonged fatigue and headache. Use extreme caution if you are considering the use of any drug that has not been prescribed for you.

Sex can be better

When you can't feel parts of your body, or have a reduced sexual response, pleasure is often found in more subtle sensations. This paraplegic woman in her thirties observes:

I'm very present when I'm having sex. I'm not thinking about peanut butter sandwiches. I don't know if I would have been that way without a disability. I know that what I've experienced has really helped me to be present. I can imagine that my disability has actually enhanced my overall experience.

Sexual experience can also be better for your partner. Studies have found that many women prefer a slower, more romantic style of sexual sharing and that genital intercourse is not their first priority. A disabled man may be a more satisfying lover in many ways because he may not be as physically or emotionally driven to accomplish intercourse.

Roberta Travis, writing in *New Mobility* magazine, says that the best lover in her experience was a paraplegic man:

He was completely in touch with his body (and mine) in spite of limited sensation, a moderately functional erection and inability to ejaculate. It just didn't matter since neither of us cared to focus on these so-called "negatives." He immersed himself in the moment of intimacy, all fears and pretenses swept aside. He was not, like so many men, primarily penis-oriented and in a hurry to climax.[23]

The physiology of sexual function

Sexual function varies greatly according to the disability, its degree and type. The stage of a degenerative disorder such as multiple sclerosis, the level and completeness of a spinal cord lesion, nerves attacked by the polio virus, the area and extent of an infectious disease of the brain or spinal cord—all are examples of what will differently determine sexual function. The better you understand how your body works, the more realistic your expectations will be of your sexual capacities. Know your body, and you will be freed of unnecessary frustrations and more open to the many enjoyable options which remain available to you.

Some physiological features of your disability will not change. A spinal cord injury, depending on the level and completeness, will affect penile or clitoral sensation and response. Weakness and spasticity from advanced muscular dystrophy, cerebral palsy, or ataxia may disrupt the ability to rotate the pelvis. Examples like these are a fact of your body and its disability.

Sometimes, your physiology can change, even for presumably stable conditions. Take the example of this forty-year old spinal cord paraplegic:

> I gained a capacity for ejaculation some twenty years after my spinal cord injury. I can't say what changed. Perhaps my own belief, since I remember very clearly my doctor telling me at the age of eighteen, just after my injury, that I was not capable of ejaculation. It was a shattering piece of news, and I wonder how much my very acceptance of his statement limited my actual ability.

Belief is a very powerful thing; this is being increasingly proven scientifically. Psychosomatic doesn't just mean in your head. Clear and measurable connections exist between what we think and our body chemistry.

Those who experience muscle spasms will need to identify sexual positions that are less likely to bring them on. For women, spasticity of the perineal muscles can interfere with vaginal penetration. Lying on your back with the knees bent or on your side are positions that are less likely to promote the occurrence of these spasms.

Orgasm is a response which men and women generally associate with peak sexual experience. Stages of the sexual response cycle are marked by increases in blood flow and muscle tension. Changes in the body you might experience include erection of the penis in men, enlargement of the clitoris or vaginal lubrication in women, sex flush (blood flow to the skin), an increase in heart rate and blood pressure, a focusing of the mind to the body, and a deep quality of relaxation.

Orgasm is very much a matter of where you put your attention. Sexuality researcher Mitch Tepper says:

> Orgasmic sex is about being in the moment and forgetting about quad bellies, atrophy, catheters, and making embarrassing sounds. What's right is what works now.[24]

What kind of sexual response you are capable of depends on the nature of your disability and nerve damage. It is also a question of time. Most spinal-injured men will be capable of erection within six months of injury, some sooner. Both women and men recover varying degrees of sensitivity and response after injury. In the case of a progressive condition such as MS, loss of response—and interest—is not unusual and might come and go over time.

In a 1995 Kessler study, twenty-five women with SCI were asked to attempt to achieve orgasm in a laboratory setting. Partners were allowed to provide stimulation if needed. They found that level of injury was less of a factor, and that education was significant:

> *Neurological pattern of injury did not preclude the ability to have orgasm; thus both women with complete and incomplete injuries should be considered candidates for sex therapy aimed at improving their ability to achieve orgasm. Women who experienced orgasms were significantly more knowledgeable about sexuality and had a higher sex drive than did women who did not experience orgasm. Sexual education would seem to be an important factor in overall sexual responsiveness and satisfaction.*[25]

There are two ways in which genital arousal takes place in the body. A psychogenic response is brought on by sensual thoughts—the presence of your partner or fantasies, for instance. Psychogenic response relies on a connection from the brain to the lower thoracic/upper lumbar area. For example, those with complete spinal cord injuries at or above these levels, sensual thoughts are unlikely to produce erection in men or clitoral enlargement and lubrication in women. With impact below this area or incomplete lesions, the psychogenic response is likely to remain.

Reflexogenic stimulations work from the other direction. They travel a direct route from the genitals to the cord and back. They can occur in the presence of varying types of genital stimulation, intended sexually or not. Some men experience reflexogenic erection during catheterization or from the weight of bedding. Persons with complete lower lumbar and sacral injury to the spinal cord will not have a reflexogenic response.

Most people with spinal cord conditions have some degree of sexual response. The area of the spinal cord between T10 and L2 is where sexual responses is processed. So people with conditions above T10, in which messages from the brain cannot reach this area, are less likely to have a psychogenic response, and more likely to have reflexive responses. The reverse is true when the effect on the cord is below L2. It is more difficult to predict response when the cord is affected between T10 and L2, particularly when the impact is incomplete.

Discovering your capacity for orgasm is a matter of experimentation, time, and patience. Your body might even go through changes over longer periods of time after a disabling trauma. In this case it is true that practice makes perfect. If orgasm is difficult or seems doubtful, don't give up trying. You'll discover how best to stimulate yourself and what kinds of sensations are possible. The right moment might arrive when you least expect it.

Sexual options

If genital sex with orgasm is impossible, difficult, or painful for you, what's left? There are many adaptations to any situation and options to consider. You are a sexual *being*, not a sexual body part.

What's possible for a disabled lover?

What sexual activities remain possible? Start with kissing—an extremely enjoyable and underrated pastime. Don't limit yourself to each other's lips. The face, the ears, the neck, the shoulders, the back—so many places that even the most severe disabilities leave capable of sensations—are extremely erotic. For example, many men have failed to appreciate the pleasure of having their nipples licked.

Touch alone is very powerful. A gentle touch of a hand on your face, or the slow exploration of each other's body is very erotic. Caressing expresses loving feelings, and promotes the relaxed, take-your-time approach to lovemaking which helps a couple reach deeper levels of passion and intimacy.

Sensual massage—in which you incorporate erogenous zones such as nipples and genitals—is an excellent way to sidestep the pressure of performance. There are books that illustrate techniques of massage possible for people with limited grip strength by using vibrators or gloves. You can take turns with this and allow each other the absolute luxury of receiving totally, knowing that you will be able to return the favor. Sensual massage is a great way to find those previously undiscovered areas of sensitivity.

There are usually many undiscovered places. Try the palms of the hands, inside the elbow, or behind the knee. There are thousands of nerve endings in places like this that light up when kissed or touched but which many people take for granted. Research has shown that when parts of the body lose sensory function, the brain turns up the volume elsewhere. Parts of the body still with feeling become more sensitive.

> *My chiropractor and my massage therapist both say that my upper body is much more sensitive than other people they work with. They share*

the theory that it is a compensation for my paraplegia, that the rest of my
body became more sensitive because of the lost sensation in the lower
part.

When the woman is disabled, she usually still has the option of sharing genital intercourse, even if she might not perceive sensation from it. There may be a need for additional lubricants. Water-soluble products such as K-Y Jelly should be used rather than petroleum-based lubricants, which can promote infection. Men having intercourse with a disabled woman might experience less friction as a result of weakened vaginal muscles. Yet the reverse may also be true: a woman with spasticity could have very active vaginal muscles during intercourse.

Women's fear of not pleasing a partner because of lack of tightness in the vagina can interfere with pleasure, just as men can be concerned about maintaining an erection. However, less friction might extend the amount of time a couple can participate in intercourse before male ejaculation occurs; if intercourse becomes tiring, the couple can use other options to achieve satisfaction. Regardless of the muscle tone of vaginal muscles, intercourse is a very intimate experience, but doesn't have to be the final act of a lovemaking session.

Oral stimulation

Oral techniques can take on a greater role in disabled sex. Oral sex may not have been part of your sexual repertoire; you may imagine it is inappropriate or unpleasant; you may even feel it is taboo. Younger persons might not be comfortable with the idea if they have never participated in this kind of contact. Yet many consider oral sex as enjoyable a form of lovemaking as they would ever experience.

Some women report that intercourse is less stimulating than genital stimulation with the mouth, tongue, or lips. This may be exactly the forte of a disabled partner.

There has been some concern expressed that oral contact can transmit sexually transmitted diseases such as AIDS. Mitch Tepper explains:

This is considered a low risk activity for acquiring the HIV virus, but
if fluids reach an open sore in or near the mouth, it is still possible for a
virus to enter the bloodstream.

If you have concerns about disease transmission, there are unlubricated and even flavored condoms which a man can wear. Women can use a dental dam or improvise with plastic wrap. As in any sexual partnership, both partners should be aware of their health status, be honest about past contact and, if necessary, request appropriate testing to ensure each others' health and ultimate trust. Once you feel you can trust that a monogamous relationship is well established, these matters become less of a concern.

Changing your style

New sexual possibilities open up when you are willing to change your attitudes and reconsider previous beliefs. You might need to become more the giver of pleasure rather than focusing so much on your own, and perhaps discover a surprising degree of stimulation in that role. You can use sex toys, view adult videos, or read erotic material together.

If you are with a fully orgasmic partner, you can "ride the wave," drawn into the intensity of their climax. The deep, shared connection with your lover is itself an orgasmic experience, a shifted consciousness. If your attention is fully with them, and not thinking about what you aren't feeling, you have a greater chance of experiencing emotions and sensations that will be very satisfying.

While you might shift your attention to your partner, that doesn't mean giving up the idea of being the recipient of direct pleasure for yourself. Mitch Tepper writes:

> The possibility and benefits of receiving sexual pleasure still need to be pursued. Reciprocal sexual pleasure is seldom impossible.[26]

The visual experience is often amplified for the disabled lover. Choose positions where the disabled partner can see what is going on, with enough light for the purpose. Perhaps leave your glasses on or your contact lenses in place. A disabled man who cannot see what is happening might not be certain of the state of his erection. This can be discouraging and distract from the ability to relax into the moment. Many disabled men are gratified by being able to participate in intercourse at all and being able to also witness intercourse is particularly stimulating.

Anything that is pleasurable is fine. You are in the privacy of your own relationship. Whatever you choose, in any order, at any time is entirely up to you. The more you can drop your expectations and assumptions, the more possibilities will reveal themselves to you and the more satisfying your sexuality can be.

Take extra care

Sex can be physically demanding. Your disability may preclude your ability to move in certain ways. For example, without the ability to use your legs, hips, and bottom to assist in pelvic movements, the conventional work of intercourse becomes tiring very quickly. An able-bodied partner needs to understand that certain motions have a time limit. The partner can take on more of the physical work, and you can relax and enjoy, moving as your capacity allows.

Use pillows or various sized cushions to help get your bodies into comfortable positions—and within reach. Pillows can also help stabilize you so you can remain in a given position longer. The strain of needing to shift your weight or fatigue from bracing with your arms can distract from your pleasure.

Educate your partner about your ability to balance yourself and in what directions and positions you are able to bear weight. If your upper body balance is limited, your partner will need to know when not to lean weight against you, such as when sitting up, straddled together. This position can work with the proper support, possibly even in your wheelchair.

You need to change positions regularly to prevent pressure sores. This takes attention, since you may not have sensations to tell you when to move. Hugging with your partner in the wonderful aftermath and glow of lovemaking, you might not want to break the spell to shift positions. But at some point you must; this is an important point for your partner to be aware of. You can just say, "It's time," and find another lovely way to lie together.

Toys and the setting

Explore the world of sensual products, which are now quite easy to acquire without the stigma of being in poor taste. If you are uncomfortable going into a shop, there are catalog suppliers who are very discreet in their packaging.

Sensual products include:

- **Dildos.** An artificial penis which a female partner might enjoy as a supplement to whatever capability a disabled male partner may have for erection. Lesbian relationships benefit, too.

- **Vibrators.** Available in many shapes and sizes and can be sexually satisfying or used to give massage to either partner.

- **Erection rings.** Position at the base of the penis to retain blood which creates the erection, thus maintaining it.

- **Penis stiffeners.** Worn as a supplement to ease the pressure of having to maintain a full erection.

- **Books and videos.** For private stimulation, to share with a partner, or for instructive purposes.

You can make simple modifications to these products—such as a velcro strap for a vibrator or dildo—to accommodate limited grip strength that might otherwise be needed to use them.

Some couples enjoy using a waterbed, which some already use for prevention of pressure sores. Waterbeds can be difficult to get in and out of for a person with a disability, but when properly filled, heated, and padded are very comfortable. The rocking motion can contribute to enjoyment during sex.

Pay attention to the setting for romance. Set soft lights or burn candles. Choose music that will enhance the mood. Wear sexy clothes that are fun to take off of each other. Use perfumes or incense (we are biologically built to respond to sensual aromas) or surround yourselves with flowers. Remove items that could detract from romance, like prescription bottles at the bedside. Pay attention to the setting and have fun with romance.

Bowel and bladder issues

In a scene from the film *The Waterdance*, a recently injured quadriplegic man is with his female lover for the first time since his accident. During their lovemaking his catheter slips, wetting the bed. His reaction is embarrassment and frustration while she attempts to reassure him that it is not a problem. But the moment has been lost. They are caught by surprise in these new emotional dynamics of their sexuality.

Certainly loss of bladder control can interrupt the romance of the moment, but the couple in the film was facing the shock of their first encounter with the issue. When a couple develop a true intimate bond, their bodily fluids need not be repelling. We all deal with body fluids—urine, semen, menstrual blood. Many people will be barely troubled by such slips.

A brief spasm of urination or movement of the bowels might occur during particular motions. Some of the same reflexes triggered during sex also control bladder and bowel activity. Choose techniques or positions that are less likely to exert pressure on these areas, or time such activities earlier in your lovemaking before the bladder begins to fill again.

Keep a towel handy just in case. Empty the bladder as fully as possible and take care not to drink excessively before sex. A regular bowel management program will help prevent surprises.

An indwelling catheter—which remains in place continuously—can be bent over and worn inside of a condom during intercourse, taking care to not exert any tension on it. Use of an internal catheter increases the risk of urinary tract infection which can be passed on to a sexual partner. Emptying the bladder after intercourse will help prevent infections.

Women with indwelling catheters may be able to leave them in during intercourse, depending on the size of their vagina and the positions used. Some have found that a catheter is able to remain in place more easily when the man enters the woman from behind.

Men who wear a condom-like external catheter need to remove it before genital contact, cleaning the area to remove traces of adhesive and urine. Some men develop a sensitivity to latex and experience drying of the skin of the penis, or open sores, particularly on the head which is very delicate. A high commitment to cleanliness, the use of creams, or switching to a silicone type of catheter help manage this problem. It is unwise to have intercourse while the skin of the penis is irritated or broken down. A normal prophylactic condom might be used at such times.

A partner or spouse who aids you in bowel and bladder care may come to have a difficult time seeing you in sexual terms. If personal assistance duties are placing stress on your sexual relationship, take some time to explore ways to shift the responsibility from your partner by doing more yourself, if possible, or perhaps by employing a greater degree of outside attendant assistance. Perhaps there are portions of your support that you had not thought you could perform. There might be products available to aid in grip and dexterity that you were not aware of or had only thought of for other purposes, like feeding. Be creative and open-minded, and possibilities will increase.

Male erection

While there are many other ways of being sexual, it is the desire of most men to be able to reliably participate in intercourse. It is psychologically gratifying for a man to perform intercourse. As much as their partner might not begrudge a limitation on erection, most partners enjoy this form of sexual contact. More to the point, it is a lovely experience to share.

How erection occurs and is maintained is complex, and depends on the physiology of the specific disability as well as psychological factors. Men with a disability experience either psychogenic or reflexogenic erections or both. More spinal cord impairments occur above the area of the spine where psychogenic erectile function is processed in the hypogastric nerve plexus between T10 and L2. This means that fewer men experience erection psychogenically, since their erotic thoughts cannot stimulate that area of the spine, but their reflexogenic processes remain intact. In either case, surface sensation is not necessary to accomplish erection.

But loss of penile sensation might limit the ability to maintain an erection if a man's expectation is that the sensation of intercourse is what stimulates erection. Loss of sensation (not always the case in a disabled man) might lead to doubts about the ability to maintain the erection, especially in positions where the man cannot see his penis during intercourse. To the degree that a psychogenic process is involved, such mental distractions will affect the ability to maintain an erection.

This is not much different from problems of erectile dysfunction that many able-bodied men experience, where the cause can be either psychological or physical. Thinking, "Can I keep it up?" is almost a guarantee of not being able to. It is simply a case of performance anxiety. The ability to clear the mind during sexual intimacy is as important a psychological skill for disabled men as for anyone else. At the same time, our desires ebb and flow with our body chemistry and the events of our lives at the time. No one is always ready for sex.

Psychogenic erection can rely on very subtle forms of touch and contact. Being subtle, these sensations might be overridden by bearing a partner's body weight or by body contact which pulls on hairs. Part of the method is to shift your attention to more subtle sensations that men with later disabilities might never have noticed prior to disability, or never thought of these feelings as being sensual. Sexuality educator Mitch Tepper notes:

> It's about getting in touch with subtle forms. I try to help people develop them with techniques such as breathing, focusing, and biofeedback.

Partners will need to work out techniques so that the disabled partner can still have the sensations that are pleasurable and maintain erection. Choose positions carefully and emphasize the kinds of touch that are arousing.

An adolescent, injured at the stage of his peak period of testosterone levels (the male hormone) and his early sexual experimentation might imagine that he would have to maintain the degree of erectile rigidity he experienced as a teenager in order to be able to enter his partner. The inability to do so is thought of as a severe failure. According to this thirty-six-year old spinal cord paraplegic:

> I have since learned that all men reach a lesser degree of response as they age, which need not impair their capacity for intercourse. Age eighteen is the point of optimal potency, but those of us injured at that time have no other point of reference.

The "stuff" method is a way to share intercourse with a lesser erection. The flaccid penis is pushed into the vagina; this is more easily achieved in certain positions. Squeezing the base of the penis will direct more blood into the shaft and head, increasing erection. Keep pressure at the base—or use an erection ring designed for that purpose—to prolong erection.

Always ask your doctor about the implications of any treatment or elective surgery you might be considering. You may well choose to surrender some sexual function in favor of reduced pain or some other benefit in order to extend your independence. Just be fully informed.

Methods to induce erection

There are a number of methods that reliably produce erections. Most men and their partners need to experiment to find the best solution. The invasive nature of some of these approaches is another reason to explore other sexual options rather than be overly reliant on penile intercourse.

Vacuum pumps have been used for erectile dysfunction over the last twenty years. A plastic tube with either a motorized or manual pump creates a vacuum which draws blood into the penis. An erection ring fits at the base of the penis, holding in blood to maintain the erection. The health of the skin on and around the penis needs special attention from regular users of the pump, particularly those who use catheters. Check regularly for irritation. Sexuality researcher Dr. Marca Sipski of the Kessler Institute for Rehabilitation in New Jersey says that:

> Rings should not be used for more than thirty minutes. Gangrene of the penis has been shown to occur in men who have fallen asleep with the rings on.

Prostaglandin—marketed under the name Caverject—is a drug which is injected into the corpa cavernosa, the area of the penis which fills with blood and therefore produces erection. Men are trained in making the injections themselves prior to sex. The drug causes blood to flow to the corpa cavernosa, and the resulting pressure constricts the area which allows the erection to last longer. Erection occurs in about twenty minutes and lasts generally no more than two hours, depending on the dosage. One needs to take great care with cleanliness and must avoid veins in the penis which could bleed excessively if violated by the needle.

There is a danger of over-stimulation. Priapism is a condition in which blood held too long in the penis can begin to clot. In general, an erection which lasts more than four hours is worthy of concern. This is a serious enough event to require immediate medical attention. An overdose or the excessive use of injections can cause permanent damage.

Recently a drug has appeared that does not require injection. Sold commercially under the name of MUSE, a suppository is placed into the urethra through the tip of the penis. It has not been found to be as effective as the injections.

The oral drug Viagra is a relatively new treatment for erectile dysfunction. Viagra has some known potential side effects such as transiently changing one's vision; it can pose health risks when taken with medications containing nitroglycerin; it doesn't work for all men; and it is expensive and some insurers or HMOs do not pay for the drug.

Nevertheless, Dr. Michelle Gittler of Schwab Rehabilitation Hospital in Chicago says:

> *I can only tell you that my guys who rely on reflexogenic erections swear by Viagra.*

There are also permanent, surgical solutions. Penile implants are available in various forms. One is a solid silicone rod which provides an immovable, semi-erect solution. Another is a flexible silicone rod so the penis can be adjusted downward for comfort away from sexual activity. A self-contained implant will become firm when it is squeezed or bent, and return to a flaccid state after a period of time. Lastly, an inflatable prostheses—the most expensive—allows manual control of the degree of erection as needed. There is some risk that the pump—also implanted under the skin—may leak or that pressure sores could form inside the penis.

Since these are surgical alternatives, there is always some risk from the invasive nature of their installation and the presence of a foreign object inside of the body. Discuss these options in detail with your urologist, and take the time to speak with others who have experienced them. Mitch Tepper comments on the dangers of implants:

> *There is some risk of erosion from the inside. The rod can stick through the end of the penis or back near the testicles. There is more risk of complication from implants than from any of the other options. Even if you take it out, there is damage to tissue, and it may be difficult to go back to using injections or any other method. The ability to get the same erections as before surgery may be reduced.*

A couple should discuss how these solutions will affect their sense of intimacy. Will the partner feel that the artificial erection has less to do with how appealing she is? On the other hand, a greater sense of security about their erection can allow men to focus more on the sensuality of the moment. The range of positions can also expand as there is less need to prevent the overriding sensations mentioned earlier which can counteract erection.

Birth control

Disabled women need protection from pregnancy as much as able-bodied women. Some special considerations need to be made for disabled women, especially those who have limited sensations in the genital area. Find a gynecologist familiar with your disability who can advise you on the fine points.

Menstruation is usually interrupted in women after a spinal disease or injury, but usually returns within six months as the body recovers from its shock. Women who are close to menopause may find that their menses will not start again.

The pill is the most effective birth control method, but there is a risk for disabled women of thrombophlebitis—blood clotting as a result of poor circulation in the legs from not walking. Women who experience spasticity are less exposed to this problem since muscle contractions assist in the movement of blood. Your gynecologist can perform a test for susceptibility to clotting.

Some professionals feel that the risk of clotting plus the inability to recognize problems because of limited sensation are cause enough for disabled women not to use the pill. Guidelines developed by Planned Parenthood of New York City specifically recommend against them. Others say that with today's lower dosages, the risks are minimal, and that if clotting has not occurred within six months after disability, it is unlikely to occur with the pill. You must also consider interaction with other medications you might take.

Progestagen injections provide protection for 90 days with a very high success rate. Progestin subdermal implants are also highly effective and can remain in place for up to five years.

An intrauterine device (IUD) presents an increased risk of infection. Disabled women need to pay extra attention to warning signs such as:

- Pain
- Cramps
- Fever
- Vaginal discharge
- Light spotting (bleeding)
- Changes in menstrual cycles
- Increase in spasticity

Those with reduced sensation should check the placement of the IUD often to ensure it is in place. Risks include pelvic inflammatory disease, ectopic pregnancy where a fetus begins to develop outside the womb, and perforation of the uterine wall, which is rare.

Again, there is disagreement on the wisdom of using an IUD. Its placement and removal can cause autonomic dysreflexia, typically an issue only for women with spinal cord injuries above the sixth thoracic vertebra. Women who use anticoagulants should not use an IUD. Excessive blood flow could occur during menstruation.

Diaphragms and vaginal condoms are effective about 90 percent of the time. A diaphragm also needs to be checked carefully for position, particularly for women who press on their bladder to assist in manual voiding. Extended wearing of a diaphragm also increases risk of infection. Women who used one prior to injury should be refitted to account for weight change and reduced muscle tone.

A vaginal condom requires the use of a spermicidal foam or jelly. Users of a Foley catheter who leave it in place during sex need to take care that the condom is not torn by the catheter.

Sponges and caps are moderately effective and available without a prescription. Like the IUD, diaphragm, and condom, they require sufficient hand function to insert and position. Sponges are more effective in women who have not already given birth.

Natural methods of birth control involving timing and abstinence are statistically the most unreliable. Some women opt for sterilization, having already had their children or knowing they choose not to be mothers. This is very effective, but entails some surgical risk.

Pregnancy and parenthood

Can disabled women conceive and have babies? Yes, in most cases.

Can disabled men make babies? Increasingly the answer is, "Yes."

Until recently, not many paraplegic men were producing children. But now men with spinal cord injuries are increasingly able to make babies. Likewise, spina bifida will affect the ability to produce children according to the scale of the disability and what mechanics of the reproductive system are affected by the disability. The question of childbearing seems to come up more with regard to spinal cord injury, thus its emphasis in the following discussion.

The Baylor College of Medicine study on women with disabilities found that the medical profession is not serving women well with regard to pregnancy. Providers and the women themselves often operated under the false belief that women with spinal cord injury should avoid pregnancy. Recent ten-year studies have found that women with spinal cord injury are giving birth more often, yet:

> Very few clinicians have experience managing pregnancy, labor, and delivery in women with SCI. Unfounded assumptions of poor outcomes may influence clinicians to behave as though risks are greater than they actually are. If the chance of a positive pregnancy outcome is considered slim, or threat to the mother's life too high, clinicians may encourage women who want to have their babies to have unnecessary or undesired therapeutic abortions.[27]

This paraplegic woman reports being given incorrect medical advice:

> I was thirteen when I broke my back. (I'm a complete paraplegic.) I remember being told by my blushing sixty-year-old doctor that I could have children, but only by caesarian section. I have since found out that that is totally untrue.

Women in the Baylor study reported having trouble finding obstetricians or midwives willing to assist them in what were considered high risk pregnancies. The Baylor report says that their own study and previous findings confirm:

> Normal labor and delivery are possible, even routine, and generally pose little or no added risk to the mother or baby.[28]

Physicians and midwives do need to understand issues faced by women with disabilities including autonomic dysreflexia, urinary tract infections, skin breakdown, spasticity, and the effect on a fetus of medications they might be using.

Before you start trying to have a child, address health and emotional considerations. You'll probably wonder what it's like to be a parent with a disability. If you are a woman, you'll want to consider the consequences on your own health of becoming pregnant.

If you are disabled by a genetic condition, you will want to fully understand the odds and consequences of passing such a condition on to a child. This does not mean you should choose not to bear children if there is a chance of passing on a disability. People with disabilities have historically been told that they should not be parents—much less sexual—because it would be wrong to bear a child with a disability. This attitude is widely viewed by people with disabilities as discriminatory. You have the right to bear children, and such testing for genetically passed disability is available to you for your own information. The decision is yours.

Can you parent?

Disabled people are raising children with great success, adapting creatively to child-rearing just as they do to their mobility needs. Children naturally adapt to your parenting style.

Meeting the physical needs of parenting means finding additional ways to adapt to a disability. Slings, seat belts, and velcro come in very handy for securing a child in your lap. Adjustable-height tables make it easy to lift your child from a lower position, then raise the child to a higher level for changing diapers and so on. For parents with limited hand use, buttons and snaps on children's clothing can be replaced with velcro, and loops placed on shoes to help pull them on. A modest degree of family support or paid help might be used during stages when physical demands are greater.

The cultural aspects of parenting can be challenging. Once your child is in school, relationships with other parents and the community are a source of important support, information, and local advocacy. But other parents might not support your need for access to their home, or schools might plan events you cannot attend for lack of access. Some people think that the child takes care of the parent, an assumption that is deeply insulting to parents with a disability, who work as hard as any other on behalf of their children.

Through the Looking Glass is a group in Oakland, California, operating on a five-year grant from the National Resource Center for Parents with Disabilities. At an October 1997 conference, a task force met to review a recent national survey of 1,200 parents with disabilities conducted by Berkeley Planning Associates in Berkeley, California. Here are some of the results:[29]

- 36 percent of disabled parents reported that their medical providers' lack of disability expertise caused problems in prenatal and birthing services.

- 31 percent reported medical providers' attitudes caused barriers.

- Disabled parents reported needing assistance in: recreation with their children (43 percent), traveling outside the home with their children (40 percent), chasing or retrieving children (39 percent), and lifting or carrying children (33 percent).

- Transportation affected more aspects of parenting with a disability than any other issue. 79 percent reported transportation as a problem which interfered with or prevented routine as well as critical parent-child activities.

- Cost was the most frequently identified barrier to childcare (30 percent), followed by lack of transportation (20 percent).

- 48 percent reported adaptive parenting equipment was too expensive. 32 percent reported adaptive equipment was unavailable or not yet designed.

- 57 percent reported using personal assistance services for help with parenting. 54 percent reported services were not available when needed. 46 percent reported services were unreliable.

- 43 percent reported difficulty finding housing.

- 32 percent reported facing discrimination.

- 14 percent reported pressure to have a tubal ligation. 13 percent reported being urged to have an abortion.

The children

Children of disabled parents tend to be more independent, learning to do appropriate tasks for themselves that are strenuous for the parent. For example, very young children develop the ability to climb onto a wheelchair and maintain their balance. These children also get the chance to have a deeper compassion for all people, drawing a lesson from the perspective they gain through their parents.

Don't be surprised if you find a lack of support for your decision to have a child. Society still imagines that a disabled parent puts a child at risk by not being able to respond to an emergency or chase a child into a place where a wheelchair cannot go. Your family, friends, church members, or colleagues may withhold their support. In *Spinal Network*, a woman with mild cerebral palsy, is quoted as recalling:

*I was told quite bluntly by many that I had no right to have a child. I
was told I was selfish; I was repeatedly told that I could not hold, care for,
or look after the baby.*[30]

Children of disabled parents don't know the difference. To them, a wheelchair is totally normal. They know that their parents function fully and love
fully—doing all they can to provide a healthy upbringing.

Donnie Herman—son of Paul, a paraplegic, and Anne, a quadriplegic—was
asked at the age of ten if he would like to see his parents cured. "Cured of
what?" he answered.

Getting pregnant: male ejaculation

A man's inability to produce a usable ejaculate is one weak link in a couple's
ability to bear children. For example, among those with spinal cord injuries,
an injured woman is usually capable of conceiving, carrying the fetus and
giving birth. The challenge rests with the man with a spinal cord injury. Sexuality research has focused more on male sexuality and the two issues of
sperm retrieval and quality.

Depending on the type and level of impact on the spinal cord, a disabled
man may or may not be capable of ejaculation. The response from the head
of the penis travels to a given portion of the spinal cord—between T10 and
T12—independent of nerves traveling to the brain. It is a completely reflexive process.

Semen and sperm are two separate substances which are combined at the
very moment of ejaculation, which is initiated as a biochemical and nervous
system response. Three discrete steps take place:

1. Emission is the step in which sperm and other fluids are secreted from
   the Cowper's and prostate glands, the seminal vesicles, and from the testicles. These fluids assist the motility—the portion that are actively
   swimming—of the sperm, lubricate the movement of ejaculate through
   the urethra and out the penis, and include the sperm itself.

2. In the second stage, the bladder neck is closed to prevent semen from
   backing into the bladder during ejaculation. Disabled men with
   impaired nerve function might experience retrograde ejaculation, in
   which semen flows back into the bladder. The acid environment of the
   bladder and urine is a threat to semen, though if urine is collected and

sterilized, it can be possible to harvest semen from urine for artificial insemination.

3. Ejaculation is the forcible expulsion of the ejaculate, and the third step of the process. This occurs via the second to the fourth sacral segments. Complete injury in this area will usually preclude ejaculation.

For men with a spinal cord injury, there is less frequency of pregnancy. In a study at the Miami Project to Cure Paralysis, only 10 percent of men with a spinal cord injury who were able to ejaculate during intercourse succeeded in impregnating their mates.[31] In men injured at a younger age, the maturation of their testicles may have been hampered. In others, it is possible that irreversible structural atrophy can occur as a result of their disability. Such changes are more likely to occur within six months of injury, if at all. There is a suspicion on the part of researchers that there might be hormonal abnormalities in spinal cord injured men which affect sperm production.

A severe bladder infection can cause sterility. An infection can spread from the bladder to other genital passages, and compromise reproductive capabilities. Marijuana smoking also has damaging effects on sperm. One cycle of sperm production takes three months, during which time you want to recover from any present infection, take extra care with your bladder program and drinking, and abstain from any damaging substances.

Assuming there is no physiological damage, there are products that can help produce an ejaculate. A vibrator can stimulate ejaculation. A product still in development from MMG Healthcare uses a specific frequency and amplitude of vibration to induce ejaculation; the FertiCare vibrator is available from ILTS, Inc., in Evans, Georgia. The manufacturers report a high success rate of ejaculates. Over-stimulation with a vibrator, however, can be a risk to tissues if used excessively. For example, FertiCare and MMG recommend sessions of three minutes with a pause of one minute, repeated up to five times.

With electro-ejaculation, a probe is inserted through the anus to directly stimulate the nerves which elicit the ejaculation response. Men with sensation may require anesthesia for the procedure. The duration and voltage must be carefully monitored to avoid burns. Those with higher spinal cord lesions might be at risk of autonomic dysreflexia. Ejaculation may not occur on the first attempt.

The issue is not limited to gaining ejaculate, it is also about the quality of the product. Spinal-cord injured men have been found to have a normal number of sperm; however, the sperm have lower survival rates and less capacity to make the swim all the way to the uterus and the egg. An average male has a sperm motility of 60 percent. In a study conducted by Nancy Brackett *et al* of the Miami Project to Cure Paralysis, spinal cord injured men have been found to have rates ranging from 23.5 to 30.9 percent.[32]

Temperature is a factor in potency. Consider the shape of the male genitalia, in which the scrotum hangs freely to allow the testicles to have plenty of air surrounding them for a cooling effect. Since disabled men sit most of the time, the testicles stay warmer. It has been postulated that this temperature difference compromises semen quality.

This view however, is not without its detractors. Nancy Brackett reports:

> A cohort of men with spinal cord injury who walk did not use a wheelchair for locomotion (i.e., they walked with crutches) had semen quality as impaired as that of men who used wheelchairs. Based on these studies, there appears to be no strong evidence to suggest that elevated scrotal temperature in men with SCI is a major contributor to their poor semen quality.[33]

Other factors suspected of affecting sperm motility, as discussed in the 1996 Brackett study include:[34]

- **Methods of bladder management.** Men using intermittent catheterization had better motility.

- **Infrequency of ejaculation.** Intervals of less than one week but greater than twelve weeks resulted in ejaculates with lower sperm concentration or motility.

- **Hormonal changes.** While men with SCI have been found to have the same levels of testosterone—the male hormone—as uninjured men, some study subjects had elevated levels of follicle-simulating hormone (FSH) and were found to have no sperm in their semen.

The quality of semen is apparently affected by the method of collection. In another study led by Nancy Brackett, the percentage of motile sperm was greater for study subjects who used vibratory stimulation as compared to electro-ejaculation, although the sperm counts were comparable.[35] They found that there is a larger component of retrograde ejaculate with electro-ejaculation—sperm which had been exposed to the destructive acid environment of the bladder. This seems to account for the difference.

The potency problem can be solved by collecting and then freezing ejaculate, preparing it for artificial insemination at a later time. Not all frozen sperm recover the ability to swim, so this process involves gaining several samples, and then combining them with a fresh ejaculate before inseminating the woman. In another study led by Osvaldo Padron at the University of Miami in 1994, freezing sperm of spinal cord injured men was no more destructive than for able-bodied men.[36]

In some cases, taking hormones can help produce more sperm to aid this process. There may be supplements you can take to improve quality of sperm.

Getting pregnant: other approaches

There are a number of methods for becoming pregnant—that is, when the traditional approach isn't working. They range in cost and complexity. Typically, you would start with the least expensive and least invasive methods.

Some couples are willing to invest almost any amount of time, expense, physical stress, and emotion to have a child of their own. It can be a considerable drain. A single advanced procedure can cost as much as $15,000 per try, while using vibration and at-home insemination is very inexpensive. Most who succeed say that, having had their child, it was well worth whatever they went through. Yet the success rate is not high, so there is the risk of being left exhausted and depressed—and broke! You and your partner need to fully explore your feelings about having your own biological child, and weigh what you discover against current medical options to decide what is best for you.

When the man is able to produce an ejaculate—by any of the methods mentioned earlier—sperm is collected and then the woman is inseminated by injecting the ejaculate with a needle-less syringe. When a procedure such as electro-ejaculation is performed in an office or clinic, the insemination will also be performed there. A couple can increase the odds of success by the use of drugs that stimulate the production of more than one egg per cycle, and by using standard methods to identify the woman's peak ovulation.

When normal ejaculation occurs, the sperm is sent into the cervix at approximately thirty miles per hour. With the injection method, sperm have to be helped along with gravity by having the woman lie on her back and elevate her pelvis for a period of time after injection.

Modern science offers several options for uniting a sperm and an egg. A couple can consider:

- **Intrauterine insemination (IUI).** Sperm is collected and analyzed for quality and quantity. The specimen is washed and concentrated in preparation for insemination. The woman is monitored for her cycles, and just before ovulation, a hormone is given to induce it. On the day of insemination, a fresh ejaculate is obtained, the concentrated specimen is added to it, and then injected directly into the uterus.

- **Intratubal insemination (ITI).** This method is recommended when there are two eggs in the same fallopian tube, which is where insemination normally takes place. With ITI, the ejaculate is delivered via a catheter while watching with ultrasound, and the sperm is placed as close to the ovum as possible to increase the chance of success.

- **In vitro fertilization-embryo transfer (IVF-ET).** Widely known as the test-tube baby procedure, the goal here is to generate as many healthy eggs as possible in order to harvest them before ovulation and perform the insemination outside of the body. In twenty-four hours, it is possible to observe if fertilization took place, and then replace the embryos into the uterus. This procedure has shown only a 12 to 17 percent success rate.

- **Gamete intrafallopian transfer (GIFT).** Eggs are harvested as in IVF, but rather than being combined outside in a dish, the eggs and sperm are placed back into the fallopian tubes via a catheter. The process proceeds naturally within the woman's body with a 36 percent success rate.

- **Zygote intrafallopian transfer (ZIFT).** Insemination is performed in a dish to produce viable embryos, and then placed into the fallopian tubes rather than the uterus. This procedure has a 37 percent success rate.

- **Intracytoplasmic sperm injection (ICSI).** It is now possible to extract sperm from an ejaculate, or directly from either the testicles or the epididymis—a very long, convoluted tube where sperm mature until they are stored until ejaculation. These sperm are then injected into an egg using either the IVF, GIFT, or ZIFT process. Only a few motile sperm are required for the process.

Pregnancy

Pregnancy involves major changes to the body and metabolism. Some of the possible effects for any woman include anemia, thrombophlebitis, swelling in the legs, blood pressure changes, carpal tunnel syndrome, infections, constipation, morning sickness, and so on. Any of these problems are minimized by being in good health at the beginning of the pregnancy, and making a commitment to the best pre- and post-natal care.

A pregnant woman using a wheelchair faces additional issues. As you gain weight, there will be increased ischial pressure and added risk of skin breakdown. Be certain to have a proper and well-maintained wheelchair cushion. A different product might be necessary during the later stage of the pregnancy. You will need to do pressure relief push-ups or change your posture more often to prevent sores, so some upper body exercise for added arm strength might be in order. As you gain weight you might even need a wider wheelchair, especially if you are being pinched in the hips where there is risk of skin breakdown. Take measures to ensure the health of your skin, keeping it very clean, optimizing your diet for healthy tissue and circulation.

Any medications you take for bladder control, stool softening, control of spasms, or other implications of your disability need to be completely reviewed with your doctor at the earliest possible stage of your pregnancy. Bladder infections during pregnancy present a risk to the fetus. Certain antibiotics used to treat infections can be even more dangerous to the baby. Some women use Valium to control spasms. There are cases of babies who have had to endure Valium withdrawal after birth.

Miscarriage rates are no different for disabled women than for the general population. Spinal cord injured women are at no increased risk of children with birth defects. Birth weights are typically within normal ranges. Women with multiple sclerosis or muscular dystrophy may pass on genetic tendencies to these disabilities.

You might not sense the early signs of labor if you have spinal injury above T10, and could miss the opportunity to prepare for delivery before your water breaks. Normal vaginal delivery is possible in most cases, but if you are without use of abdominal muscles the doctor might need to assist in lieu of your inability to push down. Forceps, a vacuum extraction unit, or an episiotomy—in which incisions are made to enlarge the vaginal opening—might be called for. Cesarean delivery may be necessary in some cases, but no more often than for nondisabled women.

Some doctors recommend beginning cervical checks at twenty-six weeks since there is some statistical evidence of increased risk of premature delivery by spinal cord injured women. They might even recommend hospitalization after thirty-two weeks to monitor the pregnancy as closely as possible. There is risk of dysreflexia during delivery for women injured above T6, a fact that your obstetrician should be aware of.

Disabled women can breastfeed. This is a reflexive response initiated by the baby's sucking. Some women injured above T6 experience a decrease in milk production after a time due to lack of nipple sensation.

For a woman using a wheelchair, pregnancy has its extra challenges. For this couple, it raised questions about having another child:

> My husband thinks having one child is perfect and doesn't even want to consider a second. I truly believe it is for the most part because he doesn't want me to have to go through the ordeal of pregnancy again. It was hard on me, but in a way I think it was just as hard on him to see me lose a little bit of my mobility. He thinks our son is wonderful, but doesn't see a need to risk a second pregnancy. I am still torn on the subject.

Pregnancy is a demanding experience for any woman. When you provide for special needs while working with an obstetrician and/or midwife who understands those needs, you have the best chance of a manageable pregnancy in which you maintain good health.

Adoption

Only some couples unable to have a child of their own can afford the new high-tech approaches to producing a birth. Financially and emotionally, the cost gets too high. Couples may also choose not to have invasive hormonal or surgical treatments. Adoption is a possibility, but this is not an easy option either.

Most children available for adoption are from an ethnic-minority background. In the U.S., most parents looking for children to adopt are Caucasian and—like other prospective parents—prefer to find a child of the same race as their own. The competition is pretty stiff, since able-bodied parents tend to be given the advantage by agencies. Another portion of the children have health problems or were abused. It is harder to find homes for these children. They are a challenge for any parents to raise, but all the more for a disabled parent, depending on their capacities and resources. But for some-one with a disability who feels a passionate calling to share his or her love as a parent, these issues can be resolved.

Finding your own way

Yes, there are a lot of adjustments to make, and some issues which are com-plicated in the already treacherous milieu of love, sex, and babies. But just as there are roadblocks, there are discoveries unique to sex with a disability, if you have the patience and the adaptability to find them. If you can over-come the initial obstacle of being discouraged by all the cultural messages of youth and body image and the over-emphasis on intercourse as sex, possibil-ities will expand. Your sexual nature is a gift of your existence, and no dis-ability—no matter how severe—disqualifies you from the capacity for inti-macy and sensuality.

CHAPTER 9

Spinal Cord Research

Recently there has been dramatic progress in central nervous system research. Researchers have begun to unlock the complexities of what happens when the brain and spinal cord are injured and what obstructs their ability to regenerate and recover function. Researchers are working on a variety of fronts to figure out how to promote the growth of central nervous system (CNS) tissues and to get nerve pathways communicating again.

Many of the current lines of research might translate into increased function for thousands of people with disabilities. It is likely that research into conditions such as muscular dystrophy or multiple sclerosis will provide insights on spinal cord injury. What researchers discover about spinal cord trauma may well impact treatment of other conditions involving nerve cell damage.

This chapter gives a snapshot in time of the state of spinal cord research as of this writing. We begin the chapter with a discussion about various ways that the idea of cure is seen, in the culture at large and in the disability community. Next, we look at the nature of a spinal cord injury and obstacles that must be overcome. Finally, we look at the nuts and bolts of what scientists are doing out there: the research areas that are most promising and a number of particular studies.

The fantasy of the cure

The notion of walking again is very potent, deep in the modern psyche, and used unsparingly in the media as a surefire device for tugging on emotional heartstrings.

Not that many years ago, doctors thought it was inconceivable to solve the puzzle of how to repair spinal cord damage or brain cell damage.

At the time of my injury in 1973, my doctor told me plainly that the spinal cord simply does not recover, and it never will.

However, the fantasy of walking again may yet come true. Significant advances in molecular and cellular biology in the past decade have expanded the potential to understand and influence the human nervous system. There is considerable optimism with regard to repairing chronically injured spinal cords. Researchers say it is just a matter of time and money.

The process of spinal cord research benefits other disabling conditions. Spinal cord research is not just about getting the spinal cord to grow, but about mapping the structure of the body and its systems, methods of treatment and rehabilitation, and genetic advances that overlap into many other areas of medical research. Walking gets all the emphasis in the media, when in fact there are many other benefits to be gained from central nervous system research. In the process of solving the spinal cord puzzle—which indeed seems likely to put some people back on their feet—we will also learn much about control of spasticity, bowel and bladder function, respiration, pain management, sexual function, and more.

Walking also depends on whether we are talking about acute or chronic injury and degree of completeness. Many people with acute, incomplete spinal cord injury who get treated quickly have a good chance of walking out of the hospital.

Setting aside whether a given person or group of people will walk again, the real value of this research work is that some people with disabilities will be able to function at higher levels of independence and activity than they can at this moment. Life will change significantly for those who now suffer too much pain or whose time is so occupied with self-care that they cannot commit themselves to a career or to travel, for instance. Some people can barely leave their homes or find themselves trapped in an extended care facility. Such people are much more interested in increasing their freedom and independence in any way possible than they are in walking.

Ambivalence toward cure research

Some people in the disability community have expressed concern—if not outright resentment—about the emphasis on a quest for a cure. They resent being thought of as broken and resist the notion that they should happily change to fit the popular image of what it means to be "whole." Some see the quest for cure as prejudicial, as if a person with a disability is assumed to be incapable of living a meaningful life.

In the disability community there are mixed feelings about spinal cord injured actor Christopher Reeve, who has been an extremely ardent supporter of spinal cord cure. He consistently states his intention to walk again. An article in *The Mouth, Voice of the Disability Nation*, states:

> Incurable quadriplegic actor Christopher Reeve's public begging for cure has distracted the world from demands by people with disabilities for equal rights.[1]

But the more widespread attitude appears to be one of balance. When you are injured, you get on with your life, which includes disability, while welcoming the potential for developments in research that can contribute to your quality of life.

> I think many of the anti-cure people focus too much on the semantics of the word "cure." How about "fix" instead? I have a spinal cord injury, which cannot be "cured" since I am not "sick." It is not a disease. But while I live a full life now and don't sit around whining about a cure, I fully realize that I could function better if my spinal cord was "fixed." I spend a lot of time managing my spinal cord injury—time that in the past I could use on my career, my relationships, my personal activities, etc.

> So, hey, I don't care what they call it, I am all for science and medicine attempting to allow my bladder, my bowels, my reproductive system, or my legs to function the way they were designed to.

Cure research can be a source of emotional support and hope for families, albeit with the attending danger of expectations that might not be fulfilled. Physicians tend to be extremely cautious discussing research with their patients for fear of building up unrealistic hopes. Many people find that their treating doctors are less informed on the status of research than they are themselves. Still, it's possible to be hopeful while taking what you get:

> Regarding an SCI cure, my wife and I look forward to the day when I'll walk again. We don't spend our time thinking about it, but are definitely heartened by the optimistic research.

Others seem to use the potential for cure as an excuse not to face their disabilities, to allow themselves to be cared for, and to surrender to the fears and challenges that must be faced in adapting to their disability. According to an active disabled person:

> I know folks who have my illness and live for a cure. They don't use assistive devices and spend most of their time in bed, because "a cure is around the corner."

Quite a puzzle: a spinal cord overview

The brain and spinal cord make up the *central nervous system* (CNS). The *peripheral nervous system* (PNS) carries motor impulse messages from the central nervous system to our muscles, and sensory messages to the spinal cord, which carries them back to the brain.

When injured, the PNS recovers, the CNS does not. Why the difference? The PNS and CNS systems are distinguished by two essential qualities.

- **A different biochemical makeup.** The PNS has a biological environment that supports the process of regeneration, while the CNS doesn't have the right biochemistry for growth. The CNS has been found to contain factors that actually inhibit regeneration.

- **A different physical structure.** Peripheral nerves have a system of sheaths that help direct a damaged nerve back to its "connection" as it regenerates. Central nerves have no such guiding channels. The small amount of regrowth that does occur after an injury has no idea where to go.

To understand the challenge of the immensely intricate research puzzle, we must know something about the way the spinal cord is built. Simplistically, it consists of long nerve axons surrounded by a protective coating called myelin. We need to know what happens to this system when it is injured and what would stimulate growth in a way that will restore function.

What happens in spinal cord injury?

The spinal cord is composed of millions of fine nerve fibers called axons, which carry motor impulses to neurons which in turn pass the information to the peripheral nerves and onward to muscles. Sensory messages move in the opposite direction, from nerve endings throughout the body, through the cord, and back to the brain. These nerves are like telephone cables—dense bunches of thin "wires" down which electrical signals travel (see Figure 9-1).

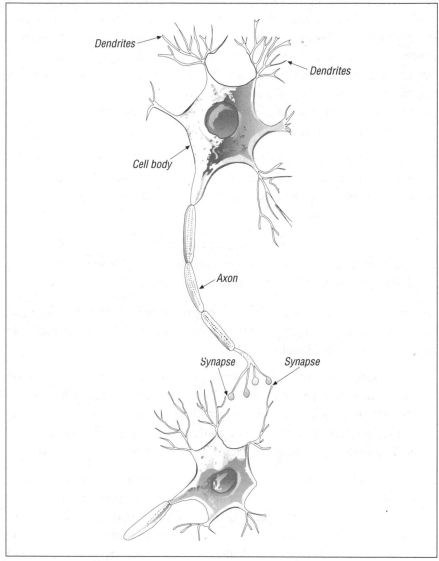

Figure 9-1. The parts of a nerve

Sometimes, in response to trauma, the body does manage to accomplish a degree of axonal regrowth on its own. Small amounts of nerve repair and remyelination have been observed. Central nerves have been known to sprout, sending out new shoots looking for a connection, but the odds are not good of linking up to a useful receptor without some help. The body really can't do this repair by itself.

As soon as a spinal cord is injured, a complex chain of events begins. The cord starts to hemorrhage, bleeding from the inside out. The cord—a soft, gelatinous material—doesn't have the basic nutrients and fuel it needs to function and maintain itself. The contents of the nerve, its axoplasm, leaks out the end, immediately shortening the broken end of the nerve and putting distance between it and its former connection. The portion of the axon which is away from the neuronal cell body dies, while the cell body and remainder of its axon survives.

Soon after trauma, the body attempts to clean up the mess in a chemical onslaught that causes further secondary damage. As Melinda Kelley, Ph.D., Associate Director of Research at the Paralyzed Veterans of America, describes it:

> Special cells called microphages and microglia help "eat" the debris and digest it. They also produce chemicals which detract from the regenerative process while they are in the area.

As damaged cells get digested by the body, some healthy ones get eaten too, spreading the extent of the injury. The body tries vainly to repair itself, but in reality causes more harm.

In only hours, the cord becomes inflamed and distorted, with the body's release of molecules called cytokines. There was once a belief that injured spinal cord tissue suffered from oxygen deprivation, but research has not supported this view, unless there is a continued physical compression of the tissue. Damaged cells produce free radicals which cause further damage.

The body has an intelligence of its own, a miraculous system of programmed response to its own conditions. One such process called apoptosis is a sort of cell suicide. When cells discover they are no longer needed by the body, they destroy themselves. Spinal cord and brain trauma tricks cells into believing they have completed their work, apoptosis begins, and further increases the degree of secondary damage.

Within a week, nerve cells begin to degenerate, and whatever regenerative efforts the body had been trying come to a stop. Eventually scars are formed by glia cells which cap the injured nerve ends. Glial scarring is thought by some researchers to be an obstacle to regeneration and an important part of the puzzle—the removal of the scarred ends to allow the axon the freedom to grow. Glial scarring was the focus of Russian experiments in the '70s, which produced very little result. Still, a number of labs have already succeeded at getting axons to grow through scarring in early efforts; there is some controversy over how much of a difficulty glial scarring actually is in solving the puzzle. Some feel the scar is the key issue to overcome, others believe that axons grow just fine in scar tissue.

Axons are surrounded by a protective material called myelin. When an axon is damaged and retreats, the myelin which surrounded it is also affected. As described by Dr. Young:

> Myelin is made by cells called oligodendroglia. Injury damages both axons and oligodendroglia. Each oligodendroglia myelinates as many as 20–30 axons. So, when oligodendroglia are damaged, they die and many axons may become demyelinated. Remyelination occurs, but many axons that survive the injury either are demyelinated or poorly myelinated.

Remyelination is a substantial part of the spinal cord cure puzzle, since a regenerated axon will not work without a restored myelin layer to protect it.

In an incomplete spinal cord injury, it is not unusual for some axons to remain intact, yet be unable to pass impulses because of disruptions to their myelin. Nerve regrowth may not be the entire challenge here. Restoring myelin could mean a degree of renewed function for some spinal cord injured persons. The majority of SCIs are incomplete injuries.

Spinal cord researcher Dennis Choi of Washington University in St. Louis has been addressing the question of apoptosis:

> A great deal is currently being learned about the molecular under-pinnings of apoptosis, and this knowledge is translating into specific strategies for inhibiting apoptosis. Overall, I would describe this research as still in early stages (cell and animal model testing). There are some theoretical concerns with the strategy of inhibiting apoptosis, that will have to be answered by further experiments. For example, the spinal cord may be better off if some badly damaged cells undergo apoptosis, rather than hanging on and getting in the way of recovery.

The degree of axonal death just after the injury is aggravated further by a loss of circulation to the area. Blood supply through a system of very fine capillaries is disrupted. Traumatized tissues are damaged by this loss of blood, but so are nearby healthy nerve tissues which have not been directly impacted, but nonetheless need a constant supply of nutrients.

Blood and all of its nutrients and factors must be present to foster regeneration. For a true recovery, a permanent vascular system must be re-established. This very fine network of capillaries must integrate with existing tissues and maintain the flow of metabolic materials into and out of the new tissues.

The first successes in axonal regeneration—while exciting—produced disappointingly small amounts of growth. Recent efforts have been more encouraging in getting axons to grow over longer distances, and are beginning to produce promising functional improvement.

The PNS has Schwann cells which promote growth and remyelination, but these are not present in the CNS. The central system has cells called oligodendrocytes which produce myelin, however they are unable to produce enough to compensate for the degree of damage involved here. At the time of injury, some Schwann cells will migrate into the area from the nerve root where the PNS meets the CNS at the spinal cord, and have been found to remyelinate some axons and promote some growth, but they don't generate enough myelin to be meaningful.

There are just not enough nerve growth factors present in the CNS to respond to trauma. The body apparently has figured that, once born, it no longer needs the capacity to grow central nerve tissue. Even worse, there are "inhibitors" that have been discovered getting in the way of the body's attempt to regenerate. As we'll see, much research is focused on combinations of factors to promote nerve growth and to defeat the inhibitors.

But there's more. Getting a nerve to grow with proper insulation is useless unless the nerve can get to the right destination. Remember that the central nervous system doesn't have the guiding channels found in the peripheral system. The axon has to reach the correct location. In animal studies, there have been cases of regeneration with no functional improvement whatsoever.

But it is not clear that specific nerves must make exact connections. There are hypotheses that the body might be able to retrain itself to use new connections however it needs to. The receptor sites needing an axonal path to the brain might also have the ability reach out and grab a new axon, rather than having to guide an axon to the site itself. All of this is very preliminary.

In some cases, the spinal cord becomes attached to surrounding tissues. This is known as tethering, and can restrict the flow of spinal fluids—which surround the cord—past the injury site. Pain and loss of function can result.

Surgery to untether the spinal cord is already being performed. Of forty people operated on at the University of Miami and reported by the Miami Project to Cure Paralysis, 79 percent showed improved motor function, and 62 percent had reduction in chronic pain.[2] For some people, untethering surgery might be necessary as part of a spinal cord regeneration therapy.

Even if we can overcome all these barriers, can we walk? Suppose we get axons to grow—possibly as many as five million are needed—by supplying the growth factors and obstructing the inhibitors. We ensure that they are protected by myelin. We provide a continuing supply of blood and nutrients to the area, and get the scarring out of the way to allow growth. We get the axonal end to grow long enough, and direct it to the right location—or train the body to reroute its messages—and form working neurons and synapses to get the message out to the muscles. Can we walk now?

That depends. Now we need to ask to what degree atrophied muscles have the capacity to receive impulses and start to produce muscle fiber capable of sufficient contraction. In other words, will the muscles work, and how strong can they become? To carry the weight of the upper body and to work continuously without early fatigue is a tall order. After only months of atrophy from disuse, the degree of lost muscle strength is considerable. After years of disuse, who knows?

Whether muscles can work again depends on whether or not there is damage to "lower motoneurons," a particular type of cell in the spinal cord. Even if the brain-to-muscle communication is interrupted, the muscles can still be receiving enough signal for muscle cells to be maintained. Without lower motoneuron signals, muscle cells die. Ironically, spasticity (often seen as a disadvantage) preserves considerable muscle tone. People with spasticity will have less work to do rebuilding muscle if the cord is regenerated. There is also no question that spastic muscles have functioning motoneurons.

Many people have contractures, in which muscles, tendons, and ligaments have shortened after years of sitting. Even if the spinal cord can be completely cured, there are considerable issues of rehabilitation involved in getting someone into the right posture, building muscle, and reteaching them the process of walking.

In the matter of osteoporosis, again there appears to be disagreement. If people who do not walk for a period of years lose strength in their bones, will they be able to support their own body weight if they were to make those bones carry their upper body? Some texts suggest that osteoporosis is not reversible.

Walking, as we've said, is not even the whole picture. What does all of this—nerve regeneration, myelin sheathing, establishment of blood supply, removal of scarring, nerve connections, and muscle rebuilding—have to do with sexual function, bowel and bladder control, pain, and many other side issues related to various disabilities? The answers are far from clear, even though so much is being learned about the detailed, microscopic world of the central nervous system.

So this—extremely simplistically—is the puzzle researchers face. One can understand the fascination of the challenge. With the availability of modern microscopes, laboratories, and computers, scientists can now study and engineer at the molecular level. They can see the processes, they can control them to some degree in the body or they can reproduce certain aspects in the laboratory. They can attempt to reproduce some of the pieces through genetic engineering. How remarkable! Surely more than a few researchers have imagined a Nobel Prize, the possibility of commercial success, or at least a place in history.

The research effort

There is a huge array of research projects geared toward disability-oriented research. It would take many encyclopedia-sized books to list them and even begin to describe their work—much less how the research fits together. Particular studies and researchers will be mentioned here to give you a sense of the variety of studies, the immense complexity, the excitement of the progress, and the skill and dedication of the researchers. However, for each project or person mentioned, there are dozens who deserve equal billing.

SCI research beginnings

The first attempt to understand spinal cord injury took place early in the century, when a Spanish neuroanatomist named Santiago Ramón y Cajal conducted experiments with dogs and cats. He showed that the brain and spinal cord are made up of specialized cells, different from the rest of the body's nervous system. He was the first explorer who mapped the structure of neurons and axons that make up the system, and is revered today by anatomists as a pioneer. He observed that, when cut, central nervous system axons made a brief effort to regrow, and then stopped. His work is the source of the long-standing belief that nothing could be done to regenerate CNS nerves.

In the early 1980s, a Montreal Institute of Neurology team led by Dr. Albert Aguayo became the first to demonstrate that spinal cord axons could grow more than the slight distance that had been observed by Cajal. Suddenly the accepted dogma that spinal cords could not regenerate had to be reconsidered. But this demonstration was still a long way from getting damaged axons to grow enough to bring about a "cure."

Dr. Wise Young, formerly at New York University and now the Director of the Neuroscience Center at Rutgers, State University of New Jersey, has been interested in spinal cord regeneration since well before it caught on in the neuroscience community. Early on, his attempts to get spinal cord research on the agenda at the Society for Neuroscience conferences met with little enthusiasm. But then Dr. Aguayo and his colleagues made the breakthrough that demonstrated that spinal cord axons could indeed grow. A few years later, Swiss researcher Dr. Martin Schwab identified a growth inhibitor and began work on counteracting it. Suddenly central nervous system research caught on, and Wise Young has been in the thick of it ever since. Dr. Young is a key spokesperson for SCI research, is widely quoted in articles and books, and has posed for more than one photograph with Christopher and Dana Reeve, the current standard bearers for spinal cord research.

Nerve regeneration: something is in the way

The first assumptions about the inability of axons to regenerate were that something was missing. Then, in 1988, Dr. Martin Schwab of the Brain Research Institute at the University of Zurich in Switzerland discovered that something prevents growth. His team found a protein which inhibits CNS regrowth after a trauma. The team has been experimenting with ways to turn off this inhibitor to allow axons to regenerate. In 1990, an antibody called IN1 appeared to block the protein. They observed about eleven millimeters of growth in a rat spinal cord. This was a major step in the research.[3]

Here was their test: In a group of sixty rats, Schwab treated half with IN1, and then sent the whole group to his colleague Dr. Barbara Bregman in Washington, D.C., at the Georgetown University School of Medicine. She didn't know which was which (a blind test). Dr. Bregman's team measured the ability of each rat to walk, including specific details like the length of their stride. Once the lab finished the tests and checked against which rats were treated and which not, they found that the treated rats had regained from 70 to 80 percent of their stride after treatment with IN1, recovering nearly full function.

But the inhibitor protein discovered by Schwab's team is apparently not the only one. Jim Salzer at New York University discovered another—a myelin-associated glycoprotein (MAG)—in the late 1980s. Actually, it was another researcher who found that the protein prevented axonal growth, and yet another who found that the IN1 antibody had impact on it. At this early stage, it is hard to know if other molecules in Schwab's test rats also had an effect on the experiment. Such is the complexity of this research, and an example of how collaborative the process needs to be.

The inhibiting proteins reside in the myelin—the fatty tissue surrounding nerve axons—in very small quantities. It is very difficult for scientists to purify and analyze the proteins in order to generate enough to be used for research. Scientists must refine the molecules down with absolute precision in order to develop a usable treatment. It is painstaking work, and an example of why this research takes so long. The difficulties of getting a quantity of usable protein for research also limits multiple laboratories from being able to participate in the work. There is not enough to go around.

Another approach to turning off the inhibitors is being explored with cellular adhesion molecules (CAMs). CAMs reside on the membrane surface of nerve cells. They foster communication between the nerve cells. For instance, CAMs help nerve cells to recognize an axon so they know where to go and do their job of creating myelin. CAMs also help override the inhibitors, and so play a similar role as the antibody called IN1.

A CAM known as L1 is known to play a role in regeneration of axons. Another Swiss researcher, Melitta Schachner, showed that L1 stimulated growth and did so in the presence of the inhibiting protein discovered by Schwab. L1 is known to be present in the developing brain and spinal cord, but goes away after birth. L1 found in rats is 99 percent similar to that found in humans, making animal studies more reliable as indicators of what might happen in humans.

L1 is found on Schwann cells—which produce myelin in the peripheral system—but not on oligodendrocytes—which create myelin in the central system. This makes Schwann cells of great interest because they might not only remyelinate the spinal cord, but could promote regrowth of the axons. And since IN1 is so difficult to produce, L1 might prove to be a more practical solution, if only because it is easier to synthesize.

Factors like IN1 and L1 can clear a path by overriding inhibiting proteins, but something more is needed to really get things growing. Dr. Naomi Kleitman, Director of Education at the Miami Project to Cure Paralysis, says,

> *Whether a nerve cell can regenerate is more a question of environment than the absolute ability of a cell in one or another part of the nervous system to be able to grow.*

The job for researchers is to create that right environment for regeneration to take place.

Growth factors

Neurotrophins feed nerves, and so stimulate growth. The brain and spinal cord already produce these growth factors, but not in enough quantity to repair a trauma. There is quite a list of growth factors being studied by researchers. Nerve Growth Factor (NGF) was discovered in 1951 by Italian researcher Rita Levi-Montalcini and Viktor Hamburger of Washington University of St. Louis. Others include basic fibroblast growth factor (bFGF), brain-derived neurotrophic factor (BDNF), and glial cell line-derived neurotrophic factor (GDNF), among many others, are commonly referred to in research literature.

According to Wise Young:

> *It is really important that we try and compare all of them. We currently do not know enough about the regenerating axons in the spinal cord to predict which one will work the best. It is likely that many of the factors play multiple roles in different tissue and at different times during development.*

Naomi Kleitman of the Miami Project talks about the presence of up to fifty growth promoters present in the peripheral nervous system.

> *Any nerve cell will respond to these if it has the proper receptor for it. We know that central nerves can respond to these as well as peripheral nerves in many cases. During the course of the life of a nerve cell, it might be receptive to a given growth factor at one point and a different one at another time.*

The one that has shown the most promise and has earned the most research attention is called NT3. In 1994, Dr. Schwab and his team used NT3 along with the inhibitor antibody, IN1. They got nerve fibers to grow the entire length of a rat's spinal column—another groundbreaking step.

In the July 15, 1997, issue of *The Journal of Neuroscience*, researchers at the University of California at San Diego reported an early success in axonal regrowth using gene therapy. They managed to get injured rats' own cells to produce growth factor right at the injury site. They used normal skin cells from the rats, and altered them genetically to get them to produce NT3. When grafted back into the animals, these new cells secreted NT3 which produced axonal regrowth. Some rats recovered a degree of walking ability.[4]

Another good piece of news in the study is that the cells continued to produce NT3 for several months. This means the cells were able to produce enough to be effective, yet were not what researchers call immortal cells. Such cells can cause cancer, since they continue to reproduce and ultimately spread where they are not wanted.

Wise Young summarizes his optimism about future progress:

> *The story is now becoming clear. There are facilitory and inhibitory proteins. In the presence of facilitory proteins, the inhibitory proteins do not prevent axonal growth. We are achieving a much better understanding of these proteins. It is a very exciting time in regeneration research.*

Schwann cells

When nerve axons die, so does their myelin. So if axons are regenerated, the myelin must also be regenerated. In the peripheral nervous system, Schwann cells promote growth of myelin and regeneration of injured nerve axons.

In the central nervous system, oligodendrocytes perform the job of myelin production. However, says Naomi Kleitman:

> *Oligodendrocytes have an additional inhibitor that is not present in Schwann cells. They seem not to be very aggressive remyelinators. For some reason, Schwann cells are really aggressive about doing what they want to do.*

Oligodendrocytes in the central nervous system also have a tendency to cross over between axons, whereas Schwann cells have the ability to myelinate along the length of a single axon.

Since Schwann cells are not naturally present in the spinal cord, researchers are particularly interested in bringing them into the CNS and using them there as a possible tool for spinal cord repair. It is already well proven that Schwann cells are also able to regenerate myelin in the CNS for both sensory and motor nerves. The challenge remains to find how to create the conditions in which Schwann cells can accomplish this regeneration in a compromised spinal cord.

Schwann cells have the ability to create a connective framework that holds cells in place as they regenerate. This framework is a latticework of proteins called an extracellular matrix. The extracellular matrix looks like a blanket that wraps around the axon and the Schwann cells. This matrix—different in some respects from the extracellular matrix found in the central system—is a key characteristic of Schwann cells, and has growth-promoting features of its own. Its major component is a protein called laminin which is also a promoter of growth. Kleitman states:

> Not all cells like it. Laminin is just one kind of protein that some cells like to grow on at certain points in their lifetime.

Schwann cells contribute to the regeneration of the nerve as well as the myelination, and so perform a double duty. They help the nerve to grow, provide a myelin sheath in a controlled fashion along the nerve, and the matrix generates a structure that keeps the whole thing in place. Kleitman explains:

> That is why these cells (Schwann) are so potent, because they basically bring their whole manufacturing system with them.

In initial trials performed by Dr. Richard Bunge, Schwann cells alone produced some growth, but only for certain kinds of nerve cells. The researchers found that the simultaneous use of a nerve growth factor was necessary to produce better results.[5] This conclusion was confirmed by Swedish researchers in 1996, led by Lars Olson, M.D. They bridged gaps in injured spinal cords of adult rats by using nerve grafts and acidic fibroblast growth factor (aFGF). Within months, this grafting procedure led to limited but definitive functional improvement in locomotor activity.

At the Miami Project, researchers are working with Schwann cell "bridges." The bridges are based on work from Brown University which produced a hollow polymer tube that can be wrapped around nerves. (Remember that the scale is microscopic.) According to Kleitman:

> We took six million Schwann cells, mixed them up with a commercially available extracellular matrix mixture, and stuck it inside one of these hollow polymers. What happened was that the Schwann cells all lined up and created a nice little pathway that you can attach between severed ends of a spinal cord.

This little pathway serves as a guide for nerve growth between two damaged axonal ends.

Schwann cells alone will not be the magic solution. Dr. Mary Bartlett Bunge of the Miami Project led a study where Schwann cells were engineered to produce the growth factor BDNF. In the first set of studies, they did a complete transection of a spinal cord, and laid down a trail of half a million Schwann cells. They found a lot more growth with BDNF and Schwann cells in combination than with Schwann cells alone.[6]

Dr. Kleitman observes:

> Almost everybody you talk to is going to talk about what combination of factors and cells we'll need to use.

The following questions still remain about Schwann cells.

- Can enough cells be placed and controlled to bring about optimal repair?
- There are a number of different kinds of nerve tissues to be repaired in the spinal cord. Can Schwann cells affect them all?
- Can Schwann cells penetrate to the areas of the cord where regeneration is needed?

At this stage, getting nerves to grow in the spinal cord is not really the problem. Now it is a matter of getting enough of them to grow long enough and establish functional connections. Dr. Young estimates that about 10 percent of connections are sufficient to support substantial functional recovery in rats and humans. Since most people still have some connections remaining across the injury site, regeneration only needs to make up the difference.

Getting the growth factors there

Regeneration of the spinal cord is not just a matter of giving someone a pill or an injection. Growth factors must be integrated into the complex, continuous metabolic processes in the body. Growth factors must get to the right place, interact with other very specific molecules, and be replenished as they are used. Rather than just putting growth factor into the body, researchers are finding ways of getting the body to produce the growth factor itself.

A University of California at San Diego team is using fibroblasts. These are cells in the skin that can produce substances which affect nerve growth. Fibroblasts have certain advantages. As Wise Young explains:

> Fibroblasts represent a very important candidate for delivery of growth factors to the injury site. Among other features, they can be isolated from the individual receiving the cells and then genetically modified in culture. This is the best way to prevent rejection of the transplanted cells when they are put back into the body. I believe that fibroblasts will be a major vehicle for delivery of factors to the spinal cord.

Making the right connections

Dr. Samuel Kuwada of the University of Michigan is performing a "molecular genetic analysis of axon guidance in the spinal cord." Neurons make connections with their appropriate target cells by relying on specific molecules that direct axons. Scientists believe that identifying and understanding these guidance molecules may help direct regenerating axons to the right place. The University of Michigan researchers use zebrafish embryos to help them generate molecules called netrins. Netrins appear to play a role in making connections during embryonic spinal cord development.

Dr. Marc Tessier-Lavigne is also exploring netrins at the University of California at San Francisco. His team's work suggests that a couple of different netrin molecules are found in the adult CNS. Their research abstract states:

> Netrins seem to attract some classes of axons and repel others. The work being proposed here seeks to pinpoint the receptors on axons that mediate the biological effects of the netrins. Candidate receptors have been identified in the past year, and their functions in development and regeneration of connections are beginning to be evaluated.

Pattern generators

Then again, maybe the exact nerve pathways don't have to be recreated. Another avenue of research has studied exactly what the pathways are that produce the unique combination of impulses that make walking possible. There is some early evidence that the body has the capacity to reroute its messages, like a telephone operator plugging into a different line. The human body has some remarkable adaptive abilities, and part of the solution to the puzzle may involve letting the body do its own thing by simply removing the impediments, and then giving it the building blocks it needs. These are known as pattern generation studies.

Walking apparently doesn't rely entirely on messages from the brain. Part of the process of walking happens below the level of the injury, impulses traveling between muscles and the spinal cord without having to make it past the injury and back to the brain. It is not clear to what degree this might be the case in humans, but Miami Project researchers have studied a person with a seventeen-year history of incomplete cervical injury who began exhibiting involuntary stepping-like movements in his legs. This study strongly suggests that there is a "central pattern generator," a group of nerve cells that synchronizes muscle activity during alternating stepping of the legs.

More on remyelination

While Schwann cells show promise of addressing the problem of lost myelin, scientists know better than to place their bets on one direction, no matter how promising. The spinal cord is not a consistently friendly environment for Schwann cells. They need to get into the heart of the cord where injured axons reside. But astrocytes—a type of cell that provides nutrients to neurons—and oligodendrocytes—the equivalent of Schwann cells in the CNS—sometimes prevent the penetration of Schwann cells.

Wise Young and his team have been hopeful about the use of O2A cells to generate remyelination. He says that:

> We have shown that O2A cells from the mouse will migrate long distances when implanted into the spinal cord to congregate in areas of demyelination.

Oligodendrocytes are the producers of myelin in the spinal cord, yet are overwhelmed by the scale of an injury. So why not just put more of them into the area to restore myelin? The challenge is to find a proper cell line or growth factor which will do the work of generating oligodendrocytes in the body but not become immortal. Again, according to Wise Young:

> A number of laboratories (William Blakemore in Cambridge and our laboratory in collaboration with Jack Rosenbluth at NYU) have shown that oligodendroglia precursor cells can be transplanted to remyelinate axons in the spinal cord.

Dr. Moses Rodriguez at the Mayo Clinic has discovered a monoclonal antibody that promotes remyelination in rats that have been demyelinated by viruses, autoimmune disease, and chemicals. This work holds promise for any CNS myelin deficiencies, including spinal cord injury and multiple sclerosis.

Mapping the spinal cord

Recent computerized tools like CT (computed tomography) scans and MRI (magnetic resonance imaging) have fostered a revolution in medical care and research. SCI scientists are getting a highly detailed, three-dimensional look at the spinal cord thanks to this technology.

Projects are underway which are designed to map the cord, including work at Purdue University and at Washington University in St. Louis, Missouri. At Purdue University, they are gathering information produced from 3D images, and making this material available as a database through computer networks researchers can access. Dr. William Snider of Washington University believes that mapping the cord is critical to the process of achieving regeneration. He says:

> We think understanding how axons first find their targets in developing spinal cords applies to the situation after injury. A regenerating axon will likely have to retrace the same incredibly complex path to reform working connections.

A map of the spinal cord will also be a valuable diagnostic tool in the emergency room. The extent of injury will be much clearer to doctors, thanks to the ability to see a three-dimensional image of the injured cord. Researchers also benefit from being able to better witness the effect of their therapies.

Preserving and restoring muscles

We've already discussed the need for lower motoneurons to be present for muscles to retain the ability for recovery in the case of a spinal cord regeneration. Research is also addressing the question of producing sufficient muscle mass for walking.

To determine whether muscle tissues could contract if the cord were repaired, a physician might perform certain simple diagnostic tests for the needed lower motoneuron activity. They would use reflex testing—tapping with that little hammer we have all seen as a stereotype of a doctor's checkup—or they might use an electrical stimulation device to see if muscles respond to a direct impulse. This would be evidence that muscle cells have not died, and so imply that lower motoneurons are in place.

If muscles are to be preserved and possibly restored in the future, at the time of injury the lower motoneuron nerves need to be preserved or replaced before substantial muscle death occurs. According to Wise Young:

> Neuronal replacement was considered science fiction until recently. The big discovery occurred rather quietly about a decade ago.

This was when researchers discovered that they could culture stem cells—which have the ability to turn into almost any kind of cell—from the central nervous system and that these cells can survive. Several researchers have reported they can induce these stem cells to differentiate into motoneurons. This suggests that it is possible to replace lost motoneurons in the spinal cord. But it would be necessary to get the nerves to grow all the way down to the muscles, a slow and difficult process.

You can accommodate a degree of motoneuron death. Explains Young:

> Muscles probably follow the same 10 percent rule that applies to the central nervous system in which only 10 percent of the axons in the spinal cord are necessary and sufficient to support substantial function. Individual muscle cells can increase their bulk many times. A weightlifter, for example, can increase a muscle width by five to ten times. This results more from expansion of individual muscle cells than from the production of more muscle cells.

In other words, there can be a degree of muscle cell death from lost gray matter in the spinal cord where motoneurons reside, and it can still be possible to build enough muscle strength for functional use.

Fetal cells

Fetal cells are also more technically referred to as embryonic tissue. Cells from a human fetus have advantages that make them of interest to researchers and give them the potential to be helpful from a wide collection of conditions. People with Alzheimer's, Parkinson's, Huntington's, diabetes, leukemia, epilepsy, and other conditions are believed to be in a position to gain from embryonic cell research. There have already been early successes with Parkinson's disease.

Fetal cells are considered "plastic." Since they come from a human fetus in early development, they have a unique capacity to mature into any kind of cell. They grow and divide very quickly, and lack the markers which set off an immune reaction to foreign bodies. When they are inserted into another body, they are not seen as invaders, so rejection is less likely to occur. They integrate well with existing tissue.

The missing growth factor needed for axonal growth is present in fetal cells. These cells play a role in fetal development of the spinal cord, but "turn off" after we are born. Therefore another avenue of research has been to transplant fetal cells in the hope of switching the nerve growth capacity back on.

First U.S. human fetal cell trial

A landmark study into spinal cord therapy was performed at the University of Florida at Gainesville. In 1992, they did transplants on fifteen cats whose spinal cords had been severed. The fetal cells reunited the separated ends of the cords. Eight of the cats regained the ability to walk. One of them did so well that a researcher described its recovery as "almost acrobatic." It was able to climb stairs, and exhibited only minor signs of its injury.[7]

The University of Florida researchers have ten volunteers with syringomyelia in a study that will look at the implant of fetal tissue into a human spinal cord. In 1997, surgeons at the Karolinska Institute in Denmark performed the first such surgery, in cooperation with neurosurgeons and researchers from Denver's Craig Hospital. In July of that year, the researchers at the University of Florida performed an implant procedure on the first American human subject, a forty-three-year-old male.

The goal of this research was not to produce a spinal cord cure, but to conduct a much more preliminary exploration. Many spinal cord injuries exhibit the development of fluid-filled spaces in the spinal cord at the injury site. This condition, known as syringomyelia, is often a source of additional pain and spasticity, and even loss of function above the level of injury. There is a standard surgery for the condition to relieve the fluid pressures. Many people require repeated surgeries to relieve the pressure.

During the course of this standard surgery, the UF researchers inserted the fetal cells. They are interested in seeing if the cells help to plug the space where fluids continue to collect. Researchers want to see how long it takes for the fetal cells to have an effect, how much tissue is needed to produce the effect, and what kind of immune reaction the body has to the tissue. These are all important initial tasks that must be addressed before researchers can approach the larger goal of studying functional recovery in humans.

The Danish researchers identified one notable advantage. Having used immunosuppressive drugs at first to aid in the acceptance of the fetal cells, they discontinued the therapy and found that the cells were able to survive on their own.

Ethics of fetal tissue

Use of fetal tissue is clearly a delicate topic in ethical and political terms. One of President Bill Clinton's first acts of office in 1993 was to remove the five-year old moratorium on fetal cell research which had been imposed during the Reagan/Bush era. The only fetal cells that had been allowed to be used were those from spontaneous abortion (miscarriage). Spontaneous abortions are often the result of conditions that render the tissue unusable in the first place.

Ethical concerns revolve around the idea of women having abortions for pay in order to generate tissues for research. There are federal laws in place that already address some of these questions. Women considering an abortion may not be approached about tissue donation until they have already made their decision and signed their paperwork; there is in fact no guarantee that the tissue would even be suitable. Women may not be paid for fetal tissues. There are criminal penalties for such activities.

The fear that research will contribute to a rise in abortions seems an unlikely concern. A National Institute of Health panel found that after thirty years of research into embryonic tissue, such research had not affected women's reasons for seeking an abortion.

In the hope of circumventing these complex ethical questions, there are efforts at hand to genetically produce cells with the same features as fetal cells. If these efforts succeed, actual fetuses will no longer be necessary for the therapy.

Other transplantations

Researchers are experimenting with many kind of cells, from both human and animal donors. Cells are studied for the various features we have seen— a capacity to stimulate growth, to resist or suppress inhibitors, to multiply and go to the right place, and so on. The variety of possible sources for cells is huge.

In a recent study by Dr. Geoffrey Raisman, at the National Institute for Medical Research in London, cells have been taken from inside the nose. These olfactory ensheathing cells succeeded in stimulating the recovery of a small spinal cord injury in rats. These cells are of interest because they are easy to collect, and are continuously produced in the body, providing a generous supply. They are also the only type of cell in the central nervous system capable of regenerating themselves. There is also hope that they can act as a chaperone, helping newly generated axons to cross that difficult boundary between the peripheral and central systems. This is the point where axonal growth often stops, and one reason why growth has not reliably led to functional improvement.

The Canadian Spinal Research Organization (CSRO) is working with the enteric nerve system in the human intestine. It contains a wide variety of nerve cells that are being cultured for transplantation into spinal cords to observe their ability to survive and create new connections. Supported by CSRO, Dr. Richard Borgens at Purdue University has already found that enteric cells implanted into an injured spinal cord reduce secondary inflammatory damage in the weeks and months following injury.

Controversial treatments

In Tijuana, Mexico, a group of neurosurgeons are working with embryonic cells from the blue shark. Although they report improvements in the sixteen human subjects they have worked with, they have not documented their research in a detailed fashion, making American researchers uncomfortable. Rather than conducting a carefully documented research study, the Mexican clinic is interested in offering what they believe is a useful cure, and are able to do so without the constraints placed on physicians in the United States by the Food and Drug Administration. Anyone considering participating in such undocumented research should go to every possible extreme to understand the work and its risks before considering an unregulated procedure.

Another controversial treatment for SCI is called omentum transposition. The omentum is a band of tissue in the abdomen of mammals which seals off abdominal injuries. A surgical procedure partially detaches the omentum, reconnecting it at the injury site. Removing it seems not to have a negative effect on the abdomen. The theory is that the omentum tissue—which is rich in blood vessels—may supply the damaged nerve cells with vital oxygen, and possibly secrete chemicals that stimulate nerve growth.

Initial animal trials seem to show some functional improvement if the operation is completed within three hours of injury. Little or no improvement is shown when the procedure is done six to eight hours after injury. Scarring at the cord has been observed as a result of omental transplant, as well as abdominal complications. Clinical trials for people who have had a chronic spinal cord injury had been scheduled and then canceled. This research has not been scientifically documented, so there is considerable skepticism regarding its value.

Treatments at the time of trauma

While the search goes on for an ultimate solution to regenerating the spinal cord, there have already been early accomplishments which help reduce the extent of damage to the cord at the time of injury. Methylprednisolone and gangliosides are examples of drugs which have been found to reduce the inflammatory process that occurs after injury. While not a cure per se, these drugs are the early product of a continuing scientific effort which, it is hoped, will bear much greater fruit as the process continues.

Methylprednisolone (MP)

A milestone in practical treatment occurred in May 1990. The results of the National Acute Spinal Cord Injury Study (NASCIS-II) showed that the drug methylprednisolone (MP) was found to reduce the extent of spinal cord trauma when given within eight hours of injury. Improvements of up to 20 percent have been measured, compared to people who were given no drug. MP also compared favorably against another drug in the test, naloxone.[8] The use of MP with spinal cord trauma is now standard in emergency centers throughout the United States.

The effect of MP is significant, according to Wise Young:

> For someone with incomplete spinal cord injury and treated with methylprednisolone, the likelihood of the person walking out of the hospital is high. For example, athletes Dennis Byrd and Reggie Brown both walked out of the hospital. While people should not develop unrealistic expectations, they should also not become unduly pessimistic.

MP is an anti-inflammatory agent in common use for other purposes, such as a treatment for flare-ups of multiple sclerosis, lupus, severe asthma, and other conditions. This was the first time that treatment of any kind was found to have an effect on the spinal cord.

Scientists are not certain how MP actually has this effect, but they suspect several things may be going on.

- Inflammation is an automatic response of the body to injury, releasing various enzymes and beginning a natural, destructive process designed to clean up foreign bodies—dead spinal cord cells in this case. MP is already known to function as an anti-inflammatory, so it limits secondary trauma by reducing the swelling of injured tissues.

- Nerve tissues have a one-cell-deep endothelial protective layer. When breached by injury, fluids in the nerve are allowed to escape, and external fluids invade. MP seems to reduce the permeability of this layer.

- Along with various other chemical changes, MP apparently increases blood flow to the injury site, bringing in important nutrients and healing factors while also helping to carry away damaged cells.

MP might also play a role in regeneration. Future spinal cord treatment might itself be inflammatory, so the tissue would need protection. Naomi Kleitman of the Miami Project points out:

> Chances are good there would be some injury to the cord from putting cells in. If I were undergoing that, I would want MP at the time of surgery.

GM-1/Sygen

In June 1991, early results were published which suggested that GM-1 (monosialic ganglioside, known commercially as Sygen) also contributes to the reduction of spinal cord damage if administered within seventy-two hours.[9] In ways similar to MP, Sygen may protect cell membranes, reduce cell destruction by the body's natural response, and alter the general chemical environment. The study also speculates that Sygen stimulates beneficial enzymes at the injury site.

Dr. Fred Geisler of the Chicago Institute for Neurosurgery and Neurological Research spoke at the National Spinal Cord Injury Association conference in Chicago in August of 1998. He reported preliminary findings that showed statistically positive improvements in subjects with a range of severity. In all cases, MP had been given for the first three days after injury, and then a six-week course of 100-200 mg of Sygen per day was begun within seventy-two hours for half of the study population. The group receiving Sygen recovered more rapidly, but after six months the extent of recovery was similar for both groups.[10] The study used the Benzel classification system to measure the outcome, which categorizes locomotor ability. Improvement in hand function for people with cervical spinal cord injuries would have little impact on the study results.

While Sygen is being studied for its usefulness at the time of trauma, gangliosides have also been found to stimulate the growth of nerve cells. Sygen might therefore play a role in supporting the action of nerve growth factors.

Drug cocktails

Determining the proper dosage and delivery method for drugs at the time of trauma has proven to be difficult. As with any drug, there is the danger of unacceptable side effects, so the toxic levels must be determined. MP, Sygen, or any other drug each have their own ways of acting at different times during the injury process, so timing matters.

A cocktail, or mix of drugs, might prove to be more effective than a single drug. Researcher Linda Noble, Ph.D., of the University of California at San Francisco, says:

> *Mother Nature didn't put us together so simply that one substance would just do the trick. It seems logical that it's a much more complicated system and that it's going to most likely require a cocktail.*

Interactions between the drugs also are important to study. Sygen and MP have been found to be antagonistic to each other. Researchers are studying another drug called tirilazad mesylate, which they suspect might prove to be a better partner in the mix.

MASCIS

The Multicenter Animal Spinal Cord Injury Study (MASCIS) is funded by the U.S. government's National Institutes of Health. MASCIS is following up on the initial work with MP and other pharmaceuticals. These drugs have shown potential. The task now is to determine dosage, extent of follow-up therapy, and so on. This is a huge job, requiring thousands of experiments, well beyond the capacity of any one laboratory.

Linda Noble is a member of the MASCIS team. She says that the project is a very important development.

> *It forced us to develop the best experimental model, putting it in all of the participating labs, and then following very specific guidelines for experimental design. This has never been done before in spinal cord research.*

Such research is very slow, and for good reason. According to Noble, the issue is reproducibility. What is done in one lab must be capable of duplication in another to prove consistent results. The only way to do this, and so find out the specific behavior of a drug or a therapy, is to closely control the conditions.

> *It's a very precise cookbook of instructions. It's very demanding on technicians and very time-consuming. Because the process is so meticulous, it is fairly slow.*

Established at a time when spinal cord research was uncoordinated and marginally supported, MASCIS represents an important step in making the research more efficient. MASCIS represents a newfound cooperation between laboratories and scientists, and makes it possible for answers to be found that an individual lab could never have pursued on its own. This project is an important evolutionary step in the history of the research effort.

Hypothermia

Another method being explored to limit secondary damage at the time of injury is to lower the body temperature by two or three degrees, intentionally inducing hypothermia. This reduces the release of free radicals and glutamates which destroy healthy cells not affected by the trauma. This treatment is counter to common sense, which would dictate that the body needs optimal circulation in order to respond to injury and recover itself. However, in the case of spinal cord trauma, it appears that interrupting the destructive process of secondary damage is of greater value.

W. Dalton Dietrich, scientific director of the Miami Project, says:

> If you can cool the body by a few degrees, and then on top of that, provide a neuroprotective agent (such as MP or Sygen) or growth factor, you may see further dramatic improvements in the treatment of persons with acute SCI.[11]

Large-scale controlled studies have not yet been performed on this question.

4-Aminopyridine (4-AP)

The first effort to have an effect on the chronically injured spinal cord—well after the trauma—involved a drug called 4-Aminopyridine or 4-AP, sometimes referred to as Fampridine. Animal studies have shown that some nerve axons that survive a spinal cord trauma nonetheless fail to conduct an impulse past the injury site because of damaged myelin, the insulation of our spinal nerves. 4-AP appears to improve the function of demyelinated nerves. It does not actually restore myelin, but instead helps existing axons with otherwise complete connections to relay impulses.

Dr. Andrew Blight of the University of North Carolina discovered the effects of 4-AP on the spinal cord. It was initially used as a treatment for multiple sclerosis and in the laboratory to study neurons and axons. The loss of myelin surrounding nerve axons allows potassium to intrude, among other effects, interfering with the passage of nerve impulses. 4-AP is a "potassium channel blocker" which limits potassium from interfering with conduction in demyelinated nerves. By blocking the potassium, 4-AP increases the ability of these otherwise healthy axons to pass on an impulse. Since the greater portion of spinal cord injuries are incomplete—and presumably there are myelin-deprived but undamaged axons present—this could be a hopeful therapy for some people with central nervous system disorders.

Clinical trials performed in Canada in 1995 showed improvements in both motor and sensory functions following injections of 4-AP. Some of the subjects were more than a year post-injury. The degree of improvement varied. A man in Canada was able to consummate his marriage as a result of 4-AP treatment, yet other trial participants showed no reaction whatsoever. According to Dr. Blight:

> One third of the people with incomplete spinal cord injuries have experienced an improvement in quality of life in a variety of ways. In some people with significant preservation of motor function, the types of benefits include reduced pain, spasticity and muscle stiffness, increased or more normal sensation, and some improvement in motor functions, such as hand grip or walking efficiency. There are also consistent indications of improvements in bladder control and male sexual functions.[12]

Researchers were surprised to observe the reduced pain and spasticity. If anything, they were concerned that pain and spasticity would increase since 4-AP amplifies nerve signals.

All responses were temporary, yet scientists also found that benefits sometimes lasted for as long as four days, even though the drug was no longer present in the blood. Further research is exploring how it is that 4-AP continues to operate in the system.

4-AP works by increasing the excitability of axons, allowing them to better pass on the voltage of a nerve impulse. It also increases the amount of neurotransmitter at the synapse of the neuron, helping the impulse to transmit itself better across the nervous system.

The search continues for a therapy which will permanently restore myelin, either by stimulating the body to remyelinate its own axons or by implanting new cells which would take hold and reproduce. That discovery would cancel the need for the effects offered by 4-AP. In the meantime, human clinical trials of 4-AP are underway at the time of this writing.

Since there is some progress in the use of transplanted cells to remyelinate axons, physicians need to know whether there are intact axons present that would respond to such treatment. Toward this end, 4-AP could serve a diagnostic role, because if someone responds to the drug it means there are intact but demyelinated axons present.

There is no question that recovery from a spinal cord injury will involve many different factors, as described by quadriplegic research fundraiser, Marco Saroni:

> It's obvious that a cure is going to be complicated. There will be pharmaceuticals like growth factors, inhibitors. There will be surgery techniques, medical supplies, drug delivery, and a huge rehab effort. All of that is happening in parallel.

Acorda Therapeutics

Acorda Therapeutics, the first commercial venture established specifically to develop a spinal cord therapy, was established in 1995 by Dr. Ron Cohen. After working at another biotechnology firm, Cohen took a sabbatical to investigate what area of the industry would be exciting and had business potential. He found about twenty different spinal cord research fundraising entities spreading their money around to various universities and research labs with no coordination of the effort.

> The academic laboratories are designed to make discoveries, not to develop them into something useful. A commercial entity is needed to conduct more extensive animal studies, conduct toxicity studies to make sure the therapy is not harmful, and then figure out how to make a pure medicinal grade product. Only then can you proceed with human trials.

At that time, no major pharmaceutical companies were showing interest in spinal cord therapy. They consider the market too small and were not convinced that the research would be fruitful. Another factor in deciding to pursue spinal cord research was the superb animal models developed by Wise Young and his team. Acorda's capacity to test as many as 3,000 animals per year owes its thanks in part to this animal model.

Cohen gathered together the key players to discuss the issue, and found them frustrated with the lack of organization and cooperation between the various funding groups and research labs. These scientists understood that research is of no value unless there is some way for its findings to be approved by the FDA, manufactured, distributed, and sold. These are tasks that happen in the commercial realm, so the spinal cord research community supported Cohen's efforts to establish Acorda.

Acorda is privately financed, but has also received some institutional support. Acorda provides funds to its laboratory contractors, and is poised to license therapies from the laboratories as they become available. Licensing will provide royalties to the universities where the labs are located, helping them to continue their work. Meanwhile, Acorda gets the right to produce and market the therapy. The first product Acorda intends to market is the drug 4-Aminopyridine (4-AP), which helps existing myelin-compromised axons pass on a nerve impulse. The Canadian Spinal Research Organization gained the patent rights for 4-AP, and in 1995 licensed them to Acorda.

Who's paying for the research?

Spinal cord research has not been the kind of popular cause that attracts large amounts of money. Muscular dystrophy has the emotional image of disabled children, a well-known celebrity in Jerry Lewis, and a huge annual telethon to promote their fundraising. AIDS has the fearsome quality of an epidemic and the political and cultural intrigue of our society's struggle with the acceptance of homosexuals. Cancer and heart disease happen on such a large scale at such extreme cost that large contributions by government and individuals seem modest in comparison.

What would it take for spinal cord injury to become a more popular cause? Unfortunately it took the injury of Christopher Reeve, who now brings his fame as an actor and the remarkable coincidence of his film role as Superman to the fore, aggressively promoting spinal cord research. Suddenly the likes of Paul Newman and Robin Williams—close friends of Reeve's—are showing up at the fundraiser dinners.

The government has not been making the optimal investment in SCI research through the NIH, instead placing their emphasis on cancer and AIDS research. Lobbying efforts by the disability community have been focused on matters of employment, transportation, accessibility, and civil rights rather than on spending for cure research. In 1993, only $30 million was being spent by the federal government on spinal cord research. Sounds like a lot of money, but it is a tiny amount compared to what is spent on cancer research. When you compare it to the $6 billion dollars SCI is said to cost our economy each year—as estimated by the U.S. Centers for Disease Control—it is mere pocket change.

Spinal cord research is now getting more money, but many would say far from enough. The task of fundraising remains left to a variety of groups who raise money any which way they can, from individual memberships, corporate donations and endowments, parties, golf tournaments, and the like.

The organizations

Since the 1970s, a variety of groups have formed and re-formed for the purpose of advancing SCI research. One of the first, begun by the wife of a spinal-injured man, was the Bermuda Conferences on Spinal Cord Injury Research, which has given an award every other year since 1972.

In the late 1970s, the Paralyzed Veterans of America (PVA), the Spinal Cord Society (SCS), the Paralysis Cure Research (PCR)—formed by spinal-injured people—and the Help Them Walk Again Foundation were active. The Help Them Walk Again Foundation organized one of the first scientific meetings on spinal cord injury in 1979. The Spinal Cord Society funded much early research and earned national attention when its computerized walking demonstrations using functional electrical stimulation were featured on the television show *60 Minutes*. Its founder, Dr. Charles Carson, was honored as a hero by President Reagan in a State of the Union address.

What was once a shifting melange of groups has now consolidated into a few key entities which have grown and become more stable. Even more, where once they tended to be isolated and competitive, now they are cooperating and coordinating their efforts. These organizations include the American Paralysis Association (APA), the Miami Project to Cure Paralysis at the University of Miami School of Medicine, the aforementioned PVA and the Canadian Spinal Research Organization (CSRO).

These groups have become a primary source of information regarding research, through publication of newsletters and press releases, and through conferences. They also have a presence on the Internet, maintaining sites on the World Wide Web that provide current updates on research and funding.

While Christopher Reeve has been the impetus for some wider awareness and increased funding, his public presence has begun to wane, as most human interest stories do in the media. You can help by supporting one of these groups, participating in their events, inviting friends and family to contribute, and writing Congress to encourage increased funding of the National Institutes of Health.

Variety of studies being conducted

There is a dizzying array of research projects being conducted under the auspices of these groups. Each season the APA, the Miami Project, and others all publish newsletters. The newsletter pages are graced with the faces of scientists next to their microscopes or banks of mysterious electronic devices, with summaries of their projects in very detailed terms. This is not reading for the average non-scientist, but it sure gets across the scale of talent at work. A few random examples:

- Dr. Robert H. Brown of Massachusetts General Hospital is working on a "non-viral vector for the targeted delivery of neuroprotective proteins to spinal cord motor neurons." The intent is to limit cell death from free radicals just post-injury.

- Ron McKay, Ph.D., of the National Institute of Neurological Disorders and Stroke has been following up on a discovery made in the early '90s. Stem cells in the brain and spinal cord have a unique ability to multiply and mature, giving added hope to the possibility of transplantation of cells.

- Jack Diamond, Ph.D., of McMaster University in Ontario, Canada, is exploring the "functional consequences of primary afferent intraspinal sprouting." Injured nerves often send out fresh sprouts that can't find a useful connection. This research attempts to find a use for the degree of regeneration that already takes place in the injured spinal cord.

- L.J. Stensaas of the University of Utah has studied the spinal cord of the newt. He found that "astrocytes"—cells normally found in nerves that provide nutrients—play a role in removing degenerating nerve axons, and then act as a base for growth of new fibers.

- Dr. Amy MacDermott of Columbia University is looking into the "selective excitotoxic death of GABAergic dorsal horn neurons." Some people with spinal cord injuries become extremely sensitive to touch, which is often painful. Dr. MacDermott feels that there is a chemical process which over-stimulates sensory nerves, and he hopes to develop a pharmaceutical treatment to minimize pain from this cause.

- Dr. James Guest, completing his doctoral dissertation at the Miami Project, demonstrated that human Schwann cells support regeneration and myelination in adult rat spinal cords.

- Jian Zhou, Ph.D., of the University of Texas in Dallas addresses the "structural analysis of neurotrophin receptor signaling in neurons." This work intends to better describe the process of how signals are delivered through nerves by neurotrophins, which also support the nourishment and growth of nerves.

Reading these newsletters can leave you wondering how all these detailed studies fit together. They don't. There is intentional overlap, and various solutions are being explored for any given piece of the puzzle. One finding might shed light on another, or certain projects may suddenly add up to a solution that hadn't been considered (just as the discovery of penicillin was an "accident").

There seems to be more cause than ever to hope for some answers that will make a difference in the daily life of people with CNS disabilities. Hundreds of brilliant, highly educated, and trained people are working hard, and it is difficult to imagine that they won't make a difference in our life on wheels.

Who else benefits from SCI research?

There has been a great deal of emphasis on spinal cord research here, but SCI research will benefit people with other disabilities such as spinal muscular atrophy, stroke, traumatic brain injury, multiple sclerosis, Guillan-Barre syndrome, myesthenia gravis, and Alzheimer's and Parkinson's diseases. Elderly people with severe osteoarthritis can suffer the degradation of the spinal column itself, which can ultimately impact the cord. There are dozens of vascular, neurogenerative, and congenital diseases that impact the spinal cord. Spinal cord tumors can occur in cases of metastasized breast or prostate cancer. People affected by all these conditions can benefit from this research.

When combined, people with these conditions far outnumber those with traumatic spinal cord injury. But SCI happens more commonly to young people, while these other conditions often appear later in life. Older people with other conditions will become wheelchair users. But their survival is often short, for example, once a cancer has spread, whereas a young person with a spinal injury is likely to live a normal life span. That difference in longevity makes the long-term costs of spinal cord injury greater, cold as that might sound. The fact is that there are plenty of forms of human suffering, all with their advocates and scientists clamoring for money from the same corporate and government sources. The fact that young people are being injured with a lifetime ahead of them is part of what justifies the amount of work done on spinal cord research. Fortunately, many others will get the chance to benefit.

Electric walking

The first "cure" effort to get wide public exposure involved simulating walking by using electrical impulses to make muscles contract. In 1970, scientists at the Rancho Los Amigos Hospital near Los Angeles and another group in what was then Yugoslavia got a paraplegic standing up with this approach, known as functional neuromuscular stimulation (FNS). In 1973, a test subject at the University of Virginia walked forty feet, and a Vienna project got two people walking as far as one hundred meters using crutches. In the U.S., Dr. Jerold Petrofsky was a key player at Wright State University in Ohio, and now leads the Petrofsky Institute where FNS is featured.

FNS is a subset of functional electrical stimulation (FES), which is used in many other applications where electrical impulse devices are used in places other than the muscles. A heart pacemaker is an example of FES, using electrical stimulation to balance the beating of the heart. FES is used for pain management, hearing enhancement, as an aid to male ejaculation, muscle strengthening, wound healing, and scoliosis correction. These uses are already accepted practice, and many other applications are either at the basic research level or as far advanced as clinical trials.

As with much "cure" research, FNS for standing and gait control has been over-dramatized by the media. As a walking device it is still at a very early stage, and limited to a narrow population of qualified, potential users. At the moment it is very exhausting, although participants in trials have shown improvements with hard work and regular therapy and practice. No one is yet able to use it full time for their general mobility, but instead find that a wheelchair is more efficient and less tiring.

Yet researchers have accomplished a great deal, including subjects who have been able to walk up and down stairs using only the hand railing. Some have gotten far enough to use it for brief walking tasks such as walking down the aisle at their own wedding. Several current projects are designed to achieve hands-free standing. This is all meaningful progress, but FNS for walking still has a way to go before it is a valid alternative to wheeling, if ever.

How muscles walk

How a muscle is normally stimulated in the body is a very complex sequence of events. Muscle stimulation is not simply a matter of how much electricity to send to which part of a muscle. This is a very detailed matter of how the impulse intensity rises and drops, and the maintenance of the impulse during a contraction.

The body, it turns out, does not simply send a continuous stream of electricity to the muscle, but rather a stream of pulses. A continuous current quickly exhausts a muscle. Muscles also have different roles to play. Some are for posture, and some are for movement, each displaying very different electrical profiles. Matching the natural pattern of stimulation is one of the key challenges of FNS for walking, so that such a system can be used productively without over-stimulation of the muscles. The system must mimic the body's miraculous design, which makes the most efficient use of its muscles to minimize fatigue.

Walking involves thousands of simultaneous signals going back and forth between muscles and the brain, a tremendously intricate coordination of sensations and contractions. The most sophisticated systems presently use only fifty electrodes, though that number is sure to grow. At present, the only possible stimulus is to make the muscle contract—the user gets no sensory feedback to know where their muscles are.

Electronics is one half of the system, the other half is bracing. In the past, some people were fitted with heavy leg braces, which only added to the weight that they had to balance, lift, and propel using crutches. This load made more work for the electronics, too, so part of the effort has been to develop lightweight bracing. The development of the Reciprocating Gait Orthotic, or RGO brace, has been helpful thanks to its more lightweight design.

People who have been research subjects with early systems have been concerned with appearance. Most people don't want to go out in public all wired up and braced in a way that attracts unwanted attention. Lightweight braces and small power and control devices that can be worn under the clothes are being developed to make FNS more practical and desirable.

Locating the electrodes

There are several methods of stimulating the muscles. Some designs use tight-fitting, stretchable pants that contain the electrodes. This is the most discrete method, but placing electrodes on the surface of the skin is the least effective way of getting the signal to the muscle. The signal has to pass through layers of skin and fat. This approach has the disadvantage of stimulating muscles in groups, with much less individual control. There is also some risk of irritating or burning the skin with the stronger current it takes to reach through the skin to the muscles.

The alternative to electrodes on the skin is to implant electrodes directly into the body, so they can contract specific muscles. Electrodes are either sewn to the surface of the muscle or a cuff design is wrapped around the tissue. Another type is implanted deep into the muscle, and can be inserted by a modified hypodermic needle without the use of a surgical incision. Implants bring with them the risk of infection, and can break or slip out of position.

Once the electrodes are implanted, the wires either come back out through the skin to be hooked to external stimulators, or the stimulators can be implanted as well. External stimulators are easier to upgrade than implanted stimulators, as the technology continues to develop. However, electrode wires coming through the skin need daily care.

Parastep

As of 1997, the FDA had approved the Parastep System, produced by Sigmedics of Northfield, Illinois, and originally developed at the University of Illinois Medical School and the Michael Reese Medical Center in Chicago.

The user operates controls on a walker, with buttons for sitting, standing, movement of the left and right legs, and intensity of the contractions. The Parastep System uses twelve externally applied electrodes. A small number of people are using the system with lofstran crutches—the type with the forearm loop. They use more of a swing-through gait, rather than the individual stepping that would be seen using a walker.

Parastep users like John Targowski, a student at the University of Michigan, report a variety of benefits. John values the increased muscle bulk from electrically stimulated contractions:

> I like to keep the size of my leg muscles in good proportion to my upper body. Although other paraplegics might take some offense, I really don't like the typical appearance of huge arms and chests attached to stick legs. Secondly, I am an optimist and a future thinker. Soon, spinal injury will be curable or at the very least, treatable. When this time comes, I want the bones, muscles, and tendons in my legs to be ready.

Who can use it?

A very narrow population of people are even able to use Parastep. To be a candidate you must have sufficient upper body strength to lift yourself into a standing position, enough muscle power in your legs for the FNS system to be able to lock your knees strongly enough to support your weight, and good range of motion. This usually means a lot of work in the therapy gym to build the upper body, increase balance, do aggressive stretching to correct contracture of the muscles from sitting, and to build more muscle tissue using FNS bikes and exercise devices.

Other characteristics that would disqualify you for FNS include significant spasticity, cardiac disease, epilepsy, severe scoliosis, symptomatic osteoporosis, obesity, or autonomic dysreflexia. FNS is used primarily by people with spinal cord injury, but can be used by some people with multiple sclerosis, spina bifida, or stroke. A specialized system is in use to correct the foot drop problem common as a leftover of stroke.

In a study conducted at the Continental Rehab Hospital in San Diego, ninety-one people passed the early screening and were able to stand with Parastep. Only fifty completed the training, some because of personal demands. Thirty-one of them were able to walk an average of 324 feet. Twenty-one of these people have used Parastep in their homes and community. Researchers found there was not a strong correlation between success and the level of the injury. In other words, having an injury at T12 did not especially ensure greater success than a level of T6, although no one higher than T4 achieved independence with the system.[13]

Open/closed loop

An open-loop system is controlled entirely by the user, often with switches mounted on the handle of a walker. The FNS controller only sends signals to the muscles according to your commands.

A closed-loop system tracks and processes information to help the system make some of its own decisions. As computer chips get smaller, more powerful, and require less energy—the Parastep runs on eight AAA batteries—designers are able to increase the intelligence of the system. The angle of the knee or ankle can tell the system where the leg is in the process of taking a step. A closed-loop system can know to control impulses to specific muscles depending on the degree of contraction. It could sense how much weight is on the foot, so that when the right foot is firmly on the ground, for instance, the left leg could be made to lift and the knee to bend.

Some combination of automatic and user-defined control is the goal. Researchers are very aware that the results could be disastrous if the system takes a step for you when you don't want it to.

Not a cure yet

FES/FNS is not being promoted as a replacement for a wheelchair. It is a limited option, requires a lot of effort to use it, and still has a lot of development work left to increase its attractiveness. It also should not be thought of just in terms of walking. Standing, in and of itself, is valuable for preventing bone loss, to promote circulation. For many people it is a great psychological boost to be able to stand. Some systems are geared toward assisting in transfers from a bed, wheelchair, bath, commode, chair, or sofa. The ability to stand temporarily in the kitchen to reach a shelf or at a job can have worthwhile benefits. Again, just as with spinal cord regeneration research, you should not be excessively caught up in the image of walking again.

Getting a grip

In August 1997, the Food and Drug Administration approved the Freehand System from NeuroControl Corporation of Cleveland, Ohio. It is an implanted FNS device that restores hand grip and release ability to quadriplegics.

The Freehand System is a surgical option, involving a five- to seven-hour operation under general anesthesia. Incisions are made at the upper arm, forearm, and chest. Eight electrodes about the size of a dime are sewn onto the appropriate muscles. In some cases, tendon transfer surgery is also performed to transfer function to chosen joints using muscles that can be most effectively contracted by the Freehand system. Tendon surgery can also increase your ability to extend your arm at the elbow or bend your wrist.

Many quadriplegics with a level of C5-6 still have sufficient shoulder and upper arm and elbow function to use the system. The shoulder is used as a switch, making subtle, largely unnoticeable movements to initiate movements in the hand and fingers and to lock the grip position. An external sensor attached to your chest reads your shoulder position, sending the information to an external controller mounted on the wheelchair. Then a signal is transmitted to the implanted stimulator which activates the appropriate combination of eight electrodes implanted in the muscles of the forearm and hand.

Two kinds of grip are possible with this device. Palmar prehension is a cuplike grasp in which the thumb and fingers close toward each other for grasping cups, balls, or a game piece. Lateral prehension brings the thumb to the side of the index finger while closing the fingers for holding a pen or an eating implement. One might be a candidate for one or both grips.

First you would undergo therapy to strengthen muscles using FES exercise to build tone prior to the surgery. Most of this can be done at home. After the implant, the arm is kept immobilized in a cast for up to a month to heal from the surgery, during which time you will probably need additional assistance with daily living tasks. Then another process of therapy and training will take place before you would get full use of the implant. You must stretch and strengthen the muscles, and learn how to use your hand again. It will be odd to use your hand without sensations, and you must learn to pay extra attention to the temperature and safety of the material you will pick up. The entire process can take up to twelve weeks.

The internal stimulator is similar to pacemaker devices which have been implanted in heart patients for the past twenty-five years. It is made of inert material that is unlikely to produce an immune system rejection response from the body.

The first Freehand user had the implant surgery in 1986, and the company says that the person is still using it successfully in 1997. There is no long-term data available about how long the system will last. The internal stimulator has no batteries, and is designed to be long lasting, but eventually will age. It is probable that the technology will improve well before the device breaks down. Either situation will require additional surgery. It is conceivable that someday more than two types of grip will be possible.

At the time of FDA approval in August 1997 there were twenty hospitals around the United States that performed the implantation surgery. Costs vary among centers and physicians.

The ability to grip is far more significant for these people than being able to walk. Their independence is multiplied now that they have a greater—or newfound—ability to feed themselves, to write, operate a telephone, and perform many other basic daily activities without assistance. They are also saved the cost of a major portion of the attendant support they no longer need, or dependence on sip-and-puff or voice-operated control devices which have a limited usefulness and a capacity to break down. Hopefully, insurance companies will recognize the direct savings of covering the Freehand System. Their savings would be almost instant.

Who are the researchers?

The day of the lone scientist who makes a historic discovery are pretty much over. Hidden knowledge that could be found that way has been found already. Dr. Ron Cohen of Acorda Therapeutics says:

> There is a huge public misconception of the Louis Pasteur type of scientist alone in his lab who finds a vaccine and then finds a child to try it on and saves the child's life. There was a time when that was the only way it could be done, when there were no large pharmaceutical companies. We only heard about the famous ones who succeeded, but for every one of those there might have been hundreds who came up with what turned out to be quack remedies that might have even killed people.

Times have changed, indeed. Researchers are now trained in years of intensive study and clinical internship. People are increasingly specialized in pursuits such as molecular biology, genetic engineering, or microsurgery. Such specialization naturally requires people to work in teams, each applying their focused knowledge according to their appropriate role in the process. Research today is necessarily a collaborative process.

Researchers also have access to a tremendous amount of previous experience and information, now all the more accessible via the Internet and dedicated medical information services like Medline. Computers have expanded the precision and capabilities of testing and measurement equipment many thousand-fold, making it possible to see into worlds that were previously closed to the microscope. Calculations done in a moment by a computer would have taken months—or years—by hand.

Researchers now operate under much more stringent regulatory and ethical standards. Compared to the history of medical research, wanton experimentation is all but completely ended. Researchers go to great extremes to verify the value of human trials before they proceed. The FDA demands that they offer extensive proof of their studies before permission is given for human trials. There will always be risk with experiments, but when the initial groundwork is done well, the likelihood of life-threatening reactions to testing are very low. These, at least, are the standards you should apply to any research project that you might consider participating in as a subject.

Living by the grant

Researchers rely heavily on grant money from many sources. If they conduct work that proves fruitless or unverifiable, they run the risk of not being able to acquire additional funding. Remember, learning from what doesn't work is different than having a failed experiment. The test is not always whether they produce a usable therapy, but whether they gain valuable information toward that end. Either way, researchers are very motivated to work in a highly organized fashion. It affects their ability to keep working by means of qualifying for grant money.

The only way that these labs can exist is to pursue funding from different sources, with many projects going at once. It is not unusual for several donors to contribute to the same research, though when future licensing or other commercial interests are involved such funding is carefully defined according to who would be entitled to possible commercial fruits of the work.

Commercial funding, such as that by Acorda, inevitably overlaps government money. The government does not mind investing in research that might result in a commercial product. It helps the economy, so Washington does not regard this as a conflict of interests. Says Acorda founder Ron Cohen:

> But when it comes to overlapping with another company, the lab will not take funding for the same project because the companies won't agree to that.

PVA's Melinda Kelley says that:

> Most people don't know that the National Institutes of Health fund most of the biomedical research in this country—at least that done at academic institutions and medical centers. It is not the case that labs are usually funded by companies.

The motivated scientist

Researchers are often the unheralded heroes, working on extensive studies that are highly detailed, challenging, and time consuming. Some of them could probably be out in offices and hospitals treating patients and making much more money, but chose the course where they feel they can make the most difference. They seem to be more interested in taking pride in their work than in following the money, which they have to beg for through the grueling process of grant writing and approval. Their motive is compassion; results are their reward.

Linda Noble, researcher at the University of California at San Francisco, says:

> I was a physical therapist, and when I was an intern I chose spinal cord injury as my specialty and spent a lot of time with these patients. I was very frustrated by the situation they were in, that they didn't get answers. I decided the best thing for me was to work in the area of spinal cord research.

Dr. Richard Borgens of the Center for Paralysis Research at Purdue University studied limb regeneration in salamanders as a graduate student. He won an award for the work from the National Paraplegic Foundation, and encountered a room full of chair users at the award ceremony. He found himself uncomfortable as a person who could walk among so many wheelchair riders, having never even seen a quadriplegic. The human character of his work became clear, and he says:

> People with spinal cord injuries gave me an important professional start—and I still strive to repay the debt.

What about the animals?

Not all research can be performed on cells in dishes or simulated on a computer. Some tests require a working biological system that parallels human beings, such as that in rats and dogs. Spinal cord research is not just about how to get a nerve to grow, as we've already seen. It is about the immensely complex system of chain reactions that occur in the real environment of living physiology. It is about the response of the body to a substance you might place into the system by any of a number of methods. It is about finding out that there are other factors at play which might not appear until you try what seems like a viable approach. This living research can only be studied in animals.

According to the American Academy of Neurology (AAN), less than 1 percent of research animals are dogs or cats. Ninety percent of research animals are rodents, such as rats and mice. AAN points out that more than ten million unwanted animals are put to death each year in animal shelters, and only 1 percent of that total are released for research. In fact, most research animals are carefully bred for their purpose. AAN also points out that animal subjects have produced benefits for the veterinary community as well, benefiting animals as well as humans.[14]

While some animal rights activists might draw comparisons to human experimentation in Nazi Germany, remember that such atrocities were performed with no concern for the experience of the subjects, often without the use of anesthetics, watching suffering of the deepest kind in order to "learn" from it. In the present, highly regulated setting of medical research, government inspectors make surprise visits to determine the conditions of animal research. Besides, says AAN:

> Treating research animals humanely is not only the right thing to do, it is a matter of self-interest. Scientists know that mistreatment can distort test results and ruin years of painstaking, costly work.

Using animals for research is widely supported by physicians, 97 percent of whom responded to an American Medical Association study with support for their continued use.

The AAN says that "medical progress is simply not possible without animal research, and millions of people will pay the price if it is curtailed." They are concerned that animal rights activists will compromise promising research into Parkinson's and Alzheimer's disease, traumatic brain injury, meningitis, spinal cord paralysis, stroke, epilepsy, and many others. The AAN says that animals are used "with the dignity, gentleness, and respect to which they are entitled."

There was a time when research was sometimes carried out indiscriminately without concern for the suffering of the subject animals, but that time is past. There are very strict guidelines that laboratories must follow, and those who do not conform risk being forced out of operation.

Linda Noble of UCSF notes:

> You have to be very careful about how the experiments are done and that you make sure you have people working in your lab who understand that they are working with living creatures entitled to as much care as you would give to a human patient. That's exactly how we work. Being a good scientist means that your use of animals is kept to a minimum. It's very clearly thought out. The quality of care that spinal cord injured rats get is superb. We basically run an intensive care unit. We are monitoring our animals all the time. My goal is to help the human population and I can't do it any other way.

You might find that the issue of using animals in research raises conflicts for you, as you attempt to balance your desire for less pain and greater independence in your own life with an ethical and moral position regarding the treatment of all living creatures. This person with a spinal cord injury sympathizes with what animals were undergoing, but doesn't want research to stop:

> I eat meat and wear leather, so I feel it would be hypocritical for me to take a stand against animal research. I also feel that if animal research ever results in a cure for SCI (or any other disease), or helps relieve human suffering in any way, I will thank and honor the animals that were used to bring this about.

Research relies on the use of animals for its work. As much as we might prefer not to inflict suffering on any living creature, this work cannot take place without them. Since researchers are motivated by compassion for humans and a desire to end suffering, they are going to use animals in their research with respect, and keep their suffering to the absolute minimum possible. Researchers who mistreat animals deserve to lose the right to conduct research. The research community has demonstrated that it takes its ethical concerns seriously in the process of doing this remarkable work—work which appears to have so much potential to improve the lives of everyone, including people with disabilities.

Being a research subject

Before any research can be approved for use, clinical studies must be performed. At first, animal subjects are used, but ultimately human trials will be necessary. You might well be a candidate to participate in studies of therapies before they are approved for public use. This is a complex and very critical decision to make, one that demands you be informed and think carefully about the risks that might be involved.

By their nature, research studies entail a degree of risk. The very point is to observe the effects—positive or negative—of the tests. The reason to participate in such a study is to help scientists develop useful therapies, not to get treatment before it is publicly available. There is no guarantee that the tests will be beneficial for you. The motive of most test subjects is the benefit of future persons who will use the therapy if it proves of value. That might include you.

Clinical trials

A clinical trial is a tightly designed plan, prepared by doctors and scientists. The government's Food and Drug Administration (FDA) might participate in its development, as might a commercial entity interested in being the producer of the drug. This is a very precise project, defining specific criteria and methods.

It used to be that any researcher could go out and try the next "miracle cure" on anybody they could convince to go along. Doctors were under no restrictions in their experiments, and there were plenty of "snake oil salesmen" out pitching the latest elixir to cure any ailment you might think of. Even Coca-Cola was first promoted as a curative.

Of course, people often suffered and sometimes died in the process of this uncontrolled approach. Today the standards are very high, if only because a scientist who does not work within a very prescribed process risks wasting years of work if his or her data is not found responsible and consistent. More to the point, the scientists conducting the study will be just as concerned with your well-being as with their reputations and legal liability.

Most trials employ a Safety Monitoring Committee which reviews the study as it progresses. They have the power to end the study at any point if they find that the therapy is not effective or is causing harm rather than help.

The hospital, clinic, or school conducting the study will also have an Institutional Review Board which has seen and approved the study protocol in advance. They receive regular reports and have the power to suspend a study.

Withdrawal

You have the right to withdraw from a study at any time, but it may be possible that abruptly ending a therapy could itself be dangerous. You must understand that when you agree to participate you must follow the instructions absolutely and report any effects to your supervising physician. If you are considering withdrawing, discuss this with the doctor whose job it is to be your consultant, helping you to make the final decision. He should then advise you of the safest way to end the therapy and/or resume your previous treatment.

Placebos

Many studies involve use of a placebo, an inert substance given to some subjects rather than the actual drug being tested. This is to reveal whether some of the results observed might be because a subject believes they have been given a beneficial drug. It is now increasingly understood that attitude and belief can have a real impact on the physical—the so-called mind-body connection.

It is important to compare people who are getting the drug to people who are not to understand what real impact the actual drug is having. In some studies, you might consistently receive either the active drug or the placebo. In others, you might be getting one or the other at any one time.

It is not possible to request that you be given the active form of the drug. It would alter the results of the study if you knew which you were getting. Again, your reason for participating is to assist research, not just to gain early access to an unproved treatment.

You might be asked to cease taking a drug therapy that has already been prescribed for you. Drugs interact with each other in the body, and the needs of the trial might require that you end your current treatment. You must balance the possible risks of going off of your present therapy against the potential benefits of your participation.

Blind studies

Clinical trials are generally either single-blind or double-blind. If you are in a single-blind study, you do not know whether you are getting the active drug or the placebo, but your doctor does. In a double-blind study, neither you nor the doctor knows. However, other investigators involved in the study have that information. If you were to have a severe reaction to treatment, it would always be possible to find out what you actually received.

Phases

Clinical trials are performed in three phases:

- **Phase I.** Sometimes referred to as a "safety study," its main purpose is to test dosage. This is the time of greater risk because less is known about reaction to the drug. High doses might be given exactly to measure side effects. Only a few persons are used at this stage.

- **Phase II.** More people are included in the study, now that there is some sense of what the appropriate dosage should be. Now it is possible to begin to observe the effectiveness of the treatment. Several rounds of Phase II studies might be performed before the team feels ready for Phase III.

- **Phase III.** Many more subjects are studied, often at a number of participating institutions. This is the time to validate the discoveries of the first two phases, and prepare statistical data to use in the process of gaining FDA approval for the potential commercial introduction of the therapy.

Money

Some trials pay their subjects for their participation, and some don't. There might be certain procedures which you would need to pay for, and you should check with your health insurer to see if they would be covered. There could be travel and accommodation expenses during periods in which you might need to stay near a medical center for initial tests and observation if you live away from where the study is centered. Or your usual doctor might be able to participate and conduct some of the procedures.

On the other hand, you might benefit from additional coverage due to your participation in the study. You could be seen more regularly by doctors, and in effect be getting more aggressive care of your condition at no extra expense.

You should not pay a fee to participate in a clinical study. These are always performed with funding from public, charitable, or commercial sources. The group conducting the study should not be in a position to profit from the actual study. They might, however, profit from future licensing or sale of the drug if it attains FDA approval.

Risks and benefits of participating

Some risks of participating in a clinical trial:

- Adverse reactions to the drug
- Possible harm from receiving a placebo rather than active treatment
- Physical discomforts from tests
- Disruption in your personal schedule to be present for tests and examinations

Some benefits of participating:

- Possible improvement in your condition
- More frequent monitoring by doctors during the study
- Improved coverage of expenses
- Personal gratification for your role in assisting the study

Questions to ask

You have the right to ask any questions you have about the study and your role in it. You should seriously reconsider your willingness to participate in any study in which your questions are not fully and patiently answered. Among the things you should know are:

- If you live a distance from the study center, how long will you need to be available to them and at what stages of the study?
- What kinds of tests will you be asked to submit to during the study?
- How long is the study expected to last?

- Is there a possibility that you will be receiving a placebo?

- Will your usual doctor participate or be informed about your role in the study?

- Who will know that you are participating in the study? Is your participation anonymous or simply confidential?

- What risks are already known about the substance or therapy being studied?

- What are the potential benefits the study hopes to demonstrate?

- Are there any results already known about the drug, good or bad?

- How many others are participating in the study?

- Will you need to go off of your present drug therapy?

- What, if any, portions of the study will you need to pay for?

- Who will pay for treatment if you should experience an adverse reaction?

- Who is financing the study?

- What forms will you be asked to sign, and what legal obligations do all the parties agree to?

Inclusion still the priority

For the foreseeable future, we will remain a human community with a significant population of people who have physical disabilities of various sorts. Regardless of the modern miracles that continue to be pursued by science, everybody is entitled to full inclusion according to their true capabilities. We need to support research that can improve quality of life, but not at the price of continuing to cast people with disabilities in the role of damaged goods. Maybe some people will walk again, maybe not. Either way, we mustn't let any hope we place in research prevent us from continuing the progress disability advocates have made in removing social and physical obstacles which now prevent too many people from living to their full potential.

CHAPTER 10

Politics and Legislation

The history of disability includes much recent progress. Knowing more about movements to secure disability rights can make you more aware of how various laws may impact you, and perhaps make you more inclined to take an activist role yourself.

In this chapter, we examine recent U.S. history, beginning with the Rehabilitation Act of 1973, the Independent Living Movement, and the Americans with Disabilities Act. We also look at access to education (IDEA), Social Security, community care, controversies surrounding assisted suicide, access to transportation, and law enforcement. The chapter closes with a look at remaining challenges.

Rehabilitation Act of 1973

The Rehabilitation Act of 1973 protects people with disabilities from discrimination by the federal government and their contractors. The key provision of the bill is Section 504, a small bit of text that almost went unnoticed. According to Joseph Shapiro in *No Pity*, it was "no more than a legislative afterthought."[1]

Section 504 said that no federal agency, public university, federal contractor, or entity that received federal funding could discriminate "solely by reason of handicap." Federal funding is pervasive enough for this to have far-reaching effects. This was a historic first, and it happened without any lobbying from the disability lobby, no hearings or debate. It was the first legislation to address disability civil rights.

Section 504 got noticed soon enough. Disability activists realized what a potent tool was suddenly in their hands. Unfortunately, the government did too, as the Department of Health, Education and Welfare (HEW) estimated that compliance would cost billions of dollars. The Secretary of HEW, Joseph Califano, and President Carter were concerned that alcoholics and drug addicts would seek protection under 504, a concern that continues to haunt the Americans with Disabilities Act these days.

They began to consider ways to dilute the regulations, spurring protests. Demonstrators held a candlelight vigil at Califano's home and two days later occupied his offices in Washington, D.C. Protests were not limited to the nation's capitol. Concurrent—and also short-lived—demonstrations took place in New York and Los Angeles, but San Francisco would prove to be the site of greatest drama.

In 1977, a group of protestors occupied the San Francisco offices of HEW, an action which was to last for twenty-five days. After garnering support from media and state legislators, the message was sent to Washington that separate but equal was not acceptable. Califano finally gave in on April 28, signing the regulations without change.

The protest was not only a cause for wheelchair users, as people with hearing and vision impairments, mental retardation, and other disabilities came together at the protest and learned about each other's needs. The San Francisco 504 protest had a unifying impact on the disability scene which would enlarge its political scope. It also helped people learn new pride in themselves, regardless of their disability. Mary Jane Owens was present for the full twenty-five days in San Francisco. She felt that everyone there discovered their true importance and beauty, expressed by this memory:

> One image from the 504 sit-in still moves me. One night we each decided to make a wish. The last one to speak was a bright and perky young woman who wore braces and used crutches. She said, "If I'd been asked before to make a wish, it would have been not to be a cripple. I wanted to be beautiful. But now I know I am beautiful just the way I am."[2]

From law to reality

Having Section 504 in place was no guarantee that change would take place. People with disabilities and their families still had plenty of work to do to ensure that the provision would be enforced.

Disability civil rights differs from other quests for equality in one particularly crucial aspect: it costs money. Disability civil rights means building ramps, enlarging bathrooms, widening doors, adding elevators, using tactile surfaces for people with vision impairments, setting aside seats in theaters, paying personnel in corporations to manage disability services, and much more that represents real out-of-pocket costs. There would prove to be a lot of resistance to paying the premium.

Take the farming town of Rudd, Iowa, informed they had to make their public library accessible at a cost of $6,500 although no one in town used a wheelchair. They were not pleased to feel they were forced to spend money toward no good purpose. This sentiment arose in many other scenarios, including places like fire stations, in which the case is made that a person using a wheelchair would never be a fireman, so why should they have to spend the money?

But the cost of access is often vastly overestimated. Architect Ron Mace, quoted in *No Pity*, describes North Carolina education officials who believed statewide access would cost $15 billion dollars.[3] It turned out to be $15 million. Many accommodations cost nothing, such as relocating a class to another room, allowing use of private bathrooms until larger stalls are built, or raising a desk to clear someone's knees. The initial reaction of business and local governments was to assume that construction and expensive equipment was the only way to address the needs of people with disabilities. Experience has proven them wrong.

College campuses would make the same argument as the town of Rudd. "We don't have any students in wheelchairs," they would say. In hindsight, we know that this was a question of "if you build it they will come." Now that colleges are widely accessible, thousands of students wheel their way across campuses, supported by an array of disabled student services, including attendant support, sign interpreters, and access to technology. 504's impact has been broad indeed and is turning out to have been well worth the investment. Many of these people would otherwise be collecting Social Security or other forms of public money, but now are working, paying taxes, and spending money in their communities.

The Independent Living Movement

In 1972, the Center for Independent Living (CIL) was incorporated in the showroom of an ex-automobile dealership in Berkeley, and the national Independent Living Movement was born. It shared the philosophy of rehabilitation professionals that a person could be seen as a whole, but objected to the medical view of that person as a "patient" who can only benefit from a structured medical setting. Today the preferred terms are "client" and "consumer." Clients use services as part of their efforts to live optimal lives.

Word of the Independent Living Movement began to spread. People with disabilities around the country, hungry for control over their lives, began to call and visit. Berkeley students who worked at the center would return to their hometowns after graduation and start CILs of their own. The Berkeley CIL became the model and the training ground for what came to be a nationwide network.

Says Mary Lou Breslin of Berkeley's Disability Rights and Education Defense Fund:

> *This concept of a center where people would make their own decisions—and it wouldn't be run by social workers—was a breakthrough phenomenon.*

The early CILs had to hustle for money, combining any sources they could: a university affiliation, corporate sponsorships, and grassroots fundraising. Judy Heumann led a campaign in Washington to get federal funding for independent living centers included in the Rehabilitation Act. 1978's Title VII includes Independent Living Provisions so people could apply to the federal government for funds to start a CIL. Says Breslin:

> *It enabled little communities that would have had a hard time finding seed money to provide core services—things like attendant referral, peer counseling, and housing assistance.*

There are now more than four hundred Independent Living Centers in a range of sizes across the United States. Many qualify for federal funding, though this is still only a portion of their budgets. There is a national association. An annual conference allows staff from the centers to share ideas, get the latest on political issues, and gain from others' experience in establishing and managing programs.

Your local CIL might offer any of a wide array of services, such as personal assistance referrals, housing referrals, employment services, transportation, financial counseling, legal assistance, peer programs, deaf, blind, and mental disability services, and political advocacy. The Independent Living Movement has helped many people with disabilities of all kinds to pursue their best possibilities and has fostered a growing political constituency.

The movement is not without its challenges. There continue to be funding issues. After having been spawned by people who were reacting *against* the government's lack of support for disability issues—such as its foot-dragging on Section 504 of the 1973 Rehabilitation Act—many of the larger CILs find themselves reliant on federal funds. It is often a political balancing act where they must take care not to bite the hand that feeds them.

The greatest conflict on the CIL scene is between advocacy and services. The pioneers of the movement are not usually running the CILs anymore; CILs are often staffed by people who see what they do as a job and are not inclined to go occupy an office building to fight for someone's rights.

Yet there seems to be a shift back towards advocacy. Gina McDonald, president of the National Council on Independent Living (NCIL) said in an interview in *Mouth* magazine:

> There used to be a time when you'd say (to a CIL), "Who's your advocacy person?" and they'd say, "Well, we don't really have time to do that." Yet they have three independent living specialists. Now some of the centers are going back to say, first we'll do our advocacy, then look at everything else.[4]

How to reach people with disabilities continues to be a challenge. There are a variety of reasons why people might not choose to contact a CIL. Those who are working and independent tend to feel they don't need support groups or advocacy training. Those who have good resources may feel they can accomplish more on their own. The audience who shows up tends to be those with lower incomes who are desperate for community, or desperate for assistance in acquiring needed benefits. Even many of those never find their way to a CIL. Dr. Marcel Dijkers, director of research at Detroit's Rehabilitation Institute of Michigan, says:

> Probably less than 5 percent of people even know the CIL exists. To a degree, people choose not to participate. Once they're discharged, the first thing they want to do is go home and rest up from what we put them through. Four months later, when they're ready to see what's outside their apartment, they've forgotten about CIL.

In a program in Ann Arbor, Michigan, the local CIL has developed a relationship with the University of Michigan rehab unit. They get involved with people from the very beginning of their rehab experience, providing peer support and valuable information. Once the person is released—with considerable adjustments yet to be made—they are not about to forget about the CIL, thanks to the very close contact they had during their inpatient days.

The Americans with Disabilities Act

The Americans with Disabilities Act is a civil rights act. It does not guarantee you a job, for instance. It guarantees that you cannot be discriminated against for a job based on your disability. It says that employers must provide "reasonable accommodation" for you to do a job you are otherwise equally qualified to perform. If you can show an employer how you can do the job using a certain adaptive device, for example, they cannot refuse you the job in favor of an otherwise lesser candidate. Of course, the ADA does not automatically stop such events from taking place. It means you have recourse. In such situations, you can take legal action because your civil rights have been violated.

The ADA mandates access to all public services, not just those covered by Section 504, because they receive federal funds. Now the local city hall has to be accessible. Activities—from school board meetings to the city picnic—need to accommodate people with disabilities as of January 1992.

You are entitled to access to the commercial milieu, where you are protected from discrimination "in the full equal enjoyment of the goods, services, facilities, privileges, advantages, or accommodations of any place of public accommodation." That includes your bank, shopping center, transportation terminals, theaters, and so on. There needs to be a clear path to restrooms, drinking fountains, telephones, and elevators. (Not all buildings under three stories are required to install an elevator.)

The ADA also addresses public and private transportation, and requires telecommunications options for people with hearing disabilities. As of July 1993, telephone companies are required to provide telecommunication devices for the deaf (TDDs).

But, according to Mary Lou Breslin, the disability community finds itself caught in somewhat of a contradiction:

> We spent so many years during the development of Social Security
> programs having to prove that disability equated with inability to work. If
> we were denied benefits, we would have to go in front of a judge and say,

"I'm a quadriplegic, therefore I can't work." Now the same judge has to look at the same quadriplegic who is trying to get accommodation on the job. We've sent out extraordinarily conflicting messages, between the old charity/rehab model that is still completely entrenched in our culture. We see the person who has left a job over lack of accommodation suing in the courts at the same time that they have an SSI claim going. The judges are saying that you can't have it both ways.

These contradictions are all part of the continuing process of our society's adjustment to the new disability paradigm. There is no question that the Americans with Disabilities Act is a dramatic victory, a sweeping social change, and a means by which the independence of people with disabilities will surely continue to grow.

The 1998 National Organization on Disability/Louis Harris Survey of Americans with Disabilities, a nationwide survey of one thousand Americans aged sixteen and older with disabilities, finds that:

Adults with disabilities are more likely to say that they have heard of the ADA than in 1994, but a substantial minority are still not aware of it. Among those aware of the ADA, most think that it has not had a significant impact on their life.[5]

- A larger proportion of respondents than in 1994 (54 percent versus 42 percent) think that laws have been passed in the last ten years to give more protection to people with disabilities.

- Just over half (54 percent) of adults with disabilities have heard of the Americans with Disabilities Act (ADA), a significant increase since 1994 (40 percent).

- One in three (35 percent) respondents thinks that the ADA has made his or her life better, as opposed to worse (1 percent) or no different (58 percent).

IDEA

In 1973, Marian Wright Edelman, who would eventually serve in the Clinton Administration, was a children's advocate. 750,000 children were not attending school, and she was amazed to discover that many of them were disabled. This was a population she had not considered.

As Shapiro writes in *No Pity*:

> *Schools had simply turned them away, saying they were unable to educate them. Children were rejected if they had developmental disabilities like mental retardation. But even intellectually superior students were left uneducated, because conditions like cerebral palsy made it difficult for them to speak or because muscular dystrophy, spina bifida, polio, or paralysis forced them to use wheelchairs and the school building was filled with stairs.*[6]

Edelman led a parents' campaign to pass the 1975 Education for All Handicapped Children Act, now known as the Individuals with Disabilities Education Act (IDEA). The provision has passed important court tests, including the Supreme Court allowing a lower ruling to stand which claimed that all children were entitled to an education regardless of disability or cost.

The initial response of schools amounted to just another variety of warehousing, as children with disabilities were parked in separate rooms. Parents had to further the fight with demands for full integration of their children in the same classroom with nondisabled students. There was growing evidence that this approach enhanced the ability of these children to learn—even raising the IQs of children with retardation—as well as improving their social skills.

As with any new policy, there is resistance to IDEA and the need to fight for fair compliance. Not all schools are doing a good job of providing the services needed by disabled children. Some teachers resist, feeling that they are already overburdened, and that the specialized needs of such children are beyond the capacities of their time, resources, and skills. School boards do not always support having children in their local school, sometimes busing children elsewhere when they feel the program is more important. Parents find themselves fighting to get their kids in the neighborhood school, making neighborhood friends, as is their right under present law.

Resistance to inclusion happens not only with cognitively challenged children—although they have undeniable rights in the public schools. Even fully cognitive and intelligent children are still struggling for full inclusion in the education system. Using a wheelchair alone can be a problem in some settings where the school system has not embraced the IDEA and followed through on its implementation.

The term "special education" used to mean being segregated into a separate setting with limited educational demands. Now special education indicates that a properly trained teacher works with therapists, family, and/or administrative staff to develop an Individual Education Plan (IEP) and establish short- and long-term goals. In the end, the school makes a placement recommendation, which could include a separate program or integration into a normal classroom. It is at this point that parents and schools sometimes clash. Some parents opt for home schooling instead of the school's recommendation.

The quality of early education defines much about the quality of children's future lives. The best chance of children with disabilities for independence and the ability to make a contribution to our society is equal access to education at all levels. Education remains one of the key issues for the disability community and the parents who are vocal and passionate advocates for their children.

There is still much work needing to be done to ensure access to basic education. The 1998 NOD/Harris Survey found:

> While adults with disabilities continue to make progress in higher education—they are now just as likely to have completed at least some college as other adults—they continue to lag behind in getting a basic education, with one in five failing to complete high school, compared to only one in ten nondisabled adults.[7]

Social Security

The Social Security Administration (SSA) provides Social Security Disability Insurance (SSDI). Your eligibility for SSDI depends on your ability to demonstrate disability; the amount you can collect depends on the amount you have paid through tax deductions from your work life to date. If you are under 18, the determination is made according to your parents' account(s). If you qualify, you can collect monthly checks which are not taxable.

In 1972, the Supplemental Security Income Program (SSI), an amendment to the Social Security Act, guaranteed a minimum income to elderly, blind, and disabled individuals who could not sustain gainful employment. Just as meaningful, SSDI recipients were made eligible for Medicare, a federal health insurance program, and SSI recipients were made eligible for Medicaid, a program administered by the states that covers medical expense.

At first glance, disability benefits would seem a blessing. Indeed, this money has made a great difference, but there is a growing movement for Social Security reform. The problem comes if you want to work. The SSA has designed the programs with the intent of providing incentives for people with disabilities to work. However, it turns out that these benefits are a trap for some people who could otherwise be earning their own living, particularly for those with lower income potential.

According to the Government Accounting Office, 42 percent of people with disabilities would like to work, and 33 percent of Social Security beneficiaries have the potential to work. The 1998 NOD/Harris Survey of Americans with Disabilities finds an even higher percentage of Americans with disabilities between the ages of sixteen and sixty-four wanting to work:

> *Employment continues to be the area with the widest gulf between those who are disabled and those who are not. Only three in ten working-age adults with disabilities are employed full or part-time, compared to eight in ten nondisabled adults. Working age adults with disabilities are no more likely to be employed today than they were a decade ago, even though almost three out of four who are not working say that they would prefer to be working. This low rate of employment has, in turn, led to an income gap that has not narrowed at all since 1986, with one in three disabled adults, compared to just one in eight nondisabled Americans, living in very low income households with less than $15,000 in annual income.*[8]

Trial work period

You are allowed a trial work period of nine months—which do not have to be consecutive—plus an additional three, during which you can still collect your benefits, no matter how much you earn. But when the time is up, the benefits cease. If you work a month here and a month there, you might be surprised to find you have used up your trial period, so be careful how you use that time.

There is an "extended period of eligibility" (EPE) during which you can collect a benefit in a month when you make less than $500, or go back on regular benefits if you must go off work altogether. Timed from the beginning of trial work, the EPE is thirty-six months.

Medicare and Medicaid benefits are another part of this formula. You must collect Social Security disability benefits for twenty-four months before you qualify to begin with. You can maintain your Medicare benefits during the EPE, and in some cases can continue Medicare on your own beyond that time. You might pay some premiums yourself, which will be deducted from your check if you still receive benefits.

Social Security offers some Vocational Rehabilitation (VR) services, which could contribute to education, counseling, equipment, or job placement, among other benefits. The Social Security Administration (SSA) is experimenting with a program to allow you to choose approved outside providers of VR who could be paid by SSA.

You are allowed to deduct some expenses, including access modifications, some attendant care (getting dressed for work, for example), transportation, or even the cost of a service dog. Money you have to spend to be able to work can be subtracted from the calculation of your monthly income.

So if you are able to get and maintain a good paying job with health coverage, the twelve month period is a blessing which allows you to make all the money you want and still collect your tax-free disability income. You could do this on a contract or part-time basis while still covered on Medicare, which could attract an employer to give you a try, and hire you full-time with benefits once your benefits lapse. It could also give you time to start a business, in which case forty hours of work per month also counts as a trial work month.

Unfortunately, there is a large population of people with disabilities who do not fit this description.

If you don't make enough

The problems really apply to people with lower income potential. When you make $200 a month, that counts as a trial work month. Do that nine times—earning only $1,800—and you lose your benefits. At the end of trial work, you need to be at a level of $500 of gross income per month to be considered as doing "substantial gainful activity." This is when you will be considered ineligible for that monthly check. Certainly this is not enough to live on. Unless you can make a lot more than $200 a month—or $500 after trial work—getting a job is probably not a very attractive option to staying on disability.

Part-time work is often the only option for people with limited stamina or occasional need for time off to tend to demands of their disability, such as an exacerbation of MS. Part-time jobs do not offer medical coverage and are not a reliable long-term source of sufficient income for independence. Yet part-time jobs are a way to stay active, participate in the community, and take pride in earning at least part of your income. Although the government booklet "Red Book on Work Incentives" states that "the SSI and SSDI programs should not be viewed as permanent sources of income," the present system all but completely closes off other options for many people.

Dr. Ed Nieshoff, a quadriplegic rehabilitation physician in Detroit, Michigan, says of the system:

> There's a huge disincentive to work. People think, "I can stay home and make $600 a month, or I can go to work 160 hours a month and make half again that much after taxes." They say, "The hell with it. Why bother?"

PASS

The Social Security Administration established the PASS (Plan to Achieve Self-Support) program in the early '70s to help people work rather than collect disability benefits. It allows people to set aside money to pay for expenses related to pursuing work, whether finding a job or starting a business. The money can be deducted from income and not counted during determination of benefits or against trial work months.

There have been mixed reviews. In *New Mobility* magazine, Irving Laibson describes his struggles with his PASS program. He relied on PASS to begin a business and line up clients. But when he was ready to start work, PASS deemed him out of compliance because he had existing clients! He lost the clients and his business failed when the PASS operating money fell through. Yet in the same article, Barb Knowlen describes her activities as a consultant helping people to develop PASS plans, stating that seventeen of her clients earn more than $20,000 per year and no longer receive disability benefits.[9]

PASS might be of value to you, but make certain you do very complete research into the program requirements and—as with any bureaucratic process—provide full information on forms, document conversations, and keep good files.

It's a messy bureaucracy

All this discussion assumes you are approved for the benefits in the first place. There are plenty of stories of people who have had to struggle with a complicated bureaucracy to get benefits, dealing with people who might not provide full or accurate information. In the mid 1990s, as part of a federal government cutback, Social Security staff was reduced, overloading the system further.

It can be just as hard to get Social Security to *stop* the money as getting it in the first place. When you complete a trial work period, Social Security Administration is likely to keep sending you checks. No matter how efficiently you fill out their forms reporting your income, they are so immensely overloaded that they could keep sending you money for months to come.

Once they finally get to your case, they'll come calling to get that money back. If you are not very careful about which months qualify against trial work and cash those checks—perhaps for groceries or rent—you can easily find yourself asked to pay back thousands of dollars you don't have. Just because it was the fault of the system's inefficiencies does not excuse you. At best—after a lengthy and complicated appeal process for which you might need to pay an attorney—they will allow you to pay back the money in monthly payments. The system is a mess, and it needs to be changed.

Reform

The case is being made that the Social Security system will save money if it allows people a longer period of time to retain their medical coverage once they are off disability benefits. With more people at work, less money will be paid out as benefits, and more taxes collected from newly employed people. Rather than defining Social Security as an all-or-nothing system in which you either rely entirely or not at all on government support, reform proponents are urging a system that allows people to contribute to their own support, while having a safety net that provides healthcare and lets them work with a reduction in benefits rather than a total cancellation.

Proponents say that the present system wastes taxpayers' money, since entitlement benefits go to some people who would prefer to contribute to part of their own income. They say that if people can maintain their healthcare benefits, they are more likely to continue work rather than returning to the benefit rolls. They say that reforms would result in large savings to the Social Security trust fund.

Reform is no small political challenge. There is a tremendous amount of attention focused on the Social Security program. There is widespread belief that it will be bankrupt about a quarter of the way into the 21st century unless something is done to increase income and/or curtail expenditures. There is talk of raising the age for senior benefits and limiting Medicare spending. Disability reform has to compete with many other Social Security reform proposals.

Medicare is also thought to be in fiscal trouble, so the suggestion of extending Medicare coverage is another formidable political challenge for the disability community. But suggested reforms will not increase the numbers of people on Medicare—they would be getting it anyway if they stayed on disability. Instead, reforms are designed to increase the ability of people to get off of Social Security and Medicare.

The disability advocacy community is concerned that people with disabilities will be scapegoats in the current Social Security debate. People want independence, not a handout. But as long as the money is there, it should be used wisely, capably administered, and delivered through programs which truly promote work, rather than require people to risk being left poor and medically unprotected.

Community care

Many people with disabilities require assistance for basic tasks, including getting washed and dressed, getting into or out of their chair, or bowel and bladder management. Personal assistance services (PAS) make independence and daily activity possible for many people with disabilities. The lack of such home support can mean the difference between life in the community and residence in a nursing facility.

Many programs exist to provide personal assistance. Universities and cities often provide referral and funding for personal assistance services. A large number of privately owned agencies provide such service, often funded by benefits. Some users pay out of their own pocket. And then there are the very large numbers of people who rely on family or friends for home support. Even when a personal assistant (PA) is found through an agency or a private advertisement, a close personal relationship can develop.

Personal assistance is not about caring for someone in the sense that that person is "sick" or "needy." It is about providing a service, on the terms of the person receiving the support, for him to be allowed to make his own choices and control his own life. You can't replace a filling in your own teeth, so you hire a dentist. Some people with disabilities can't get dressed, so they need to hire the service. This is an important shift in society's view of disability. It is key to the change from the medical model to that of control, independence, dignity—and community presence.

This shifting of the model is what makes the concept of de-institutionalization and access to personal care in the community a charged topic.

Medicare benefits

People receiving Social Security Disability benefits become eligible for coverage under Medicare, a federal program. When it comes to home support, Medicare pays only under specific circumstances. One must be "homebound," a term with a specific definition. To qualify, absences from home must be "infrequent and for relatively short duration" and "require a considerable and taxing effort."

This definition was established at a time when there was some abuse of the program, particularly by home support agencies who were providing benefits too leniently. The homebound clause was put into law to clarify the boundaries in order to control the program. But this was before the ADA and the advent of modern power wheelchairs. Now people are much more able to get out, but are beginning to find that going out can mean losing their home support benefits.

Vicki O'Neal is a thirty-two-year-old former teacher whose story is described in the September 1997 issue of *New Mobility* magazine.[10] Now a C5-6 quadriplegic, she has recovered from her car accident in 1993 well enough to be mobile in a power chair, but needs help with dressing, transfers, and bladder and bowel care.

Once her home support—provided through an agency—was in place, she began volunteering at the local elementary school, going out to the health club to work her upper body, and taking in the occasional movie. But when the agency found she was leaving home regularly, they cut off her services, and sent her into the world of lawyers, administrative appeals, and letter writing. She has since regained her benefits, but others have not or choose to stay home rather than risk being left on their own.

The Health Care Financing Administration (HCFA), which runs Medicare, is aware of the problem. At the time home support was added to Medicare, it was considered a generous benefit, which eventually involved no time limit or co-pay. They had to hold to existing regulations, and as with any political process (changes must be approved by Congress) it took time to study the issue and invite comments from the range of interested parties—consumers and agencies alike. As of this writing, a proposal before Congress would change the homebound definition to allow for sixteen hours outside of the home per month.

While hardly ideal, sixteen hours would be an improvement. But Bill Hatch, an attorney with the North Carolina Governor's Advocacy Council for Persons with Disabilities suggests considering homebound status in terms of what someone could do *without* home support services. Quoted in the *New Mobility* article, he says "They're identifying them at the wrong time. Anybody can get out of the house with enough services."[11]

For now, the rule is that you can have home support services covered under Medicare, but only if you stay at home.

Medicaid

Medicaid is a federal government program. Social Security gives money to the states for healthcare programs. Each state must conform to certain regulations, but has the freedom to design their own programs. Much of this money goes to nursing home care.

Some people with disabilities—including young people—currently reside in nursing facilities. They are not there by choice. They are there because most states don't allow them to use the money for community-based care. Federal guidelines don't require them to do so.

ADAPT (American Disabled for Attendant Programs Today) is working to get 25 percent of Medicaid long-term care funds redirected to pay for a nationally mandated attendant services program. ADAPT has gone as far as physically barricading young quadriplegics from hospital staff rather than allowing them to be transferred to a nursing home. Meanwhile ADAPT seeks community-based options that social workers or family might not have pursued.

The Medicaid program allows states to provide funds for home support through a waiver application process, but it is a difficult, long process that few individuals venture into, if they even know the process exists. When such a waiver is offered, the programs often require the involvement of a professional nurse or social worker. People are never allowed to receive money directly and manage their own care.

In the concept known as Cash and Counseling, people manage benefit funds themselves, with the program providing support to help them use it effectively. Ultimately, people get to choose what they need for themselves, rather than being at the whim of a case worker who might not have the time—or motivation—to fully understand their needs. At present, Cash and Counseling is in the stage of demonstration projects only.

Researchers Kevin Mahoney and Lori Simon-Rusinowitz write that fear of misuse of public funds used to rule policy decisions.[12] "State and local administrators," they write, wanted "to avoid becoming embroiled in allegations of fraud" similar to those suspected in the Social Security program. But lately:

> Program officials have come to share the concerns of disability rights advocates about public program rules that may foster dependency in the name of consumer protection.

Officials are even beginning to recognize potential financial benefits for the state. According to Mahoney and Simon-Rusinowitz:

> Disabled clients might obtain much the same services at lower cost, a broader clientele might be served, or more intensive services provided without increasing total program expenditures.

Economics and politics might well come into line with the best possible quality-of-life needs of people with disabilities.

MiCASA

MiCASA is the Medicaid Community Attendant Services Act of 1997. This bill was introduced at hearing in 1998; it did not pass that Congress, but there will be a new version of the bill for the 1999 session. Its goal is to shift Medicaid from a philosophy of institutional care to allowing people choice. The bill would amend the Social Security Act, creating a new category of benefit called Qualified Community-Based Attendant Services. It would give people personal control of these funds for their own support, a first in such programs.

The 1997 MiCASA bill states:

> *A state shall permit an individual who is entitled to medical assis-*
> *tance with respect to nursing facility services or intermediate care facility*
> *services for the mentally retarded and who qualifies for the receipt of such*
> *services to choose to receive medical assistance for qualified community-*
> *based attendant services in the most integrated setting appropriate to the*
> *needs of the individual.*

Tasks at hand

In order for community-based services to succeed, people using the services will need some training. Those receiving direct payments will become employers and managers. Many people who might have no experience in a position of authority will now be hiring and directing an employee whom they can also fire. MiCASA would require states to offer them training on how to be an employer.

Employing an attendant is a complex relationship. Personal assistance is an extremely intimate interaction between two people. Success is more likely when there is mutual respect, possibly some shared interests which promote a friendly connection, and a well-defined set of responsibilities for both employer and employee.

Handling money is another area in which some people will need support. They can choose to work with a fiscal intermediary who can guide them on how to manage their Medicaid monies. There will also be some paperwork to do—such as reporting hours worked and tasks performed—that could prove to be more than users care—or are able—to deal with. An intermediary can guide them through this territory, and help them in general to advocate for themselves.

What happens if an attendant does not appear on time? For a quadriplegic who needs to have his bladder emptied, this can be a severe emergency. Providing a twenty-four-hour emergency backup service is very difficult for attendant referral agencies, particularly given how hard it already is to attract enough people to work at the generally low attendant wages. The more aging and disabled people are out in the community, the greater the need for emergency backup. This must be addressed for a program to win support, much less work, in the long run, and is addressed in MiCASA.

The Robert Wood Johnson Foundation grants

Cash and Counseling demonstration projects are being conducted in a number of states to test this approach and measure the differences between community and facility-based care. A group of such demonstrations is being supported by grants from the Robert Wood Johnson Foundation, which finances healthcare issues. The U.S. Department of Health and Human Services is participating in the evaluation of the project.

State agencies and universities in Maryland, New York, New Jersey, Florida, Arkansas, Ohio, Oregon, Minnesota, Missouri, Montana, and California are involved in the project. They will look for candidates in their respective state to participate in the demonstrations. Some people will actually get out of institutions and back in the community, with a chance to prove that these monies can be better spent.

Assisted suicide controversy

Some people with disabilities have had strong reactions against the idea of assisted suicide. Disability activist Diane Coleman testifying on April 29, 1996, before the Constitution Subcommittee of the Judiciary Committee of the U.S. House of Representatives said:

> *Assisted suicide proponents have reinforced public prejudice and fear regarding disability, labeling it "pitiful," "helpless," "hopeless," "miserable," and inherently "undignified." This is an insult to our lifestyles. Experienced people with disabilities have learned that there's more to life than toileting independently.*

> *Medical rehabilitation specialists report that quadriplegics and other significantly disabled people are dying wrongfully in increasing numbers because emergency room physicians withhold aggressive treatment. Disabled people who use ventilators report that they are increasingly asked by medical personnel to consider "do not resuscitate" orders and withdrawal of life support. In the absence of a constitutional right to physician care, a right to physician-assisted suicide is not the answer.*

There is just cause for this concern. In a study that polled caregivers as well as people with disabilities, people were asked if they thought life was worth living with a severe disability. Most people with disabilities said, "Absolutely," even those with extreme limitations and pain. The majority of caregivers thought otherwise, thinking that they would rather not continue to live.

If doctors and nurses think that this is a life not worth living, then what kind of decisions will they make about assisted suicide? How objectively can they counsel a person, and to what lengths will they go to improve a person's quality of life rather than simply offer them a "dignified end?"

Yet this is no easy choice for doctors. They swore the Hippocratic Oath, which says they will take no action which would cause harm. Assisted suicide is a very complex ethical question for the medical community.

Jack Kevorkian's patients

The image of the doctor who compassionately helps a terminally ill person to have control over their passage does not necessarily fit the reality of what does or will happen. Proponents of assisted suicide argue that it is merciful, and should be available for doctor and client to choose in the context of a responsible and humane relationship.

Dr. Jack Kevorkian is the person most identified with assisted suicide and a spokesperson for it. Most of Dr. Kevorkian's "patients," however, were not terminally ill. Many of them had disabling—not terminal—conditions such as multiple sclerosis, ALS, or Alzheimer's disease. Some were in pain, some were despondent about their disability, and felt that their lives were already over, so they asked for a "merciful" end. A few examples:

- Janet Adkins was 54, in the early stages of Alzheimer's, and her personal physician believed she had ten good years left to live.

- Marjorie Wantz was 58, reportedly experienced pelvic pain. An autopsy revealed no apparent disease in her body.

- Sherry Miller was 42, had multiple sclerosis, and felt she was becoming a burden on people.

Did these people receive appropriate medical care? Could their pain have been managed with medications, surgical measures, or even biofeedback and relaxation therapy? Were fears of being a burden on others exaggerated in their minds for lack of proper counseling? To what degree were these people left to suffer simply because they were denied proper medical care or information?

Dr. Kevorkian apparently feels that there are other justifiable reasons to take one's own life aside from painful, terminal illness. An article by Georgea Kovanis in the *Detroit Free Press* quotes Dr. Kevorkian:

> *In December 1992, Tate, sitting in a wheelchair and barely able to speak, showed up at a press conference with Kevorkian, who pointed to her and said: "Marguerite Tate has no quality of life. Everyone can see that. Look at her!"*[13]

The problem with his statement is that there are plenty of people using a wheelchair and unable to speak who are doing quite a lot with their lives.

Many in the disability community question whether Jack Kevorkian is motivated by fear of or hatred for those with disabling conditions. In a written statement to a 1991 court proceeding against him, Kevorkian wrote:

> *The voluntary self-elimination of individual and mortally diseased or crippled lives taken collectively can only enhance the preservation of public health and welfare.*[14]

Not Dead Yet

Concerns over assisted suicide have led to the formation of a group called Not Dead Yet. They have demonstrated in Washington, D.C., and participated in the preparation of an amicus brief which was presented to the U.S. Supreme Court. They are concerned that a legislative acceptance of assisted suicide will compromise the ability to get other legislation passed which will provide for full access to people with disabilities. Why spend money on home care, revise Social Security, enforce the ADA, provide full access to education, or require the insurance industry to provide coverage with a pre-existing condition when it is easier just to let people choose to die? This is the specter that scares the disability community.

The courts have been equally questionable in this regard. Numerous rulings have denied people with disabilities access to suicide prevention services that would otherwise be offered to an able-bodied person. Simply by virtue of their disability the court deemed that their lives were not worth saving.

However, the U.S. Supreme Court made a unanimous decision handed down on June 26, 1997, upholding a Washington state law which prohibits assisted suicide.

Not all agree

The disability community is not unified on this issue. There are people who view this as a matter of personal freedom, such as this disabled woman who argues that access to information is what will protect people:

> I think people could protect themselves if provided a means to educate themselves on ways to ensure their choices for medical options are carried out… like living wills and power of attorneys—whatever it takes. Or revealing the numerous ways relatives may be pressured to discontinue treatment. Or discussing how many people die because they cannot afford treatment.

> I'd be even more concerned that I would be kept alive in conditions I find intolerable so a doctor or hospital can make an extra buck off my insurance.

> I support "assisted suicide." I don't support the government or religion or do-gooders interfering with my decisions on my health. Just give me the information on my condition and a prognosis. Don't control me, control the people who want to make decisions for me.

And this man with a disability, writing in an Internet discussion:

> It's time for people to put aside their knee-jerk, emotional responses, and try to learn what right-to-die means. The vast majority of messages here have indicated that the writers don't understand—they are worried about phantom Nazis, euthanasia, and other ideas that are, in fact, the opposite of what right-to-die means. The whole idea of right-to-die is that the individual makes the decision, not someone else.

> The bottom line is this—when it comes down to my private life-and-death decisions, I don't want Pope John Paul II, Dr. Kevorkian, Pat Buchanan, Bill Clinton, Bob Dole, Andy Rooney, Rush Limbaugh, Howard Stern, or any of you, dear readers, forcing your views on me.

Another point of view:

> What scares me to death is anyone who presumes to interfere for me in my own treatment—including my choice of when and how to die. My choice is none of your business.

Yet the concern remains that people are choosing suicide because they are in a state of depression and despair as a result of not being given access to information, benefits, or medical care that would affect their quality of life. Hopefully the current debate will produce a broader awareness of where our true values lie, and dignity and quality of life will be preserved for everyone, disabled or not.

Transportation

Limiting the mobility of chair users exacts a great cost in independence. So it is no surprise that the disability movement is focusing a lot of their attention on matters of transportation, both local and national. Access to education, jobs, and public facilities of all kinds don't do much good if you can't get there. Without transportation, much of the hard-fought-for benefits of the ADA turn out to be of no benefit at all.

According to the 1998 NOD/Harris Survey of Americans with Disabilities:

> Inadequate transportation is considered a problem by three out of ten (30%) adults with disabilities (17% "major problem," 13% "minor problem"), but by only one out of six (17%) adults without disabilities (7% "major problem," 10% "minor problem"), a gap of 13 percentage points.[15]

There have been some strides in access to airline travel. In 1986, Congress passed the Air Carrier Access Act (ACAA), and followed with enforcement regulations in 1990. Among other requirements, airlines:

- May not refuse access to a person with a disability, unless the carrier can demonstrate a clear safety risk

- May not limit the number of disabled persons they carry

- May not require that an attendant travel with you, except in certain circumstances, in which they may not charge for the attendant's fare

- Must check and return your wheelchair as close as possible to the door of the plane

- In planes purchased after April 1992, must provide movable armrests, include onboard storage for one folding wheelchair on planes that hold one hundred persons, and include an accessible restroom on aircraft with more than one aisle, among other things

- Must permit service animals to accompany you on the flight
- Must train their staff in dealing with disability needs

As with most disability legislation, this has helped, but air travel on wheels continues to have its challenges. There are plenty of reports of damaged chairs—particularly power chairs—and frustrations with getting comfortable seats. Some bulkhead seats—where the greatest leg room exists—are not available to people with disabilities. For example, only passengers able to assist in emergencies are allowed in bulkhead seats near exit doors. This narrows the selection for people who are unable to stand, and who need all the more to have leg room for comfort and to be spared the embarrassment of people having to squeeze by and climb over them to get to neighboring seats. Different airlines do varying jobs of guaranteeing bulkhead seats for people with disabilities.

Air travel is frankly out of the range of what many people with disabilities can afford. Intercity trains such as Amtrak were required to provide one accessible car per train as of July 1995. They must comply fully by July 2010. Yet that is a limited option, serving only the cities where the tracks happen to go, with accommodations for a small number of chair riders. Nor does private transportation solve the problem; some families do not own cars. The bus is the option that people really need.

From an article in the October 1997 issue of the disability rights magazine *Mouth*:

> One rural Pennsylvanian who uses a power chair must pay a taxi company $200 in order to visit his mother's grave. The same trip by Greyhound would cost less than $10.[16]

Greyhound requested and received a Congressional extension for ADA compliance. One could understand the great expense and logistical complexity of making the Greyhound fleet accessible. Unfortunately, in the meantime they have bought seven hundred new buses with no lifts, apparently trying to beat the deadline of the year 2000 after which they will be required to purchase only accessible buses. Before the exemption, the cutoff would have been in 1996.

While Greyhound claims to be in (technical) compliance with the ADA, this is because of the exemption they gained. Greyhound says that they have spent millions on compliance, and indeed they have taken measures to make bus stations accessible. They allow personal assistants to travel free of charge. The problem remains that an accessible station doesn't do much good if you can't get on the bus, and people should not be forced to rely on a companion if they are otherwise able to travel independently.

Greyhound also established an ADA hotline number for people with disabilities to call to arrange for special needs. This is supposed to include assistance on and off the bus, and time set aside for early boarding. People who have called the number complain about being asked detailed questions—including their race and hair color—which then are not relayed to the station.

Daniese McMullin-Powell had an experience with Greyhound when she traveled to Washington, D.C., for a meeting between the U.S. Secretary of Transportation, Rodney Slater, and members of ADAPT. A man came on the bus with the driver to help her off, abruptly tried to grab her under her arms, when she interrupted to ask if they had received training:

> *The driver said "No." I said, "The people at the 800 number said you did." Charlie, the bus driver, told me he has worked for Greyhound for ten years and has never had any such training. One of the persons helping me off lost his grip twice and I have two bruises on my arms and body.*[17]

ADAPT members went on forty-one Greyhound trips to test the level of service. Despite claims by Greyhound CEO Craig Lentsch that their current policy of assistance was working, ADAPT members found:

- 36 percent had to recruit their own help, since employees would not or could not assist them.

- 25 percent were dropped or otherwise hurt in the course of being helped. In one case, the injury was a broken rib. Another rider being assisted in a special chair for loading had a support strap placed around her neck.

- 18 percent of wheelchairs were damaged.

- 58 percent were refused help off and on the bus at accessible rest stops.

In some cases, people were simply refused rides, even with tickets, or told to schedule their trip at another time for Greyhound's convenience. In one case, the driver called 911 for help removing a disabled passenger. Around the country came story after story of rudeness and lack of training from drivers and managers, of promises made via the 800 numbers that were not kept, and refusal to allow time or provide assistance at rest stops.

ADAPT had had enough. On August 8, 1997, a group of protesters from ADAPT confronted the CEO of Greyhound in a four-hour occupation at the Dallas, Texas, corporate offices. The executive eventually met them, but ended up leaving the room in a huff rather than directly answering their questions regarding his intention to provide access to buses.

On August 8 and 9 there was a protest action against Greyhound in forty-four cities across the country for failing to provide appropriate services for people with disabilities. Disability Rights and Education Defense Fund (DREDF) attorneys played a role in the process, which finally led to new regulations published by the Department of Transportation in September 1998. They established a number of requirements for over-the-road buses (OTRBs), including:

- Until October 2000 (2001 for small companies), boarding assistance must be provided and wheelchairs transported with forty-eight-hour advance notice.

- As of October 2000 (2001 for small companies), an accessible bus must be provided with forty-eight-hour advance notice.

- Beginning October 2000 (2001 for small companies), all new buses purchased or leased must be accessible.

- Half the fleet of large operators must be accessible by October 2006, and the entire fleet by 2012.

- At rest stops, OTRB companies must provide time and assistance to leave and re-enter the bus to use the facilities.

- Employees must be trained in the use of bus lifts, and the company must maintain lifts and other access equipment.

- Passengers who have requested service with proper notice can be compensated up to $700 if service is not provided in a timely manner.

Law and enforcement

A million pages of legislation is worthless unless someone follows up. If the disability community were to rely on public authorities to enforce Section 504, the FHAA, IDEA, the ADA, and any other disability rights laws, progress would be very slow in the actual removal of barriers to independence.

As Mary Lou Breslin of DREDF explains:

> *You have to be able to define what constitutes discrimination for the purposes of trying to solve it. It means that things that happen in the real world have to be subject to some kind of penalty if they violate the law. You have to figure out what the law is supposed to say and supposed to do.*

Because the ADA is a federal law, most ADA complaints need to be filed with the Attorney General's office at the U.S. Department of Justice. Employment discrimination complaints go to the Equal Employment Opportunity Commission (EEOC). Individual lawsuits may be filed to stop discrimination. Employment discrimination cases are the only cases in which compensatory damages may be sought under the ADA.

The U.S. Department of Justice has not been aggressive on their own. In spite of hundreds of complaints filed under the ADA—and a mandate to pursue investigations on their own—Justice has only filed charges in four cases. It is true that they have worked out agreements without the need for litigation, and part of the mechanism of the ADA should be making people aware of how to comply without going all the way to court. Yet disability activists have trouble believing that all but four of the large load of cases were acceptably negotiated. They want to see Justice take more of a proactive hand. In their view, being overloaded is not an excuse.

Where architectural barriers are concerned, law has accomplished a tremendous amount. Mary Lou Breslin also remembers the old days:

> *I'm very impressed with the amount of access that has been achieved with these laws, particularly when there was so much opposition to them for such a long time. It went from nobody realizing that architectural barriers were an issue and that they served to exclude people to it being an accepted part of the landscape.*

The effort has paid off, but the job is far from over. Many physical obstacles remain or continue to appear in new construction, but relatively little has been accomplished in the more challenging task of removing attitudinal obstacles.

Remaining frontiers

The political challenge is far from over. Making people with disabilities aware of the issues and getting them involved is part of the challenge. For example, the 1998 NOD/Harris Survey of Americans with Disabilities finds low voter registration levels:

> Only six out of ten (62%) adults with disabilities were registered to vote in the 1996 Presidential election, compared to almost eight out of ten (78%) among the nondisabled population, according to the Current Population Survey, representing a gap of sixteen percentage points. One in four (25%) adults with disabilities has been offered voter registration services from a government or community agency in the last five years.[18]

Many issues remain. Despite the huge accomplishments in making the public setting more accessible, increasing options for transportation on public buses, trains, and airplanes, and all of those blue parking spots, there are still some pretty big fish to fry in the political milieu.

Healthcare remains a tremendous challenge for people with disabilities. Insurance companies are still able to limit coverage for pre-existing conditions, either by increasing premiums or by limiting certain options. Especially in view of the high rate of unemployment for people with disabilities, being able to get coverage often means having to surrender any hope of work in favor of being eligible for Medicare.

There is, indeed, far more going on in the realm of disability politics than can possibly be covered in this book. But you can bet that at every level—from the local school board to the Supreme Court—disability issues are being pursued as people insist not only on their rightful control and independence, but on being seen as whole people rather than objects of sympathy or care.

People with disabilities have accomplished tremendous change, showing courage, resolve, and more than a little creativity in making their point. We've come a long way from "ugly laws" of the 19th century, which prohibited people with disabilities from appearing in public in some cities, to a world where the disability access symbol has become a ubiquitous feature of the public setting. Plenty of people have gotten the message: people with disabilities are full members of this society. We can count on an increasingly active and sophisticated disability community to continue the hard work of making sure that everyone else gets the point, too.

CHAPTER 11

Getting Out There

So far, this book has focused on understanding your disability and preparing for as active and independent life as possible. Now it's time to consider some of the many options available to you.

In this chapter, we look first at getting around physically: wheeling technique, transportation, accessible public spaces, and long-distance travel. Next we discuss how adaptive technology can expand your possibilities, including using computers with various input devices, voice synthesis, environmental controls, and ergonomic considerations. Then we turn to education, employment, volunteering, and advocacy work. We end the chapter with a look at the variety of sports and recreational activities you can consider.

Wheeling style and technique

You are going to become an expert at driving your chair. It is the nature of the body to gain coordination simply from the act of doing—the more you perform a particular task, the better your nervous and muscular systems adapt to that task. All of us can remember learning a skill that was awkward at first, whether it was tying shoes, playing a musical instrument, or cutting vegetables. Even if you have never had the use of your arms, you gained dexterity with your head and mouth, perhaps as a painter or computer operator. This "practice makes perfect" principle applies to driving your wheels.

You will develop a refined sense of how to operate your chair. The push and pull of the wheels or the control of a joystick will become second nature—nearly as unconscious an act as walking for those who are able.

Optimal wheeling

In order to become adept at maneuvering your wheelchair, you need the right chair, properly adjusted for your needs. When you have the right chair and have learned the basics of getting around in it, time, practice, and experience will lead naturally to expertise in making your chair do what you want it to. Style and grace will distinguish you as a true master of your wheels.

One principle you'll learn to recognize is that faster isn't always better. For power chair riders, too much speed can be dangerous, for the obvious reason that you could be thrown from your wheels. Too much speed makes it harder to control the chair, as you must brace your body against the various forces and sheer momentum of traveling so fast.

For manual chair wheelers, frenetic wheeling wastes energy, is more fatiguing and even puts the body at risk, such as for developing shoulder tendinitis. If you allow brief breaks between pushes, bringing your arms back in an unrushed manner, you will do fewer pushes for the same distance and expend less effort. A well-adjusted chair with well-inflated tires will coast more easily.

Some manual chair riders wheel quickly to demonstrate their dexterity and agility to the outside world:

> Looking back, I can see how much I was invested in being the hot-shot wheelchair rider in the early years of my disability, which happened when I was a teen. Wheeling slowly somehow made me feel more disabled, a purely psychological response to how I imagined the public saw me. Surely, I seemed to think, if they see how agile and strong I am with my wheels, they won't think I'm a "cripple" and everything I imagined to be associated with that image.

Although it's only human to worry about how others perceive us, it doesn't really matter what others think or what their cultural assumptions might be in regard to disability. If you pay attention to how you appear to others, that prevents you from paying attention to what you're doing. You are less focused on where you're going and more likely to bump into something or jam a thumb on the brake.

By taking your time, you also reduce the cumulative strain on your shoulders, elbows, and wrists which could ultimately cost you the ability to use a manual chair. Some people who are aging with disability are losing the ability to push a manual chair. Slow down just a bit, and you will have more grace, more energy for your day, and preserve independence throughout your lifetime. You can certainly still have fun in your wheels:

*I have a favorite block in San Francisco with a really wide sidewalk.
It doesn't slope too steeply toward the street, but has a great downhill
slope at a moderate pitch. It's perfect because I can build up some good
speed, but not so fast I lose control. Better than most amusement park
rides!*

Negotiating curbs and obstacles

How well you can move over changes in surface levels is affected by how
your wheelchair is equipped, and, for some manual chair riders, learning the
skill of tipping back on two wheels.

Certain wheelchair features aid in negotiating curbs and other obstacles.
Larger, air-filled wheels and casters go over curbs more easily than hard,
smaller wheels. Shock absorbers or an independent suspension system also
help in getting over changes in surface level. Some power chairs with front-
wheel drive are better able to handle a modest curb. Testing standards for
wheelchairs include a specification for maximum obstacle height. Tests are
performed considering approach angle, forward or backward movement,
and whether or not the chair is in motion as it approaches the obstacle.

For manual chair riders, riding over obstacles can often be accomplished
with wheeling skill, using the wheelie technique—tipping back on the two
main wheels. Occupational/physical therapists teach the technique to chair
riders they feel have sufficient strength and balance. The chair will need to
be properly adjusted so that the axle is not too far forward, which makes the
chair prone to tipping over backward too easily during normal wheeling.

Knowing how to do a wheelie makes it possible to wheel up or down (jump)
curbs (see Figure 11-1). A highly skilled wheeler can hop curbs several
inches high. Some riders can even wheel down a series of steps, assuming
each one is wide enough to stop on and check their balance. In some situations, the ability to do wheelies might make the difference between doing it
yourself or asking for help, or save you the trouble of traveling farther along
a sidewalk to get to a ramp.

Wheelies can help even when there is a ramp or curb cut. When you
approach a ramp going upward, a good push at the base just before the
incline gives you momentum to get started up the ramp, saving you much
energy. If you raise the casters slightly at the same time, you will maintain
better momentum. You will not have to overcome the resistance of the casters against the upward-sloping pavement.

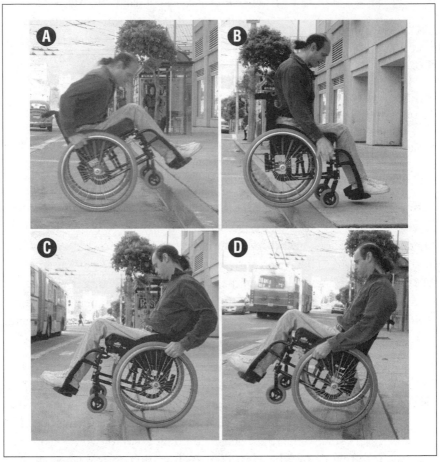

Figure 11-1. Using the wheelie technique at a curb. Photos A and B show going up a curb; C and D show going down a curb.

If you must wait for a light before crossing the street at a curb cut, don't go down the curb cut until your way is clear. That way you can use the momentum of going down the curb to help you get back up the crown of the street. Use whatever downhill energy you can, rather than wasting it by stopping at the bottom and having to push uphill with your own power. Doing a slight wheelie as you go down the curb cut will also help you use your momentum to get up the rise in the street. Techniques like this take some practice and of course depend on your strength and balance. If you are still working with a physical therapist, you can discuss developing these skills.

Another advantage of the wheelie is that it gives you an opportunity to change your position. Reclining by doing a wheelie changes the pressures on the spine and allows muscles of the upper body to relax since the back of the chair is now carrying more of your weight. As one chair user notes:

> I'm fond of tipping back against a wall and putting my brakes on because I find the change in posture to be a great relief.

Wheelie expertise offers purely recreational opportunities as well. If you can't resist the urge to show off a little in your wheelchair, doing wheelies is one of the best ways. While he might appear to balance precariously, a properly trained chair rider has great control doing a wheelie. (Assuming he isn't trying to show off excessively. Pushing that envelope can lead to embarrassing spills.) Rather than teetering on the edge of falling, the wheels are used to control balance by easily managed forward or backward movements. Popping a wheelie with a child in your lap is one of the finer pleasures of life on wheels. (Add an optional whinny sound of a horse, if you like.)

Each rider has to find his own limits and account for the dangers of any wheeling technique. Going down stairs alone entails obvious risks. Don't attempt such methods until you've gained confidence through practice with someone to check you against a fall. First, explore your abilities and limits.

Zen wheeling

Zen Buddhism is a practice in which you bring your full attention into the present moment, instead of reviewing the past or planning the future. Wheeling can be like a Zen meditation exercise. The principle of mindfulness—observing the forces at play right *now*—can be applied to driving your wheelchair. For instance, riders often encounter very tight spaces. The more patient, or present, you are, the less likely you are to bump into one side or the other, jam a finger, or damage your chair in the process.

Similarly, when you are wheeling along a sidewalk, the downhill wheel needs to be pushed a bit harder or the joystick pulled a bit to the side, to keep you on a straight line. The more aware you are of the sometimes subtle forces at play on you or your chair, the more accurately you can respond with just the right amount of effort at the right time to keep yourself traveling on a steady path. The better you observe the cracks, potholes, slopes at doorways, metal plates, and various other features of the terrain, the better you can make the fine adjustments in wheeling that they require of you.

When there is a slight rise in a section of concrete, you will want to give a little extra push to raise the front casters very slightly over it, or slow your power chair just a bit as you approach, then accelerate over it. You can also use your body weight, gently pushing against the back of the chair to slightly lift weight from the casters.

When you are pushing a manual chair up a slope, take your time and feel the forces you are working against. You can waste a lot of effort if you try to go fast, maintain a consistent speed, or always travel in a straight line. If you use your arms fluidly with the shoulders, apply your upper body weight as your balance allows, and note subtle changes in sideways slope, you can find wheeling uphill a calming experience. Sometimes you will even need to allow yourself to stop completely for a moment as you reposition your arms for the next push. The climb will be good exercise, and it will seem that you got up that slope pretty quickly because you stopped worrying how long it was going to take.

When you pay attention and your chair seems like an extension of your body, you will be amazed at the sensitivity to your surroundings you can develop. For example, you will find you are able to judge curb heights or spaces between cars in a parking lot by fractions of an inch.

Both manual and power chair riders develop elegance in the way they move in their chairs. The relationship of your awareness to your terrain and your sense in your body of what you feel through your chair is exactly the kind of integral experience taught by Zen masters. Wheeling with mindfulness will preserve your energy, reduce stress, and even protect you from the chance of an accident. You might even find that the quality of attention to other aspects of your life will improve.

Going out

Even in the smallest towns there are movie theaters, playhouses, sports events, restaurants, concerts, and other activities you will want to attend. In larger cities there might be the symphony, opera, museums, or tourist attractions.

The ADA now requires all public facilities owned by private entities to be made accessible. Public facilities include restaurants and bars, theaters and stadiums, convention centers and lecture halls, shopping centers, retail stores, libraries, museums, zoos, amusement parks, schools, social service centers (including homeless shelters), and recreation facilities such as gymnasiums, health spas, and golf courses. The language of the law is that these facilities may not "refuse service or deny participation" in an activity. They must provide access under the reasonable expense provisions of the ADA or else establish alternative service. If you cannot enter a store, for instance, it is required to provide curb or home delivery service at no extra cost to you.

Most theaters, sports arenas, concert venues, and museums in the United States and Canada now provide substantial access. This is increasingly true in Europe where, for instance, the Louvre and Musee D'Orsay in Paris are fully and easily accessible. Some facilities will even offer you a discounted entrance fee. In some cases you will need to go around to a side entrance, which should be clearly marked by an access symbol, but in general you have a good chance of getting in the front door and of being able to park nearby.

The 1998 National Organization on Disability (NOD)/Harris Survey of Americans with Disabilities found that 75 percent of adults with disabilities feel that access to public facilities has gotten better over the past four years.[1]

Seating in theaters and stadiums is more complex. There are a limited number of seats dedicated to wheelchair users, and those seats might or might not be well spaced throughout the facility. Often the accessible seating is toward the back of the theater, or away from the lower levels of the stadium or arena. This limited choice of seating can be frustrating. You also need to get tickets early, since those seats often sell out faster than the rest of the venue.

Typically, spaces are left open between or next to regular seats for a wheelchair user to park, but some riders prefer to get out of the chair to sit in an upholstered seat at a movie or concert. When that is the case, the question arises of where to park the wheelchair. If you want to sit closer to the screen at a movie, odds are you will have to allow your wheelchair to be parked elsewhere by a companion or a theater employee, particularly if it has a rigid frame. An unfolded wheelchair will be too much of an obstruction in the aisle, and even a folded chair is likely to violate fire codes which require exitways to be kept open. These restrictions might affect your choice of where to sit if you are uncomfortable being away from your chair or reliant on others to bring it to you in the case of an emergency.

Many sports arenas have begun to install a system of seats that can be folded up and out of the way to allow a wheelchair to park in the remaining space. That method of construction gives you the option of staying in your chair or not and lets chair users have more options for where to sit throughout the arena. The arena can also sell more seats to able-bodied customers as the event begins to sell out, rather than having to leave spaces empty that could only have been used by a wheelchair rider.

A key problem arises around how many people you might want to have along at an event. If you want to make plans with a group of a dozen friends, you might have a lot of trouble getting that many seats together. Chair users want the freedom to make plans with a group like anyone else. On the other hand, the facility needs to preserve the accessible seating for those who need it, limiting its use by people who can walk. When you call for tickets to an event, be prepared to hear that you are only allowed one "attendant" to be with you in the disabled seating section. In some cases, this is a policy of the ticket selling agency. If you call the arena or team offices, you might find someone willing to sell you the tickets you need.

The wheelchair seats are sometimes the best in the house. A platform might be set up at a large arena concert with the most unobstructed view in the place. It is also not unusual for a performance space to bring in wheelchair users first to avoid the crowd, which can mean you get the pick of the seats. As you attend events at local venues, you will learn their policies, how to get the best seats, when to arrive, and how to get around.

Public transportation

Having control of where you go makes a big difference in how much you can accomplish. All of the therapy and adaptive devices in the world don't mean much if you can't get to a job or run a simple errand. Freedom to move and go where you want is also central to your sense of self.

Public transportation has come a long way. In major cities, buses are now widely equipped with lifts. There are seats on the bus that lift out of the way, revealing a clamp which holds onto a wheel. There is also a seat belt. The drivers are trained in the operation of the lift and how to assist wheelchair-using passengers. The quality of service varies:

> *I have had three experiences of getting on a bus and then having the*
> *lift fail to work to get me off. The bus had to be emptied. The driver was*

> *getting no response to his calls to the maintenance department, and I missed my appointments. Once we flagged down a passing fire truck for help getting me off. I'm not inclined to trust the bus system, but realize that this is just one aspect of a huge set of problems with the bus system. No one in this city is happy with the buses.*

When you use city buses regularly, you will encounter a variety of conditions and drivers:

> *I had a lot of trouble at first negotiating with bus drivers, but over time I've learned to assert myself. I was a real "people pleaser" before my accident and so I had to develop interpersonal tools to get what I need. Seventy percent of the drivers are wonderful, 28 percent get the job done adequately, but the other 2 percent still give me grief and I have to use a stick rather than a carrot.*

Cities such as New York, Washington, Portland, and San Francisco have rail systems and subways which provide varying degrees of accessibility. Northern California's BART (Bay Area Rapid Transit) system has accessible cars and stations, but has problems with the maintenance of the elevators from the street level. In 1998, a judge ordered BART to increase its efforts and spending to ensure that elevators are kept clean and operating, and that the system in general remains accessible.

Most cities offer a paratransit service, with which you can make an appointment to be picked up and taken directly to your destination. Once you qualify through an application, the service is made available at modest cost. Unfortunately, few people are great fans of paratransit, finding that they cannot rely on the service to be on time or even to show up in some cases. For transportation to a job, paratransit is not usually a solution. If you want to get to a store or the park for a little sun, you can afford to be a little late or go the next day if the driver doesn't show up. Do some research. You might be lucky enough to be in a city with a well-run system.

There is little, if any, public transportation to choose from for many people outside of urban areas. Some will be able to rely on calling neighbors or family to get a ride and have this suffice for their transportation needs. However, greater access to public transit options might be enough to convince rural wheelchair users to move to a city.

Inadequate transportation is more likely to be a problem for those with disabilities, finds the 1998 NOD/Harris Survey of Americans with Disabilities:

> Inadequate transportation is considered a problem by three out of ten (30%) adults with disabilities (17% "major problem," 13% "minor problem"), but by only one out of six (17%) adults without disabilities (7% "major problem," 10% "minor problem"), a gap of thirteen percentage points.
>
> Seven out of ten (69%) adults with disabilities say that their disability prevents them in some way from getting around, attending cultural or sports events, or socializing with friends outside their home as much as they'd like to, compared to only 64% in 1994, and 56% in 1986.[2]

However, 60 percent of the same people surveyed thought that access to public transportation had gotten better over the past four years.

Your own vehicle

For many wheelchair users, the ideal transportation is their own vehicle—car, van, or truck. Driver's training and lessons in how to load a wheelchair are often included in rehabilitation programs or offered on an outpatient basis.

You will develop your own method for loading a wheelchair in a car. Folding chair users who drive a two-door car generally put the chair in the back seat by sliding over to the passenger side, pulling the driver seat forward, and then pulling the folded chair in by rolling it in over the rocker panel. People using a rigid frame chair remove the wheels and lift the frame—with the back folded down against the seat—over them onto the passenger seat or back into the rear seat. Those driving a four-door vehicle generally enter from the passenger side, pulling the chair in after them and securing it with the seat belt. Folding and lifting a chair in and out of a car every day can be fatiguing in the long term, causing wear and tear on the arms and shoulders.

Vans have become increasingly workable for chair users. An adapted van used to be a clunky affair, with a slow, bulky mechanical lift. The interior design was not very good looking and the quality of the ride was not very comfortable. The adapted van of earlier days was an option for those who really needed it. Quadriplegics with enough balance but not the strength to throw their chairs around, or people who needed to be able to drive from their wheelchair, found such a van their only option.

The recent advent of the minivan has changed that. There are now smaller, attractive, and comfortable vans. A number of companies specialize in minivan conversion. They lower the floor so a ramp can be used instead of a mechanical lift (see Figure 11-2), install a kneeling system to bring the van lower to the ground to reduce the ramp angle, and put in tie-down systems to keep the wheelchair secure during driving, whether you stay in it or not. The door, ramp or lift, and door locks are controlled by switches in the vehicle as well as by a remote control you keep on your keychain.

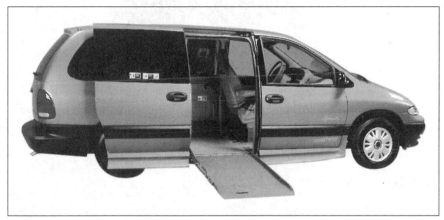

Figure 11-2. A van with a ramp

Hand controls

Hand controls on vehicles can be electronic or manual. Electronic controls manipulate the brake cylinder or engine components such as the fuel injectors, and are initiated by a joystick or other controller in the cabin (see Figure 11-3). Manual controls are mechanical devices attached directly to the pedals, usually supported by the steering column.

Electronic controls are generally used by quadriplegics with minimal upper arm strength. Installation is complex, more training is required to operate them, and they are much more costly. Programming features set the sensitivity of a joystick or button and allow people with limited arm strength to control the transmission, accelerator, and brake.

Manual hand controls brake by pushing forward on whatever control lever is used. There are no gears or linkages for the brake—the control uses a strong rod attached directly to the brake pedal so there can be no possibility of failure.

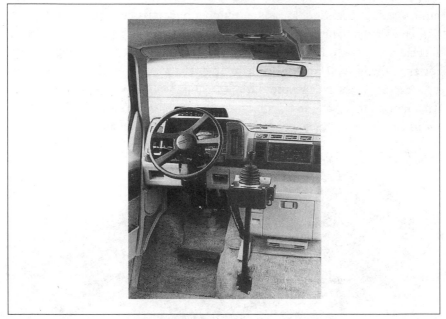

Figure 11-3. A joystick driving control

How manual controls press the accelerator varies. Some designs attach a rod directly to the pedal—particularly those designed for quick installation. Most designs use a system of gears or levers to decrease the amount of pressure your arm must exert to press the accelerator. Driving with a hand control is a lot of work for one side of the body, especially if you do a lot of stop-and-go driving.

There are three styles of manual control accelerators. One is like a motorcycle control, which you rotate; the second is pulled toward the body; the third is pressed downward toward the floor to press the gas pedal. The first two styles are more likely to cause repetitive strain injuries because you have to maintain muscular effort to use them. The third type involves the least strain, since the weight of your arm and hand can be used to maintain speed without much muscular exertion. It minimizes the amount of force needed to maintain speed and can be set for varying degrees of leverage. For any accelerator style, cruise control is recommended to reduce arm fatigue.

> *My first set of hand controls operated like a motorcycle. You would rotate the handle, which had a little extension where you could rest your palm to get more leverage. It was fine for many years, until I moved to San Francisco. I found I had to press harder to get up hills, because my*

car's acceleration wasn't so great. I started to get tendinitis in my left elbow, so I switched to the type you press down on.

There are no commercial hand control products for driving a vehicle with a manual transmission, although a few hardy souls have made their own creative adaptations to operate a clutch and gear shift while still keeping a hand on the steering wheel. For these people, the freedom to drive their favorite sports car was not something they were willing to give up.

Parking

All states issue parking permits that allow you to park in designated spaces. They are typically extra wide to accommodate opening your door fully, or to lower a lift or ramp. Parking spaces along a curb on a city street do not provide extra space, and you might not be able to use some of these spaces because your lift or ramp would have to open into traffic.

The permit is issued to the person with the disability, not to the vehicle. Anyone driving your vehicle or assisting you needs to understand that the privilege does not extend to them personally. You will get a hanging placard which is typically designed to be placed on your rearview mirror when you park. You have the option of getting special license plates which designate you as a disabled driver. Even if you have the special plates, you will still need the hanging placard for when you are riding in another car or are traveling.

Permits generally allow you to park at any metered space without paying. You must still obey time restrictions such as for rush hour or street cleaning when you could receive a ticket or possibly be towed from the street for parking illegally. Don't count on any favors because you have a disability permit. Be sure you understand what privileges your state is providing you.

Disabled parking has essentially expanded into elderly parking, as well as parking for people with heart conditions, bad knees, or temporary injuries. Doctors only have to sign the application in order for someone to get a permit. Certainly there are many people who are not chair riders who cannot easily or safely walk distances, and are fully and fairly entitled to disabled parking privileges. At the same time, there are far more permits issued in many cities than there are reserved parking spots. The competition for spaces has become fierce, and too often a chair user who needs the wider space has no parking to choose from because spaces are increasingly being used by people who can walk. Walking permit holders need to know that they should use a non-reserved parking spot—assuming it is an acceptable distance from their destination—and preserve the wider spaces for chair riders and vans. They still get to park for no charge with no time limits at meters.

Gasoline

You have the right to be assisted at service stations. It varies state by state, but in general you should get serviced at the self-serve pump—for the lower price— when there are two or more employees on the premises. If there is one person alone in a booth at a completely self-serve station, he is not obligated to come out to put gas in your vehicle. The trick is how to get attention. Here is another reason why those with special plates still need the blue placard—so you can wave it at someone to ask them to help you at the pump. Usually, you will find station owners and employees willing to help. They might even clean your windows and check your oil. If you are able to enter and exit your car without too much difficulty, you might find it easier to just get out and serve yourself.

Travel

Want to go someplace in the world? Depending on how much you want to deal with, you can go just about anywhere. Like any traveler, you'll need to get there, find a place to stay, and get around to see the sights.

Airlines

Flying as a chair rider is a bit of an art. The more experienced you are, the more you learn how the system works and the easier it is to avoid pitfalls.

First, know that you have a right to travel by air. In 1986, the U.S. Congress passed the Air Carrier Access Act. Here are some of its provisions:

- New aircraft ordered after April 5, 1990, must be accessible.
- Planes with 30 or more seats must have movable armrests on half of aisle seats.
- Planes with 100 or more seats must be able to accommodate at least one folding wheelchair on board.

- Airline personnel may not deny transportation to a passenger with a disability or limit the number of disabled passengers unless it is a matter of safety.

- You can be required to give two-day notice and check in an hour ahead of departure if you:

  — Are traveling with a power wheelchair on a plane with fewer than sixty seats

  — Require special hookups for equipment such as oxygen or a ventilator

  — Are traveling in a group of ten or more chair users

- Except in rare circumstances, airlines cannot require you to travel with an attendant. If they insist, they can choose an attendant, but cannot charge for his fare.

- Your chair must be checked and returned as close to the door of the plane as possible.

Don't ever let airlines check your wheelchair through baggage claim. Baggage handlers aren't used to handling wheelchairs and might not have procedures for dealing with them. Having a wheelchair checked this way frequently results in the wheelchair disappearing, for greater or lesser periods of time. Some travelers have reported damage to their wheelchair from improper handling. You will also be forced into dependency on airport staff to take you to baggage claim, which you might otherwise be able to reach yourself in your own wheels. You should be able to make the choice.

Instead, do what's called a gate check. A tag is put on your chair. You get onto the plane from your own chair, and it is brought back to the door of the plane when you get off. Make certain that someone on the crew knows your chair is gate checked and ask him to confirm it to the ground crew at your destination. Ground crew communicate with the plane as it is about to land; they can help make sure the wheelchair doesn't get sent to baggage claim.

Airports have many wheelchairs, but they are insufficient for a regular chair rider. Some have small wheels which you cannot push yourself. None have heel loops to help your feet stay in place. Airport chairs are generally in poor repair. Their design assumes you will be assisted. Even if airline personnel suggest surrendering your chair well before the flight, you are not required to do so. Such personnel are acting for their convenience, not yours.

Once I let someone convince me to let them have my wheelchair before I boarded the plane. They put me in an airport chair which had small wheels so I couldn't push the chair myself. Sure enough the flight was delayed, and I was stuck unable to get around. I even had to ask someone to help me to the bathroom, since the long wait was enough for nature to come calling. Now I absolutely will never give up my chair until I'm actually getting on the plane.

You will need to pass through security, like everybody else, but you can't go through the detector because your wheelchair will set off the alarm. You will have to be searched individually. When you approach the security area, be prepared to place any bags—such as a backpack—on the belt to go through the x-ray machine. Usually a security person will have seen you and will direct you to where they can check you out. They will often use a hand-held detector that makes a sound when it finds metal. You might be searched by hand, which should always be done by a person of the same gender as yourself.

Most airplane aisles are too narrow for a wheelchair to fit through. You might be able to get through the first class section to a front row seat in coach. In some cases, such as entry through the second door of a DC-10, you can get to certain seats directly from your chair. Seats in an emergency exit row will not be available to you, because of FAA regulations that such seats only can be occupied by people able and willing to assist in emergencies. That requirement disqualifies people with mobility disabilities. Unfortunately it also reduces your selection of seats with more leg room—very useful to someone unable to stand during a long flight.

Most times you will enter the plane by means of an aisle chair. This is a narrow seat that fits down the aisle, in which you must be assisted by airport staff. The typical seat has a high back and a set of straps to secure you. It is padded, but not specifically for pressure distribution. You will have to decide whether it is a safe surface for you to sit on, even for the brief minutes you will spend in it, taking into account that there might be a couple of bumps as they get you over the first hump into the door.

Recently at some airports, another design has appeared in which you don't have to be tipped back. This is easier on the person assisting you and more dignified for you. However, the seat has no upholstery, so you might need to place a cushion on it to protect yourself from pressure sores. Your wheelchair cushion might do the job.

There are some very tight turns to be made getting into the plane, and the space of the aisle is sometimes just barely wide enough to fit through. You must keep your arms in and watch closely that your clothes don't get caught on a seat arm as you travel down the aisle. The person assisting you might not be patient or attentive enough to prevent collisions with armrests as you travel down the aisle.

The staff that assists people with disabilities are not highly paid or particularly well trained. You will need to direct them, and, sadly, you should be prepared for the possibility that they will treat you like cargo. Some will be personable and cooperate with you, others will grab at you or start to carry you in without the courtesy of a warning. They will especially need guidance in where you want the aisle chair placed relative to your wheelchair for your transfer and how they should best assist you—or not—during the transfer.

> *As a strong paraplegic, I find I am mostly occupied getting people out of my way and letting me position things so I can do the transfer myself. Invariably, someone will try to push me in the chair or will begin to reach under my armpits to lift me without asking first.*

You might or might not need assistance; the issue is how to maintain control, since others will often not ask what you need. Be prepared to direct the process so it goes smoothly. Try to get to the gate early so you can pre-board ahead of other passengers. You want to avoid arriving late and being carried onto the plane through a crowd of occupied seats, unless you enjoy being made conspicuous.

Some airlines are better than others about reserving specific seats for people with disabilities. Seats at the bulkhead—structural walls at various points along the fuselage—typically afford more leg room, and there is no passenger in front to recline his seat back and limit your space. You will want to be close to the front to limit your trip down the aisle in the narrow aisle chair. Bulkhead aisle seats are your best option, if you can get the reservation agent to guarantee one for you when you arrange your flight. If the agent cannot do that, you might need to call back a week before your departure for a seat assignment or go to the airport to meet with a ticket agent. The quest for a comfortable seat can be a challenge, and sometimes comes down to the embarrassment of seeing a gate agent ask someone to surrender his seat on your behalf because airline policy prevented you from getting a commitment from the start.

On occasion, you might find yourself upgraded to the first class section. If there is an open seat, and you can get to it without the need to transfer to an aisle chair, the gate agent has the authority to switch your seat to the front cabin. It makes the airline's life easier—and you get the better food and cloth napkins, too! First class upgrades are much harder to come by these days since there are many frequent flyers who have earned upgrades through mileage programs as a bonus.

You will find that you need to deal carefully with your bladder needs when you fly. You will not have a wheelchair to use on the plane and the restrooms are small and inaccessible. Some people prefer to schedule stopovers on long trips so they can drink more freely on the plane, and then have the chance to get off to use a restroom and move around a little. Certainly you should go to the restroom at the last moment before boarding the plane to empty your bladder.

That means getting there even earlier to check in and making sure they get an aisle chair for you, with time for your bladder before you pre-board. A leg bag is mandatory equipment for most travelers, especially on long flights. This paraplegic woman typically uses intermittent catheterization:

> It's bad for me to wear an indwelling foley catheter, because it increases my chances of getting an infection. But if I'm flying a long distance I wear a foley and surreptitiously empty it into a tinted bottle.

> Otherwise I always catheterize just before I get on the plane and wear a diaper. Once I got stuck on a plane. It was supposed to be a one-hour flight from Michigan to New York, and they kept saying it would be another half hour, another half hour, so I never got off to go to the bathroom. Then they pulled away from the gate and I wasn't about to have them go back just to let me go to the bathroom. By the time we landed, I really had to go. I could have flown to Europe in the time I was on the plane.

It's an embarrassing situation, but if a flight is delayed, you might need to inform a flight attendant that there is a limit to how long you can wait, so you don't find yourself trapped in a similar situation.

Rental cars

All major car rental agencies provide cars with hand controls. They charge nothing extra, nor do they impose any additional insurance requirements for their use. Since the controls are extra equipment that generally must be installed specifically for your use—agencies don't keep cars on hand with controls always installed—you need to give them sufficient notice. It used to be that agencies needed two weeks advance notice, but now major cities have controls available to accommodate you in a matter of days. In an emergency, you might even get next-day service.

Larger agencies have special offices that handle disabled drivers. When you call the general reservation number, explain that you are requesting an adapted vehicle and ask if they need to transfer you to another extension.

The type of car you rent depends on how you put your wheels into a car. Usually agencies provide a "full-size" model, a car the size of an Oldsmobile Cutlass or Ford Taurus. They generally assume you will use a four-door vehicle, which works for people accustomed to storing their wheels in the front seat, entering through the passenger side, or if you have a companion to stow your wheels in the trunk or back seat.

Some drivers are accustomed to a two-door car, stowing the chair in the back seat by pulling it in behind the driver's seat. It used to be easy to get a two-door car with an uninterrupted bench seat in front, but now it is difficult to find such a car given the popularity of bucket seats in two-door cars. The console typically placed between the front seats obstructs your ability to slide to the passenger side and sometimes even extends enough into the rear to interfere with pulling the chair into the car. It is more difficult but not impossible—depending on the type of car and your chair—to pull the chair into the car while you are still in the driver's seat. You will have to ask detailed questions about the car you would get and perhaps employ a different method of carrying your wheelchair when you use a rental car.

When you reserve the car, reservation operators will ask which side you want the controls on. They will let you provide more detail about the control position, but these are installed at the city where you will pick up the car. If you have exacting needs, it is best to call that local agency and ask to speak to the installer. The central reservation agent can give you the phone number.

The first thing I do when they bring the car is check the position of the controls. Sometimes they are too low, and my leg blocks them from being able to travel enough to get good acceleration, or they are too far back so I have to extend my arm too far when I brake. It's dangerous to drive when the controls aren't right, so I'd rather take the extra time to make the mechanic adjust them, frustrating as it is to be delayed. Fortunately, it doesn't happen very often.

Typically, a car rental customer at an airport rides a shuttle bus provided by the agency to and from the terminal to the rental car lot. The buses are not equipped with lifts, so you will need to ask staff there to bring the car to the terminal for you. When you return the rental car, go to the normal drop-off lot and ask for someone to ride back with you to the terminal in the car. It's common for someone to be at the lot to check you in as you return the car, so it is not necessary to get out to ask a desk clerk for help.

Rental agencies do not provide permits for disabled parking. You will need to bring one with you. Out-of-state permits are generally accepted throughout the United States and Canada. If you have plates on your vehicle at home, you are still entitled to get a placard permit from your Department of Motor Vehicles. Even if you do not drive yourself, you are still entitled to a permit to be used by anyone else driving you, including during travel.

Several companies supply adapted vans in many locations across the country, including lift- or ramp-equipped models. Renting a van costs a bit more, but when you are traveling with a group it becomes affordable. Vans also accommodate some power chair users in ways that vehicles from the well-known commercial rental agencies cannot.

Trains

Trains are often less costly than airlines and can sometimes get you to smaller towns and destinations you can't easily fly into. Despite the Americans with Disabilities Act, the rail system is not truly accessible to wheelchair riders. It is one thing to get into the car and have your wheelchair secured; it may be quite another if you need a restroom or require electricity to charge your portable ventilator.

The ADA required Amtrak to provide one accessible car per train by July 1995. Accessible in this case means a wide door that can be entered from a level platform and the ability to stay in a wheelchair, secured from movement during the trip. Unfortunately, you cannot count on being able to get assistance for your bags at the station or other needs you might have. Amtrak advertises that they provide assistance in major city stations and give priority to people with disabilities who wish to reserve private rooms with seating for daytime and sleeping provisions for the night.

In May of 1998, Amtrak settled a case brought by the Disability Rights and Education Defense Fund. They agreed to change their reservations policy so that up until 14 days before departure, accessible bedrooms will be reserved for passengers with mobility impairments. They will also provide written menus and deliver food and snacks which are offered in inaccessible train cars, and will take measures to ensure that films can be viewed by all riders. They have agreed to extend the 15 percent discount for persons with mobility impairments until July 2001.

As with most travel arrangements, you deal with a centralized reservations operator. Always call the local station, in addition, to confirm that an accessible car is on the train you are scheduled for and that services are available to meet your needs. Since there are a limited number of trains with accessible facilities, you should schedule your travel as early as possible to get what you need.

Inter-city buses

Access to buses is important for long-distance as well as local travel, especially for the many chair riders who live on small, fixed incomes such as Social Security disability payments.

The Greyhound Corporation essentially has a monopoly on what is known as "fixed route" transportation by ground in the United States. Greyhound won a waiver allowing them more time to comply with the ADA and in the meantime has purchased new buses without lifts. Very few Greyhound buses have lifts, and you will find the same is true of tour buses in major cities.

There are many stories of people injured by drivers or other staff not trained to assist people onto the bus and of wheelchairs damaged by mishandling. The bus will not have an accessible restroom. Even the places they stop might not have a usable bathroom—even if drivers are willing to help you off the bus. The continuing inaccessibility of buses has a severe impact on availability of affordable transportation.

Hotels

Hotels typically have "handicapped accessible" rooms. In finer, higher-priced hotels, you can generally count on that meaning a bathroom with a wide door, room to turn around, grab bars, a hand-held shower head, and lever controls. Some rooms even have stall showers you can wheel into or multiple light switches in low positions near the bed.

Be very careful when the reservation clerk tells you they have an accessible room. Out of a desire for the business, some hotels say they have an accessible room, but that might mean only that the door into the room is wide enough for a wheelchair, while the bathroom is inaccessible. Really probe to find out exactly what they mean by accessible and how the room is equipped. Know exactly what you need, and if the hotel can't commit clearly to providing those needs, don't choose to stay there.

Since many reservations are placed through centralized operators for hotel chains, operators might not be able to answer your questions sufficiently. If you have any doubts, invest in a long distance phone call and call the hotel directly with your questions.

Beware of consolidators. These are businesses that offer rooms at reduced rates. Hotels sell reservations to a certain number of rooms to consolidators as a way of increasing occupancy rates. Consolidators might tell you the hotel has accessible rooms, but that doesn't mean that the hotel will know you are coming or that such a room will be set aside for you.

> I had an experience in New York City with a consolidator. The accessible rooms were all taken when I arrived. I had to make do with one of hotel's normal rooms, which was only usable by the hotel's removing the bathroom door.

Always call the hotel directly to ensure they know what you need and will guarantee it. Call again a couple of times before you arrive, especially the day before. The hotel should block out the room to make sure it will be available when you arrive. As hotels fill up, they start to give the accessible rooms to able-bodied guests.

Hotel rooms are often full of chairs you don't need or furniture arranged in a way that limits your movement. Beds are often placed close together, or too near a wall. That is especially a problem when the bedspread hangs off the side and can get caught in your wheels. Don't hesitate to ask hotel staff to move things around or take furniture out of the room for you.

When the only telephone in the room is on a table or shelf between beds, too little space between the beds will require you to get out of your chair onto the bed to answer the phone. Some hotels attempt to solve this problem by putting the phone on a desk or dresser rather than by the bed. Of course, you need a phone by the bed more than anywhere else because you are less mobile once out of your chair. One traveler uses this solution:

> *I take a portable telephone with me when I travel. I plug the hotel's phone cord into my set, and then I have a phone anywhere in the room.*

A portable phone is particularly useful in the bathroom. Finer hotels often have a phone installed near the toilet—which still doesn't help much if the phone rings while you're in the bath or shower.

In a rare example of hotels providing broader accessibility, a hotel in Las Vegas has installed sling lift equipment in a few rooms. Sadly, it's the folks who want to take your money in casinos who are catering to the disability crowd.

The organization Hostelling International-American Youth Hostels (HI-AYH) supplies beds for traveling students in the United States and abroad. They provide a bed, pillow, and blanket in a dormitory setting with a shared bathroom for a very low price, as little as $15 a night. There are now 380 hostels in 34 countries that provide wheelchair access, 38 of those in the U.S. Some provide family quarters or private rooms. The range of accessible features varies, since HI-AYH does not establish uniform standards. As with any hotel, call ahead and determine whether you can adapt to the facilities.

Camping

Campgrounds around the country increasingly provide accommodations for wheelchair users. They create level campsites with a firm earth surface that is easy to roll on. There is usually a paved surface for parking near the campsite. Sites are located near bathroom facilities that often include stall showers with fold-down seats. Sometimes the accessible restroom/shower unit is restricted to qualified users who get a key from the park ranger.

Some parks reserve accessible sites until later in the day before giving them out to able-bodied campers. The most desirable parks take reservations in advance, and you are well advised to plan your itinerary and make your arrangements before arriving. You are also likely to find accessible trails at campgrounds with accessible campsites.

Recreational vehicles (RVs), which you can take onto certain campgrounds, are available for rent with lifts and accessible bath facilities. Some parks are primarily outfitted for RVs with electricity and water hookups at individual camp sites. Pristine locations are less likely to allow RVs because of a desire to limit pollution and noise.

Traveling with a ventilator

If you rely on assisted breathing, you should not consider travel off limits to you, though it might involve a bit more planning and coordination, like this woman ventilator user:

> My husband and I are driving to Florida. This is something that we are greatly looking forward to. I have been ill for two and a half years. We need this time together away from doctors, hospitals, and therapists. Every hotel that we have reservations at is an accessible one. We worked closely with AAA and have everything all worked out. We have it in writing that we will be assisted with loading and unloading the car. My portable ventilator runs off the cigarette lighter in the car and has a backup twelve-hour battery. My suction machine runs on AC or DC power. My oxygen supply company has made arrangements for liquid tank fill-ups at each motel stop.

Similarly, you can make arrangements with airlines and train carriers in some cases to provide electricity for a ventilator. Naturally, you should be prepared with backup approaches should there be an emergency.

Adaptive technology

The use of computers is enhancing the lives of people with disabilities by:

- Offering access to information from home
- Accelerating participation in the political process
- Increasing employment opportunity
- Providing tools for disability-friendly pursuits such as writing, software design, or graphic arts
- Promoting participation in online communities of people with shared interests—disability-related or not

- Increasing independence for people with limited upper body strength through dramatic evolution of power wheelchairs and remote control technology

There are considerable resources for adaptive technology. Rehab centers and Independent Living Centers increasingly offer training programs and support groups on computing. The Abilities Expo takes place in four cities each year and includes an area devoted to computing.

Even if you can't easily use your fingers or hands, or can't see or hear, you can still use the technology. There is enough demand for alternative methods of using computers to encourage designers and companies to develop new accessible methods of interaction with the computer. These input alternatives include software that reduces keystrokes, adaptive keyboards, voice dictation, voice synthesis, eye movement and head controllers, switches, and puff-and-sip controls.

Adaptive technology reduces frustration. You might be able to press keys to type, but the process might be so slow, or you might make so many mistakes in the process, that you will want to give up. Your creativity and thought process are interrupted if you cannot easily interact with the computer.

Software solutions for text entry

If you have limited use of your hands, two software approaches help reduce the number of actual keystrokes required for text entry: word abbreviation and word prediction.

Abbreviation allows you to enter a small number of letters which are enough for the computer to know what the whole word should be—a sort of shorthand. Pressing the space bar might initiate expansion of the word, or the program might automatically recognize two characters without any following space. Some programs have a defined a set of abbreviations and allow a number of customizable words. Other programs allow the user to define the shortcuts. An abbreviation program can be turned on or off by the user, for times when it might not be useful. It greatly reduces the number of keystrokes you must press.

> *I really love my abbreviation software. It probably saves me a quarter to a third of the keystrokes I would have to make otherwise. At first it was a little awkward, but now using the abbreviations is totally natural. If*

I have to type at a computer that doesn't have it, I feel like I'm pressing way too many keys for the amount of text I'm entering.

Word prediction software puts up a numbered list of words on the screen as soon as a letter is pressed, suggesting what the program thinks the desired word might be. You select a word by typing its number. If the word you want has not appeared, type more letters until it does appear. The software learns by remembering the words you use the most and gives them higher priority on the list. With experience, you will usually only need to type a few characters per word.

Macro software lets you define keystrokes (usually using the Control, Alt, or Option keys) to enter blocks of standard text—for example, the closing for a letter. Many programs also allow you to automate command functions and sequences. You might enter a single keystroke to open your email program, tell it to check for mail, and enter a password. Macro software has been available for some time and is incorporated into the Microsoft Windows operating system. Macintosh system software includes AppleScript, another powerful macro tool.

Some users are unable to hold down two keys simultaneously. Functions which use the Control key, for instance, become inaccessible. There are programs which allow you to press the two keys in sequence, rather than together to achieve the same effect. On the Macintosh, this is a standard feature of the Easy Access program, integrated into system software.

These kinds of programs can typically be found as shareware that you can download from the Internet. There is a greater chance of conflicts with other software on your computer, so be sure you know what files are being installed so you can remove them if you have problems. If the program works well, it's only fair to make the small payment to the software's author which is usually requested for shareware—usually much less than you would pay for a commercial product.

Hardware solutions

The standard computer keyboard is a set of small keys that you press with your fingertips. The standard keyboard requires dexterity and accuracy beyond the capacity of many people, whether paralyzed by injury or stroke, restricted by arthritis, etc. Now there are keyboards available with large pads sensitive to touch; it is not necessary to press down on a key. Another design allows you to rest your hands directly on the keyboard and apply a slight additional pressure to select a key. There are also keyboards designed for one-handed use.

Most adaptive keyboards work in combination with abbreviation or word prediction software, or allow you to use macros to define keystroke short-cuts. Designers try to make use of all available features to ease the physical demands of computing.

Voice dictation

If you can't use your hands, you can talk to your computer and have it type what you say or initiate a command. It won't do what you say every time, but it will listen! You get to correct it when you make a mistake, a standard and critical feature of voice software.

Voice dictation technology is far enough progressed—and commercially available—to be of use now. Existing products contain libraries of up to 200,000 words and allow the user to control the computer interface—the set of commands and choices. The most difficult thing to control by voice is a cursor—the pointer or arrow with which one chooses from menus or clicks on buttons, text, or objects. Starting the cursor movement is easy enough, and you can tell it to go up or down, left or right, but getting it to stop is tricky because of a slight delay in response. It is difficult—if not impossible—to draw graphics by voice command.

> You can't get emotional when you are talking to your computer. If I am moving the pointer to a place on the screen where I want to click, I say, "Stop cursor." If that doesn't work and I say, "Stop cursor! STOP CURSOR!" it will not respond because computers don't like being yelled at! Really, it means that it just can't recognize my voice when it is so different from how I usually say the command.

It is remarkable to see a computer put a word on the screen that you speak into the microphone, normally worn as a headset. Voice systems increase in accuracy with use. You establish a personal voice file, usually during an initial training procedure in which you recite for the software so it can become familiar with your voice. Anyone can use voice systems, regardless of accent or dialect.

Early voice dictation technologies used discrete speech, with a pause required after each word. Continuous speech is a more difficult computing task. Individual words blend together in normal speech and the computer must work harder to figure out where the words separate. Dragon Systems of Newton, Massachusetts, released its Naturally Speaking voice recognition product in 1997—the first commercial continuous speech program. However, the system is not as effective for command control of the computer and so is not an entirely hands-free application. Naturally Speaking is only available for Microsoft Windows systems. Dragon Systems also offers PowerSecretary, a discrete speech product for the Macintosh. At this time, some people continue to use a blend of continuous and discrete speech software.

Voice synthesis

People unable to speak now have access to augmentative communication—a box the size of a desktop computer which functions as the person's voice. For instance, many people with cerebral palsy can use augmentative communication to help them piece together sentences with a variety of buttons, or to preprogram sentences or whole speeches. A number of people have great difficulty speaking, but enough dexterity with their hands to operate the device. People can have conversations or make public presentations using this technology.

The Trace Center at the University of Wisconsin at Madison was established in 1971 to address communication needs of people who cannot speak. In the early 1980s, they began to receive funds from the federal government for research in adaptive technology. The Trace Center has worked with computer companies to promote and integrate disability access features. They coordinate conferences and provide publications, such as a nine-hundred-page resource book. They continue to pursue research on a variety of computer platforms, including the Macintosh and UNIX. Many staff members have advanced science and engineering degrees, and play a significant role in the development and promotion of adaptive technology.

Other input devices

There are other alternatives to the keyboard and mouse for getting information from the human brain into the computer. Once it is possible to position a pointer on the screen and initiate a "click" which transfers your intent to the machine, you can do quite a lot. That includes typing, since there are programs that display a keyboard on the screen, allowing you to click on letters. A physical keyboard is no longer necessary.

The Eyegaze System from LC Technologies in Fairfax, Virginia, uses an infrared beam and a video camera. The beam is pointed at one of your eyes and makes the pupil visible to the video camera. The video camera tracks the position of the eye and moves the cursor in response to your eye movement. By allowing the cursor to rest on a command for a specified time (you choose how long), the software executes the click.

The Eyegaze System offers software for typing, speech communication, reading text, controlling household devices like the television and telephone, or turning lights on and off. The system requires the use of only one eye, but the head must be kept still.

Not everyone uses graphical interfaces that allow point and click. For people using older, text-based operating systems such as DOS, there is adaptive software. One such DOS program is controlled by Morse code—the language of dots and dashes used in the telegraph system which used to be the primary means of long distance communication until the telephone came along. It is offered by MicroSystems Software in Framingham, Massachusetts. All it takes to operate the program is the movement of one finger, or the ability to click on a mouth switch. MicroSystems also provides software for word prediction, voice synthesis, and telephone control.

Environmental control

Quadriplegics have always struggled with gaining as much independence as possible. They inevitably require personal assistance for dressing and other matters of care, but until now they also needed help operating a light switch, opening a door, answering the telephone, or turning the television on or off.

Computers to the rescue. Systems are now available that allow almost complete control of the electrical systems in your house, even for someone with no use of his arms. Such systems can be controlled by puff-and-sip control, voice command, or switches—of which there are now many types that require minimal dexterity and accuracy.

An example of how such systems work is that a menu, shown on a small display, shows programmed options, such as telephone, lights, bed, and television. You rotate through the choices and choose one, for example, lights. Another set of choices appears, for example, main bedroom fixture, bedside lamp, and hallway light. Once again you rotate through the choices and choose. For a telephone, commonly called numbers can be programmed into a speaker phone which requires no hand use. The menu will also include the operator. Some local phone systems provide special services to disabled customers, such as free operator assistance to dial numbers. Chapter 7, *Home Access*, further discusses environmental control systems.

The right system

Anything written about computer systems soon goes out of date. Speed and memory capacity increase, and relative price (dollar per megabyte of memory, for instance) has fallen at an incredible pace. No matter when you buy, there will soon be a faster, cheaper system with more features. Don't wait for the ultimate system to be created, manufactured, or put on sale. Buy what you need when you need it, shopping for the best price, service, and reliability at the time.

Find a well-informed salesperson—or computer-savvy friend—to guide you. The number of options may seem overwhelming, but once you identify what you need and what your budget allows, choices will be more manageable. Stick with what you need now, although consider ways you might need to upgrade the system in the future.

There are a variety of potential funding sources for computers and adaptive technology, such as vocational rehab and the National Science Foundation with funds available to disabled students and faculty members. Used computer equipment often gets donated to agencies or nonprofit groups who then make it available to people with big needs and small budgets. Finding funding takes research, but can be worth the effort.

Ergonomics—safety and computers

People can get hurt using computers. Injuries are typically referred to as cumulative trauma or repetitive strain injuries. Computer users with disabilities need to pay special heed, since the primary locations of computer-related injuries are in the upper extremities—hands, wrists, elbows, and shoulders. For a person with a disability, injured arms or hands are the last thing they need.

While having computer skills and using them in the workplace improves your ability to work full time and earn the same pay as nondisabled workers, be vigilant about protecting yourself from overusing your arms, wrists, hands, or shoulders. Learn something about ergonomics—the science of how to relate your body to your work—and develop a work style that does not exceed your body's ability to remain healthy.

For six years I have been living with chronic pain in my wrists and elbows from excessive computing and poor working posture. Despite periods of relative comfort and freedom, I remain prone to flare-ups which require me to limit my activities or else risk more severe pain and lasting effects. It has already cost me the ability to perform as a musician. I write by voice dictation.

I have often told people that my chronic pain problems have been more disabling than my paralysis. I could adapt very well with a wheelchair, hand controls in my car, and refinements at home. Losing the freedom—or ability—to use my arms pushes things to a very different level and demands more intensive adaptations. It also means a lower level of productivity compared to my norm. Since I still have use of my arms, it is actually more difficult to refrain than if I were quadriplegic, where I would have no choice but to use hands-free technology. It is harder to choose not to use my arms when I still have the option.

There is much available information about ergonomics now—in books, on the Internet, from consultants, and from people assigned to the job in larger companies. There is no reason for someone today to develop the chronic pain which has already struck many thousands of computer users, and caused some to give up or change careers.

Ergonomics means being comfortable and using the body efficiently. Ergonomic skills at the computer or workplace are similar to the ergonomic skills you learn for using a wheelchair—conserve energy, move smoothly, take care not to overexert and overstrain your tissues. Be aware of what you feel and don't accept discomfort. Fatigue and discomfort are messages from your body, telling you to slow down or make a change in how you use your body. When you are in pain, there is always a cause. Ergonomics as a discipline is about identifying that cause and making changes to the physical setting or work habits to prevent pain.

Muscles—even small ones—are not made to be held in continuous contraction. When you lean in toward a computer screen, work with arms extended to reach a mouse or keyboard, continuously hold a mouse button, or keep your head in a fixed position for a long period of time, you are making those muscles contract without rest. A computer screen which is too high or low will make the neck and shoulder muscles work constantly. Low level, continuously held exertions eventually become a source of pain, as you exceed the limits of muscle tissues and they begin to send out messages to cease and desist!

Sit as upright as possible without effort, letting your skeleton carry you so your muscles don't have to. Good posture becomes more complicated when fewer muscles are working in your body, or if you have a spinal curvature or other asymmetry of the body. The higher a spinal cord injury, for instance, the less of the trunk muscles are working and the greater the tendency to have to sit in rounded postures for stability. A person with such an injury using a computer needs to take care not to encourage increasingly rounded postures. The positioning system in your wheelchair plays an important role in this.

Wheelchair users sitting at desks have extra challenges. Able-bodied workers often sit in chairs that rotate on a stem, so they can turn to other areas of the desk or workstation without twisting their bodies. Wheelchairs don't rotate sideways, so you must twist the body to reach to the side. To compensate, keep objects you use most—keyboard, mouse, telephone, paperwork, stapler, etc.—close to you, within easy reach, and more in front of you than to the side. If you turn from the computer to work on some papers or make a phone call, first take the time to turn your wheelchair so you can still sit straight.

Take advantage of adaptive technology to help address the problem of cumulative trauma injuries. Why press any more keys or click any more buttons than you have to? Make an art of finding how few clicks it takes to do your work. You will be protecting yourself in the process.

Ergonomics is really about common sense: listening to your body and taking care of yourself. If you eat a balanced diet and drink less coffee and more water, you will lower your risk of injury. If you make a point to breathe, relax, and let go of muscular tension, you lower your risk. If you mix tasks and take regular breaks from computing, using your body in a variety of ways throughout the day, you lower your risk. If you make comfort a high priority, you can safely take advantage of the power and creativity possible through computing.

Education

Any school in the U.S. that receives federal funding falls under provisions of the Rehabilitation Act of 1973 and has been required for some time to make facilities accessible.

Education is a definite advantage when it comes to employment. A study by economists Douglas Kruse from Rutgers University—a spinal cord injured wheelchair rider—and Alan Krueger at Princeton University found that more than half of college graduates with SCI were employed in the study sample of nearly 6,000 persons, compared to only one sixth of high school graduates. Those with a college education earned 60 to 75 percent more than those with a high school diploma.[3]

College campuses

Most colleges and universities in this country are now widely accessible to people with disabilities. Your first priority is getting an education at the school you prefer, rather than choosing the most accessible school. Identify what you want and then see what it will take to make it work. Contact the school you are considering and ask for the disabled students services office. They will have staff available to help you with a variety of needs, from housing to financing, transportation to personal assistance services.

Some older campuses are a little harder to get around. Older buildings are not so easy to adapt. In some cases, access to a course might necessitate its relocation to another classroom. If you are a manual chair user on a hilly campus, you might consider using a power chair to get around.

Sheldon Ginns is a staff architect at the University of Michigan in Ann Arbor. In the early '70s, he was the first to investigate what it would take to provide access on campus. At the time, there were very few wheelchair riders. He found:

> Many of the changes they needed to make were not very expensive. We could add grab bars, adjust door closers, relocate certain classes, install some basic ramps, or grade up to some entrances to replace steps. The first reaction of the administration was, "Why should we do this? There aren't any students who need it." Now, of course, there are hundreds of chair users here.

Educating children with disabilities

True access to education for children remains a challenge. There continue to be reports of teachers who resist full accommodation, frustrated by lack of training or demands on their time, particularly when communication or learning disabilities are involved.

When parents complain that the school nearest home does not offer needed programs, the school district often urges parents to send children farther away. However, the extra distance means extra travel time and prevents children from developing strong social networks with neighborhood children.

> I have four children: Sarah, Collin, Laura, and Emma Rose. Two of my children have cerebral palsy. My son Collin's CP is more significant than my daughter Laura's. Our local school system, Fairfax County Public Schools, is insisting Collin go to another school forty-five minutes from home in a segregated program. My husband and I disagree and insist his needs and development are best served staying in our own neighborhood.

> My husband and I are aware that Collin has physical differences. We are also aware of how much he is like other five-year-old kids. Collin thinks that ice cream is the perfect food. He laughs when his sisters get in trouble. He loves his mom and dad, but he realizes that his buddies are way more cool. Like any other kid, Collin has his strengths and weaknesses. And, like any other parents, we know that we must "raise the bar," so to speak, to challenge him. A "separate but equal" setting has never been, and never will be, an acceptable option for the education of our son.

Children find themselves at a disadvantage in other ways in school. For example, they might miss the sex education often offered in physical education classes, which they do not attend. Accommodation is sometimes lacking in drivers' education.

What matters is that children with disabilities are educated so they can find their full potential and compete for good jobs. At present, many well-paying jobs are in the technology sector. Tony Coehlo, chairman of the President's Committee on Employment of People with Disabilities, noted in a recent speech:

> The top three occupations for young people with disabilities are laborers, operatives, and craft workers. Unless changes are made in the

education and training of youth with disabilities, we will fall further and further behind.

That's why the President's Committee has put so much emphasis on skill development programs like our High School/High Tech program to encourage students with disabilities to pursue careers in science and technology, and our workforce recruitment program to find summer internships in the public and private sectors for college students with disabilities.[4]

Success stories

On the whole, education is opening wider all the time. From major universities to local community colleges to evolving Internet-based home study options, there are ways for you to learn, gain degrees or certifications, and pursue internships.

Even if you have to put up a bit of a fight, you can reach your goals, as James Post did to finish medical school. Medical educators doubted his ability to perform as a physician with spinal cord quadriplegia. They questioned his ability to feel a pulse or palpate organs during an exam without sensation in his fingertips. However, thanks to modern diagnostic equipment and the support of a mentor—a neurologist and polio survivor who faced similar obstacles in becoming a doctor—James Post graduated with honors from the Albert Einstein College of Medicine in 1997.[5]

Employment

Vast numbers of people with disabilities remain unemployed. The 1998 NOD/Harris Survey found a substantial gap in employment for those with disabilities:

Employment continues to be the area with the widest gulf between those who are disabled and those who are not. Only three in ten working-age adults with disabilities are employed full or part-time, compared to eight in ten nondisabled adults. Working-age adults with disabilities are no more likely to be employed today than they were a decade ago, even though almost three out of four who are not working say that they would prefer to be working. This low rate of employment has, in turn, led to an

income gap that has not narrowed at all since 1986, with one in three dis-
abled adults, compared to just one in eight nondisabled Americans, living
in very low income households with less than $15,000 in annual income.[6]

Some can't work or find work because of physical issues such as pain, spasticity, limited energy, or communication difficulties. Unfortunately, there also
appears to be some discrimination on the part of employers, overt or not.
Journalist John Hockenberry—a wheelchair user—produced an investiga-
tive report shown in 1997 on *Dateline NBC*. He sent two young men to various employers asking for work. One was quadriplegic, the other walked.
The résumé of the chair rider was intentionally slightly better than the other
decoy. Witnessed by hidden cameras, several potential employers used tac-
tics to discourage the man with the disability. In one case, he was told there
were no application forms, although forms were produced for the walking
applicant. In another case, the able-bodied man was invited into a preliminary training session not offered to the chair rider.

These prospective employers might have doubted the ability of the chair
rider to perform the job, but they are at least guilty of pre-judgment without
taking the time to ask how the applicant would adapt to the tasks of the job.
In most cases, resistance is not a matter of hateful prejudice, but of simple
ignorance. When you apply for a job, try to know something ahead of time
about the tasks involved, and be prepared to explain how you will perform
them. You could also point a potential employer to resources such as the Job
Accommodation Network, described below.

There are some tax incentives for employers who spend money on accommodations for disabled employees. The Disabled Access Credit (IRS Section
44) allows companies with gross receipts under one million dollars or with
fewer than thirty full-time employees to take a tax credit of 50 percent of
their expenditures for access, up to $5,000 a year. The Architectural and
Transportation Barrier Removal Deduction (IRS Section 190) can be as large
as $15,000, although it was reduced from $35,000 in 1990. You might
improve your chances if you arrive at your job interview equipped with this
information.

One of the greatest challenges to the ability to work is the current structure
of the benefits system. Social Security disability benefits, for instance, are
tied to a person's income—and you are not allowed to make very much
without risking the end of your checks or the loss of health and assistance
coverage under Medicare. Similar income limits apply to state-administered

programs like Medicaid (MediCal in California) which serve people with low incomes. Some people with the skills and desire simply cannot afford to work. Changes are being proposed to reform Social Security to increase incentives for people with disabilities to work. Chapter 10, *Politics and Legislation*, talks about this movement and proposed changes.

People with disabilities are working more these days, even in the face of considerable physical limitations. More options are possible than either a person with a disability or an employer might imagine. More people will get the chance to demonstrate what is possible, as more workers with disabilities appear in the workplace. Some progressive programs sponsored by rehab facilities, universities, independent living programs, or large employers are designed to promote hiring of disabled workers, so they also make more opportunities available.

PCEPD

The President's Committee on Employment of People with Disabilities (PCEPD) was formed by President John Kennedy in the early 1960s to assist the business community in hiring people with disabilities.

Each year the committee holds a conference which attracts people around the country, from both government and the private sector. Seminars and lectures at the conference help corporate executives, human resources specialists, disability advocates, union representatives, and other interested parties in promoting employment of people with disabilities.

PCEPD helps employers assess whether someone is capable of performing a job. Job analysis materials help them determine employment issues such as:

- What functions are essential to the job
- What physical tasks—climbing, kneeling, lifting, carrying, etc.—are necessary
- How the job would be altered if certain physical requirements were removed or changed
- What movements through the office or field site are necessary
- What social conditions and interaction with colleagues are required
- What general skills are necessary for the job

- How previous experience might be substituted for lack of specific training or education

- What equipment, spatial arrangement, or job redesign measures can accommodate a person's ability to perform the job

Employers are sometimes hard-pressed to imagine how a person with a disability could perform a given task, but this is often because they don't know how people adapt. PCEPD helps overcome employers' resistance by demonstrating how the job can be performed, what adaptations the employer can make, and the benefits of hiring people with disabilities who are often among the most loyal of employees.

PCEPD is active on the political front. In March of 1998, President Clinton established a task force whose mission is to bring levels of employment for people with disabilities up to par with the general population. Tony Coelho, chairman of the President's Committee, is optimistic about the task force, despite the current poor state of employment for people with disabilities.

> *Only 26 percent of working age people with severe disabilities are employed—contrast that with the 82 percent employment rate of the general adult population. The employment figures for individuals with severe disabilities who are also members of racial or ethnic minority groups is even worse!*

> *Yet I for one am confident that we are going to see real progress in increasing the employment rate of Americans with disabilities.*

> *By the time the Task Force presents its final report to the President on July 26, 2002—the tenth anniversary of the initial implementation of the employment provisions of the ADA—we are going to be able to point with pride to higher employment rates for people with disabilities.*[7]

The Job Accommodation Network (JAN)

A service of the PCEPD, the Job Accommodation Network (JAN) provides information to employers to help them hire and accommodate special needs of employees with disabilities. An employer can call an 800 number to take advantage of resources, including:

- Information on adapting a job for a person with a disability

- Information on accommodating an employee with minimal expense

- Support for mobility, sensory, and neurological disabilities

- Access to a large library of material about strategies and products

- Services in English, Spanish, and French

The JAN tells employers that hiring people with disabilities expands the pool of qualified employees, and that learning how to accommodate disability reduces Workers' Compensation and other insurance costs. The JAN stresses that accommodations do not cost what employers generally expect—88 percent of accommodations suggested by JAN cost less than $1,000.

Computers and employment

Technology is creating new opportunities for working with a disability. People can work in offices or at home with a modem, voice-activated computer, and speaker phone. Adaptive technology will continue to give entry points to employment for people with disabilities.

An encouraging note was reported by economists Douglas Kruse and Alan Krueger. They found that people with spinal cord injuries with sufficient computer skills were able to earn the same level of income as an able-bodied worker. The disability was completely transparent where pay was concerned—unlike the overall population of people with disabilities who earn less for the same work than the general population. The study reports:

> *Current computer use at work appears to significantly enhance the earnings power of people with SCIs and of the general population, even after controlling for the effects of education, experience, job seniority, union status, gender, and race. Indeed, SCI workers who use a computer at work earn essentially the same amount per week as non-SCI workers, while among non-users of computers the pay of SCI workers is lower than that of non-SCI workers. Those with SCIs who use a computer at work tend to work substantially more hours per week, and are more likely to hold full-time jobs than are SCI workers who do not work with computers.*[8]

There is a tremendous need for people with computer and technology skills. Jobs in programming, data analysis, or database administration are waiting for qualified candidates. The situation is severe enough that in 1998 one of the top news stories in California's Silicon Valley was about the desire of the computer industry to allow more immigration of people with these skills because of the industry's claim that there are not enough qualified candidates in the U.S.

At the May 1998 national conference of the President's Committee, chairman Tony Coelho made these comments in his opening speech:

> *Right now, more than 346,000 computer-programmer and systems-analyst jobs are vacant in U.S. companies with more than 100 employees. These jobs pay well. Computer science graduates are receiving job offers averaging over $40,000 a year!*
>
> *A positive result of the labor shortage is that barriers of discrimination are beginning to fall. Businesses of all sizes are looking at people with disabilities to fill their needs. This burgeoning demand creates an enormous opportunity for people with disabilities who have the skills and experience employers seek.*[9]

The study by Kruse and Krueger found that people with quadriplegia, college graduates, and younger people were more likely to use a computer, and this correlated to higher levels of employment. Companies did not have to invest in training people or risk hiring someone without proven skills. Other findings include:[10]

- Only 17 percent of spinal cord injured workers returned to their previous job following injury.

- Another 10 percent said they could have returned to their previous work if they had been provided training and adaptive devices.

- Pay per hour was only slightly lower for people re-employed after injury, but hours—and weekly pay—fell by 25 percent.

- 51 percent of people in white collar jobs returned to work.

- 32 percent of people in blue collar jobs returned to work.

Larger corporations tend to be more willing to invest in hiring people with disabilities and in the equipment they need. They have the resources to commit to searching for people, sending staff to conferences such as those put on by PCEPD, and supporting accommodation needs of an employee. Ultimately, these efforts are worth the investment.

Starting your own business

Technology has made it easier to operate a business from home. A computer with a modem, a telephone, and a fax machine put you in contact with the world—including clients.

The U.S. Small Business Administration (SBA) helps some people seeking financing for a small business startup. They don't make direct loans, but if your bank turns you down, you might qualify for an SBA loan guarantee under the Handicapped Assistance Loan (HAL) program. If your application is accepted, SBA essentially promises to pay the bank if you default on the loan, removing the bank's risk. The SBA puts certain limits on the interest the bank may charge and also restricts the type of business they will approve. Gambling or real estate investment, for instance, are excluded from its list of approved businesses.

The SBA also provides information to help you start your business. Local offices provide advisers through the Service Corps of Retired Executives (SCORE) program, in which retired business executives review your plans and consult with you to help ensure success.

Temporary work

The workplace has witnessed an extraordinary shift toward contract and part-time workers. Corporations want to reduce full-time staff in order to save fixed overhead expenses of wages and benefits. More work projects are of shorter duration, with rapidly changing marketplaces and technologies. It can be difficult to predict what skills a company will need at any one time. Part-time and contract workers give companies flexibility.

Manpower Incorporated is an example of a temporary employment agency which has grown to be one of the largest corporations in the world. It maintains a list of people with specific skills and refers them to companies who call looking for those skills. Wages are paid by Manpower, who is paid a fee by the employer. Temporary job referrals can result in full-time jobs, since some companies see the service as a way of getting to know a potential employee without having to make a commitment to hire them full-time from the start.

Many people question the impact of part-time and contract work on employees and communities. Workers can wonder where the next job will come from, not earn as much as they need, or lose security by not having health or retirement benefits. However, many people like being a contract worker. You get to work on a variety of projects, meet more people, and gain a variety of skills. You also get to experience the employer before making a full-time commitment, if that is an option. If you can perform some work at home, you might be able to gain a tax benefit from deducting the costs of a home office. The flexibility of contract work can be a good employment solution for a person with a disability.

Some companies are experimenting with flex-time, in which jobs are shared and—to the degree possible—people set their own hours. This—along with part-time contract opportunities—opens up possibilities for people who have trouble committing to a full-time job because they are unable to predict physical problems such as severe infections, pressure sores, or exacerbations of MS, for instance.

The right to work

Title I of the Americans with Disabilities Act requires equal opportunity for people with disabilities, affecting all employers in the private sector with fifteen or more employees, as of July 26, 1994. The ADA protects you from being discriminated against for employment solely based on your disability. It does not guarantee you a job. You still have to qualify based on your abilities.

Federal agencies and any business receiving federal contracts of $10,000 or more were already held from discriminating based on disability by the Rehabilitation Act of 1973. Sections 501 and 503 called on the government and its contractors to take affirmative action to hire people with disabilities.

The Vietnam Veterans Readjustment Assistance Act of 1974 similarly requires government contractors to take affirmative action on behalf of covered veterans.

Advocacy and volunteering

Many people with disabilities are not employed, but still have time and skills to contribute. There are satisfying and productive options available.

There is plenty of work to do to advance the opportunities—or remove the barriers—for people with disabilities. There is no shortage of groups and associations who need help with advocacy. You can volunteer time at your local Independent Living Center or a disability-specific group like United Cerebral Palsy to advance the inclusion of people with disabilities in our culture.

American Disabled for Attendant Programs Today (ADAPT) is probably the most radical of disability advocacy groups. It has taken militant action in order to achieve access to transportation and personal assistance services in the community rather than nursing homes. There are local chapters of ADAPT in many cities around the country.

You can volunteer time and experience to a local rehabilitation hospital, which typically welcome people in a peer support role for people facing a new disability. You might be surprised how much you have to offer from your own experience.

There are always issues of importance to the disability community which require people to express support or concerns about pending legislation of public policies. Organizations such as ADAPT or Justin and Yoshiko Dart's Justice for All regularly notify people about such activities, as do politically oriented publications such as *The Ragged Edge* or *Mouth*. You can contribute with letters or phone calls to representatives, business, or civic leaders expressing your position on disability issues.

There are many other volunteer options to choose from. Visits to a local elementary school are often welcome by teachers, either to support their programs or as a way of offering children positive models of people with disabilities. Many libraries are looking for tutors to help teach adult reading courses. Local churches or agencies need help in serving many people in need, such as those who are homeless. Especially if you are feeling frustrated with your life, devoting time to your community is a wonderful way to forget your own problems and gain meaning and gratification.

The fact is that no one has the right to tell you that you can't work because of your disability. If you have the motivation, a desire to learn and develop a profession or skill, and some notion of how you would adapt your disability to that work, then go do it. Even people who should know better—like rehab staff—might discourage you for fear that you are hoping for too much. But the case has been made many times over. People with disabilities of all sorts are working as doctors, lawyers, activists, writers, publishers, artists, musicians, inventors, business owners, athletes, and almost any other pursuit you can imagine. If you want to work, then get out there and find out on your own terms what it takes.

Athletics

Sports benefit all people. Sports are fun, good for your health, and a way to meet people and feel connected. Wheelchair users participate—and excel—in a long list of sports, sometimes by means of recently designed adaptive devices. There are many sports to choose from and many organized events structured for disabled athletes. Leagues exist for wheelchair basketball, billiards, bowling, quad rugby, archery, and others. In some cases, competition is not only among people with disabilities, as in billiards, shooting, or certain classes of archery.

The National Veterans Wheelchair Games takes place each summer and includes athletes from the U.S., Puerto Rico, and Great Britain. The fifteen competitive sports include archery, basketball, quad rugby, swimming, track and field, table tennis, and weightlifting. An equestrian event is included as an exhibition.

The most substantial gathering of disabled athletes is the Paralympics, held every four years with corporate sponsorship. At the 1996 games in Atlanta, competitors from 124 countries took part in seventeen sports and two demonstration events. 64,000 people attended opening ceremonies. Quite a lot of conversion had to be performed in the Olympic village where the athletes stayed, including installing 750 hand-held shower heads, changing bathroom doors, and putting transfer benches in showers. Despite some access and transportation problems, the games came off very well.

Associations

Many associations, national and local, promote and provide opportunities for disabled athletes. Following are a few examples:

- Disabled Sports USA sponsors clinics and events in snow and water skiing, rafting, and camping, among others, and operates an adaptive ski school at Lake Tahoe in California. It holds workshops to train instructors in adaptive fitness programs.

- The Handicapped Scuba Association trains and certifies people in scuba diving—both divers with disabilities and trainers. The association also sponsors trips; some trips use a luxury yacht adapted for chair users.

- The National Center on Accessibility provides information on access to parks, operated in cooperation with the National Parks Service. It also promotes full participation in parks, recreation, and tourism and conducts research in trail design, wilderness policy issues, and the design of beach surfaces for assistive devices.

- Wilderness Inquiry provides outdoor adventures for people of all ages and abilities. Rafting, kayaking, camping, canoeing, and horseback trips are held in the U.S. and Canada. Wilderness Inquiry encourages participation of people with disabilities and recommends manual chairs with knobby tires.

- Wheelchair Sports USA oversees local groups in a range of sports and is a clearinghouse of information.

The sport wheelchair

Wheelchairs for sports such as tennis, basketball, hockey, or rugby are adjusted—or specially designed—for the sport. The chairs are invariably rigid because of the need for great agility and responsiveness. Sport chairs use wheel camber, in which the top of the wheel is angled in toward the body to expand the wheelbase at the floor, to minimize tipping. Hockey and rugby chairs have metal guards at the base because of the frequency of collisions. The racing wheelchair is a sleek, precision device with its large third wheel extending well out in front of the chair and its rider.

Archery

People with disabilities can compete equally with nondisabled participants in archery. However, some classifications specific to wheelchair users are used in events sponsored by Wheelchair Archery, USA. One class is for quadriplegic archers who use adapted equipment or might need assistance placing the arrow on the bow. Another class is for chair riders who use equipment which conforms to international rules.

People with limited use of their fingers can wear a cuff with a hook device that allows them to grasp and release the bow. The string is released by extension of the wrist, without any action in the fingers. Quadriplegic archers may also use support straps. A compound bow is a design which reduces the amount of force required to pull back on the string.

Billiards or pool

Many people shoot pool from a wheelchair. The table is low and equipment is lightweight. Billiards is a sport easily played with nondisabled competitors. Some quadriplegic players can use a cuff to hold the thick end of the stick, while having enough dexterity in their arms to position the cue and accurately strike the ball. There is a slight disadvantage in reaching far balls, but pool players have always had access to a device called a bridge, which allows them to reach the cue ball anywhere on the table. Just as a standing player must keep one foot on the floor, a wheelchair player must keep one "cheek on the seat."

The McDermott Wheelchair Billiards Tournament takes place every year, cosponsored by the Paralyzed Veterans of America.

Bowling

Some wheelchair bowlers grip and throw the ball like a standing bowler. This is more difficult in a wheelchair because of the need to keep the arm away from the wheel as you roll the ball. Since a walking bowler is using the momentum of his body to propel the ball, a wheelchair bowler must either do much more work with his shoulder (with the potential for causing tendinitis) or choose a slower style.

There are metal or wood ramps available for bowlers to use from a wheelchair. The ramp has a level surface at the top. The ball is pushed forward and down the ramp once you have pointed the ramp where you want the ball to go. Another option is a bowling stick, which allows you to direct the ball from the ground. A bowling stick, such as the Bowl-A-Cue, is a pole with four prongs conforming to the shape of the ball and used to push the ball. Another device you can use is a snap-handle—a gripper that fits in the three holes and lets go of the ball when you place it down to roll it. Most wheelchair bowlers use a 10-pound ball, rather than the 15 or 16 pounds used by most standing bowlers.

The American Wheelchair Bowling Association was formed in 1962. Competitors are required to use brakes, and ramps are not allowed in competition. The Association offers a videotape and book to help you learn how to bowl from a wheelchair (see the Appendix for contact information).

Field events

Field events include throwing javelins, discuses, shot puts, and clubs. The club is a special adapted prop that resembles a bowling pin. It is weighted at the end and can be thrown by people with quadriplegia (see Figure 11-4). There are rules about where the legs must be placed and how much contact with the seat is maintained as you position yourself to gain the best possible leverage. Gloves or assistive devices are not allowed in competition.

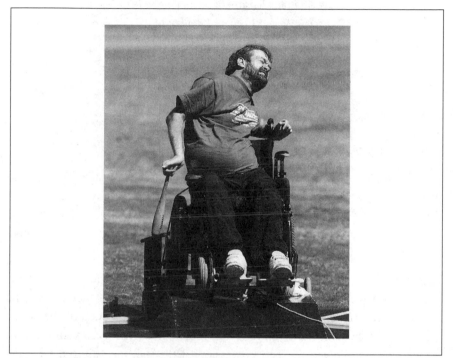

Figure 11-4. A quadriplegic man in the club-throwing field event

Juggling

Juggling can be learned with practice. You need to be willing to drop things and be patient with failure. It is worth enduring the initial awkwardness to discover how well your body can learn complex tasks and to enjoy feelings of competence and joy.

Most juggling options are limited to people with the ability to grasp with their hands, although a quadriplegic could get involved in plate spinning by putting a cuff on the sticks. You will probably start by learning how to juggle three balls. This is easily done sitting down and does not require a great deal of upper body balance. There are hundreds of possible patterns you can throw with three balls, so there is endless opportunity for exploration. A ball juggling routine can become an excellent source of aerobic exercise.

> *There are not many juggling wheelchair users, but that need not be true. At the summer International Jugglers' Association events, I am typically the only chair rider. Yet I know an occupational therapist who uses juggling in her work. Juggling could be an excellent option for many other chair riders. I have had the pleasure of advancing to the level of passing clubs in group patterns. When I began, I doubted I would ever achieve that level.*

Juggling is a growing amateur sport. Many cities have weekly get-togethers. Experienced jugglers are happy to teach the basics to anyone who shows up and asks for a lesson.

Quad rugby

Quadriplegics are generally unable to play basketball because of the grip needed to shoot the ball and the greater arm strength usually needed to loft the ball to the hoop ten feet above. In the 1970s, a group of Canadians developed quad rugby as an alternative sport. The United States Quad Rugby Association was formed in 1988.

Quad rugby is a very physical game, a blend of basketball, hockey, and football. It is played with a volleyball, which is lighter than a basketball. The object is to carry the ball across goal lines marked at the ends of the court, usually a basketball court. Players may push their wheels any number of times, but are allowed to keep possession of the ball for only ten seconds. There are many collisions, thus the rugged design of specialized rugby chairs offered by some wheelchair makers. Spoke guards are common, for protection of both the spokes and the players' hands.

Shooting

Target shooting with a pistol or air rifle can be done from a sitting position and is available to everyone with the visual ability to sight the target. There are puff-and-sip devices for firing the gun for quadriplegics who cannot squeeze the trigger with a finger. Competitive shooting is a sport which does not need separate events for people with disabilities—there is no advantage or disadvantage. You may set the rifle on a table using a tripod support, and must support the rifle without placing your arms on armrests or other supports.

Snow skiing

There are several adaptive devices for both downhill and cross-country skiing.

The sit ski is like a sled, with two tracks on the base of a shell in which you sit, strapped in. There is a roll bar at the back to prevent the ski from bearing down on top of you when you fall and roll over. Sitting close to the ground, you hold small poles or grips with metal disks to plant in the snow when you make a turn, just as you would use a pole on normal skis. The sit ski behaves like skis, responding to turns of your body.

Getting onto a chair lift with a sit ski requires the assistance of two lifters who pick you up and place you on the lift. One lifter rides with you. A buckle is attached to the back of the chair lift during the ride. Getting off the lift is the exciting moment, since you must shimmy forward to the edge and jump off to the ground while the chair is still moving. Operators slow down the lift as you approach, as when you board.

You must be certified to ski unaccompanied on a sit ski. Until you are certified, an instructor will ski with you holding a tether rope attached to the rear of the sit ski. Since it is possible to slide out of control down the hill, someone must be there to take control until you are sufficiently trained and experienced. The art of being a sit ski instructor is to shadow the skier's movements, with no tension on the tether. You don't even feel his presence unless he needs to help you gain control.

Another version of adaptive snow skiing uses a seat on two skis. It requires minimal upper body strength and dexterity to control, and sits close enough to the snow that you don't fall or roll over as you can on a sit ski.

The mono-ski is the peak experience for disabled snow skiers. It is made of a seat set atop a single regulation ski. Since you are sitting higher up, you use outrigger poles that have small skis on the end. It is possible to fall over in a mono-ski, which is why instructors do not need to use a tether. When you fall, you stop. The mono-ski requires greater dexterity and balance since it relies so much more on the use of your upper body for steering and control. The supporting mechanism is hinged or built in an X-shape which allows you to elevate the seat to a level where you can board a chair lift unassisted.

It collapses to its lower setting as soon as you are on the lift, back in ski mode.

> *The mono-ski is really cool, because it is so responsive, and it is much better being able to ski without having to be lifted onto the chair lifts. It's a lot harder to learn, though. I fell over a lot during my first lessons and really trashed my shoulders at first!*

Adaptive cross-country skis rely on the use of poles to propel yourself. A sling seat with a back is mounted on two regulation-sized long skis.

Adaptive skis have also been developed for water skiing.

Swimming

Swimming is a popular and excellent exercise option for many people, almost regardless of how severe the disability. It is a full body exercise with significant cardiovascular benefits. Because you are essentially weightless in water, you are able to move more easily. The natural resistance of the water gives muscles a meaningful, though gentle, form of workout. Even for those able only to float with assistance, it is a relief to be freed of your body weight in the buoyancy of a pool. This paraplegic woman enjoys swimming:

> *I swim three times a week. There's a pool in my building. I really love it. I do the crawl and the backstroke. It's a real sense of freedom to be able to move without the wheelchair. At first I felt self-conscious in public in my bathing suit with my bony butt sticking up in the air. But I got over it. I wear a Speedo, and also biking shorts to cover more of my legs. There are all of these twenty-somethings with perfect bodies, but I just don't care anymore.*

Your local hospital, rehab center, or recreation center might offer special opportunities or programs for disabled swimmers.

Wheelchair basketball

Wheelchair basketball is a team sport played on a regulation basketball court with the net at the normal ten foot height. Two pushes of the chair are allowed before the ball must be dribbled, passed, or shot. You are allowed to push one wheel as you dribble the ball.

There is a "physical advantage" foul. People able to use their legs may not use them to gain an advantage, such as to brake the wheelchair. Since a player can't jump or get up close to the net, those with the ability to shoot from a distance have an advantage. A trick unique to wheelchair basketball involves picking up the ball from the floor. You press it against a wheel as you are moving and let it come up as the wheel turns.

Players are rated according to physical capacity. For example, a single-leg amputee would get a higher rating than a low level quadriplegic with slightly limited hand use. The purpose of the rating system is to even out the competitiveness of the teams. No team may have more than a given number of total points when you add up the ratings of the players on the floor at any time.

Wheelchair basketball is played by many people unable to run well enough for able-bodied play, not only those with paralysis (see Figure 11-5). It is a rough game, in which players often end up on the floor. There is a significant wheelchair basketball league, with competitive play around the country. Many players practice weekly and travel to games. Wheelchair basketball is sometimes seen as exhibition play before professional games.

Wheelchair racing

One of the more well-known examples of wheelchair athletics is marathon racing. The riders train hard for the event, which involves hours of continuous racing. Wheelchair racers are the first out of the gate at major marathons, such as the Boston Marathon. The times of the wheelers are faster than the able-bodied runners.

Racing wheelchairs are extremely lightweight, finely balanced, and use a three-wheel design in which the third wheel extends out ahead of the chair. Many racers sit in a tucked posture, feet under their bodies for optimal leverage. The push rims are small so the chair can be propelled by the upward motion of the arms as well as the normal downward push.

In the late 1990s, a downhill wheelchair appeared. The front casters are very large. You lean forward and grip handles attached to the front wheels, which rotate to steer the chair. Hand brakes are mounted on these handles, using cable brakes similar to those on bicycles. You sit low to the ground. It is a bouncy ride, with speeds as high as thirty miles per hour down a mountain hillside.

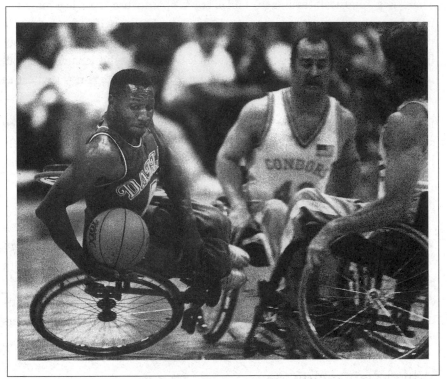

Figure 11-5. Men's wheelchair basketball

Wheelchair tennis

The basic rule of wheelchair tennis is that you get two bounces of the ball on your side of the net before you have to hit it back, as compared to one bounce in the able-bodied version. Some low quadriplegics with sufficient arm strength play tennis by using bandages or cuffs to help grip the racquet.

The art of tennis is to get into the right position, relative to the ball, so that as you swing the racket you get the most power and control. It is quite a surprise to discover you can push the chair in just the right direction and speed to be in position to hit the tennis ball, which is moving quite fast. You typically are in motion while you hit the ball, in contrast to a standing player who tries to plant his feet when taking a shot.

You will need to do a tremendous amount of upper body movement and have sufficient balance in the chair. Although increased seat dump (the downward angle toward the rear) increases your stability, it also sets you lower down. Being lower is a disadvantage in being able to hit the ball accurately into the opposing side of the court. Many players use seat belts for increased stability.

Chair riders must take care to play in a way to avoid tennis elbow, a form of tendinitis. When you hit a tennis ball, there is a considerable shock sent through the arm to the tendons which attach at the elbow. Proper technique and swing—using the body as much as possible rather than using the arm alone—help minimize the impact. New tennis racquet designs reduce vibration sent through the racquet into your arm when you hit the ball. A firm grip is important and reduces the risk of forming blisters on the hands.

Other options

This is by no means a complete description of athletic options for chair riders. Other options include:

- Boxing
- Climbing
- Dancing
- Fencing
- Fishing
- Flying
- Golf
- Hand cycling
- Hang gliding
- Hiking
- Hockey
- Horseback riding
- Hunting
- Kayaking/canoeing
- Lawn bowling
- Motorcycling
- Parachuting
- Ping-Pong

- Racquetball
- Sailing
- Softball
- Trap shooting
- Water skiing
- Weight lifting

Many, if not all, of these sports are represented by an organization which disseminates information, sponsors events, and supports development of adaptive methods and equipment. The most comprehensive ongoing source of information on athletics is *Sports 'N Spokes*, a bimonthly magazine published by the Paralyzed Veterans of America. See the Appendix for more resources.

Out there

The more you get out there, the more you learn. Even unpleasant experiences can point toward a better approach for the next time, so that you can better enjoy your life on wheels.

Resources

Disability-specific organizations

Many of these organizations also have local chapters who might provide such services as support groups and educational or therapeutic programs.

Amputee Coalition of America
900 E. Hill Avenue, Suite 285
Knoxville, TN 37915
(800) 355 8772
http://www.amputee-coalition.org

Amyotrophic Lateral Sclerosis Association
27001 Agoura Road, Suite 150
Calabasas Hills, CA 91301-5104
(800) 782-4747
http://www.alsa.org
email: alsinfo@alsa-national.org

Arthritis Foundation
1330 W. Peachtree Street
Atlanta, GA 30309
(404) 872-7100
http://www.arthritis.org

Brain Injury Association of America
105 N. Alfred Street
Alexandria, VA 22314
(703) 236-6000
http://www.biausa.org

Center for Research on Women with Disabilities
Baylor College of Medicine
3440 Richmond Avenue, Suite B
Houston, TX 77046
(800) 442-7693
http://www.bcm.tmc.edu/crowd

The International Polio Network
4207 Lindell Boulevard, #110
St. Louis, MO 63108-2915
(314) 534-0475
http://www.post-polio.org

The International Ventilator Users Network
4207 Lindell Boulevard, #110
St. Louis, MO 63108-2915
(314) 534-0475

The Muscular Dystrophy Association
3300 E. Sunrise Drive
Tucson, AZ 85718
(800) 572-1717
http://www.mdausa.org
email: mda@mdausa.org

National Brain Injury Association
105 N. Alfred Street
Alexandria, VA 22314
http://www.biausa.org

National Amputation Foundation
12-45 150th Street
Whitestone, NY 11357
(718) 767-0596

National Head Injury Foundation
1776 Massachusetts Ave. N.W., Suite 100
Washington, D.C. 20036
(800) 444-NHIF (6443)

National Family Caregivers Association
9621 E. Bexhill Drive
Kensington, MD 20895-3104
(301) 942-6430

National Multiple Sclerosis Society
733 Third Avenue
New York, NY 10017
(800) FIGHT-MS (344-4867)
http://nmss.org
email: info@nmss.org

National Organization for Rare Disorders
P.O. Box 8923
New Fairfield, CT 06812
(203) 746-6518
http://www.rarediseases.org

The National Spinal Cord Injury Association
545 Concord Avenue, Suite 29
Cambridge, MA 02138
(800) 962-9629

The National Stroke Association
96 Inverness Drive E., Suite I
Englewood, CO 80112-5112
(800) 787-6537
http://www.stroke.org
email: info@stroke.org

Spina Bifida Association of America
4590 MacArthur Blvd. N.W., Suite 250
Washington D.C. 20007
(800) 621-3141
http://www.sbaa.org

TASH-Disability Advocacy Worldwide
29 W. Susquehanna Avenue, Suite 210
Baltimore, MD 21204
(410) 828-8274 x104
http://www.tash.org

Osteogenisis Imperfecta Foundation
5005 W. Laurel Street, Suite 210
Tampa, FL 33607
(813) 282-1161

The Association for Persons with Severe Handicaps
7010 Roosevelt Way N.E.
Seattle, WA 98115
(206) 523-8446

United Cerebral Palsy Association
1660 L Street N.W., Suite 700
Washington, D.C. 20036
(800) 872-5827
http://www.ucpa.org
email: ucpnatl@ucpa.org

Disability advocacy groups

National Organization on Disability
910 16th Street N.W.
Washington, D.C. 20006-2988
(202) 293-5960
http://www.nod.org

Authorized by Congress as an advisory body to the Department of Education, NCD reviews disability-related laws and policies of the federal government. NCD publishes a quarterly newsletter and sponsors studies such as the 1998 Louis Harris Poll on disability.

DREDF
2212 Sixth Street
Berkeley, CA 94710
(800) 466-4232
http://www.dredf.org

A group of attorneys and advocates who pursue legal enforcement and remedies in selected cases.

Not Dead Yet
7521 Madison Street
Forest Park, IL 60130
(708) 209-1500
http://www.acils.com/notdeadyet/

Advocates against the policy of assisted suicide.

World Institute on Disability
510 16th Street, Suite 100
Oakland, CA 94612-1502
(510) 763-4100

A nonprofit research and advocacy group that focuses on major public policy issues. They also conduct a personal assistance program.

Hospitals

Veterans Administration Hospitals
(800) 827-1000
http://www.va.gov

Model system rehabilitation hospitals

The following major rehabilitation hospitals participate in the Model System, which collects data relevant to disability. Being a model hospital does not mean being the best, but most are large centers with many medical services gathered in one place. You should research all rehab hospitals in your area.

CARF, the Rehabilitation Accreditation Commission
4891 E. Grant Road
Tucson, AZ 85712
(520) 325-1044
http://www.carf.org

CARF will refer you to accredited rehab programs in your area.

Boston University Medical Center
88 E. Newton Street, F-511
Boston, MA 02118
(617) 638-7306

Craig Hospital
Rocky Mountain Spinal Injury Center
3425 S. Clarkson Street
Englewood, CO 80110
(303) 789-8220
http://www.craighospital.org

The Institute for Rehabilitation and Research
Texas Medical Center
1333 Moursund Avenue
Houston, TX 77030
(713) 797-5910

Kessler Institute
1199 Pleasant Valley Way
West Orange, NJ 07052
(973) 731-3600

Medical College of Virginia
P.O. Box 980677
Richmond, VA 23298-0677
(804) 828-0861
http://www.views.vcu.edu/html/pmr/sci

MetroHealth Medical Center
Department of Physical Medicine & Rehabilitation
2500 MetroHealth Drive
Cleveland, OH 44109-1998
(216) 778-3483
http://www.metrohealth.org/clinical/norscis

Mt. Sinai Medical Center
Department of Rehabilitation Medicine
1425 Madison Avenue
New York, NY 10029-6574
(212) 241-5417
http://www.mssm.edu/rehab/scrpig.html

Rancho Los Amigos Medical Center
7601 E. Imperial Highway
Downey, CA 90242
(562) 401-7041
http://www.rancho.org

Rehabilitation Institute of Chicago
345 E. Superior
Chicago, IL 60611
(800) 354-REHAB(7342)
http://www.rehabchicago.org

Rehabilitation Institute of Michigan
Wayne State University
261 Mack Boulevard
Detroit, MI 48201
(313) 745-1203

Santa Clara Valley Medical Center
751 S. Bascom Avenue
San Jose, CA 95128
(408) 885-2000

Shepherd Center
2020 Peachtree Road N.W.
Atlanta, GA 30309
(404) 352-2020
http://www.shepherd.org

Spain Rehabilitation Center
University of Alabama
1717 6th Avenue S.
Birmingham, AL 35233-7330
(205) 934-7229
http://www.uab.edu/uasom/medcenter/spain.htm

Thomas Jefferson University Hospital
111 S. 10th Street
Philadelphia, PA 19107
(215) 955-6573

University of Michigan Medical Center
Department of Physical Medicine & Rehabilitation
300 North Ingalls
Ann Arbor, MI 48109-0491
(734) 763-0971
http://www.med.umich.edu/pmr

University of Missouri-Columbia
Department of Physical Medicine & Rehabilitation
One Hospital Drive
Columbia, MO 65212
(573) 882-6271
http://www.hsc.missouri.edu/~momscis

University of Washington School of Medicine
Department of Rehabilitation Medicine
1959 N. E. Pacific Street
Seattle, WA 98195
(206) 543-8171
http://weber.u.washington.edu/~rehab

Personal assistance services

Center on Human Policy
Syracuse University
200 Huntington Hall
Syracuse, NY 13244-2340

Request the information packet: *A Checklist for Evaluating Personal Care Assistance Services.*

The Independent Living Service Center
607 S. E. Everett Mall Way, Suite 9B
Everett, WA 98208
(425) 347-5768
http://www.wa-ilsc.org

Provides a manual of information for finding and employing personal care assistants.

RRTC on Aging with SCI
3425 S. Clarkson Street
Englewood, CO 80110

Request the publication: *SCI & Personal Care Assistants: How to Find, Hire, and Keep Them.*

Functional electrical stimulation (FES)

FES Information Center
11000 Cedar Avenue, Room 230
Cleveland, OH 44106-3052
(800) 666-2353
http://feswww.fes.cwru.edu

Clearinghouse of information on functional electric stimulation.

NeuroControl Corporation
8333 Rockside Road
Valley View, OH 44125
(800) 378-6955
http://www.neurocontrol.com

Makers of FES products for hand grip and bladder control.

Sigmedics, Inc.
200 Larkin Drive, Suite F
Wheeling, IL 60090-6498
(800) 582-WALK(9255)
http://www-personal.umich.edu/~jtargows/mainmenu.html
email: fzeiss@ameritech.net

Makers of Parastep, FNS walking system. The URL is for the Parastep users' web site.

Service Animals

Assistance Dogs of America
1178 Slade Avenue
Columbus, OH 43235
(614) 459-9115

Canine Companions for Independence
P.O. Box 446
Santa Rosa, CA 95402-0446
(707) 577-1700
http://www.caninecompanions.org

Freedom Service Dogs
P.O. Box 150217
Lakewood, CO 80215-0217
(303) 234-9512

Wheelchairs and cushions

Colours
1591 S. Sinclair Street
Anaheim, CA 92806
(800) 892-8998
http://www.coloursbypermobil.com

Manual lightweight wheelchairs, including the Boing rear suspension chair, and sport models for racing, rugby, and more.

Crown Therapeutics/Roho
100 Florida Avenue
Belleville, IL 62221
(800) 851-3449
http://www.rohoinc.com

Air flotation cushions. The Quadtro allows individual inflation of four quadrants.

ErgoAir
131 D.W. Highway, #326
Nashua, NH 03060-5245
(800) 559-9856
http://www.ergoair.com
email: ergoair@empire.net

Alternating-pressure wheelchair cushions.

Everest & Jennings
3601 Rider Trail S.
Earth City, MO 63045
(800) 235-4661, (800) 708-9601

A full line of manual and power wheelchairs, tilt and recline systems, and cushions.

Flofit Medical
5455 Spine Road
Boulder, CO 80301
(800) 356-2668
http://www.flofitmed.com
email: flofit@flofitmed.com

Foam and foam/gel wheelchair cushions.

Grant Airmass
986 Bedford Street
Stamford, CT 06905
(800) 243-5237
http://www.grantairmass.com
email: grant@grantairmass.com

Alternating-pressure cushions.

Invacare Corporation/PinDot
899 Cleveland Street
Elyria, OH 44036
(800) 333-6900
http://www.invacare.com

Manual and power wheelchairs, cushions, and positioning systems.

Iron Horse Productions
2624 Conner Street
Port Huron, MI 48060
(800) 426-0354

High-endurance, four-wheel suspension manual wheelchairs.

New Hall's Wheels
P.O. Box 380784
Cambridge, MA 02238
(617) 628-6546
http://www.tiac.net/users/newhalls

Customized lightweight manual and sport chairs.

Otto Bock Reha
3000 Xenium Lane North
Minneapolis, MN 55441-2661
(800) 328-4058
http://www.ottobock.com
email: ottobockus@aol.com

Manual wheelchairs, cushions.

Permobil
6B Gil Street
Woburn, MA 01801
(888) 737-6624
http://www.permobil.se

Power/standing wheelchairs.

Quickie Designs/Sunrise Medical/Jay Medical
2842 Business Park Avenue
Fresno, CA 93727
(209) 292-2171
http://www.sunrisemedical.com

Manual and power wheelchairs, sport chairs, Jay cushions, Soneil SuperCharger battery chargers.

Supracor
2050 Corporate Court
San Jose, CA 95131-1753
(800) 787-7226
http://www.supracor.com

Honeycomb-type cushions.

Teftec
6929 Old Spring Branch Road
Spring Branch, TX 78070
(830) 885-7588
http://www.teftec.com
email: teftec@teftec.com

All-terrain power wheelchairs.

Wheelchairs of Kansas
204 West 2nd Street
Ellis, KS 67637
(800) 537-6454
email: whcharks@pld.com

Power chairs for obese users.

Home access

AARP
Product Report: Personal Emergency Response Systems
601 E Street N.W.
Washington, D.C. 20049

Publication #PF 3986592-D1290.

Advanced Living Systems
Product Search Services
428 North Lamar
Oxford, MS 38655-3204
(601) 234-0158

Has a database of products. Provides information for a small fee.

Altro Safety Floors
399 Main Street
Los Altos, CA 94022
(605) 941-1961

Non-slip flooring products.

Architectural and Transportation Barriers Compliance Board
1331 F Street N.W.
Washington, D.C. 20004
(800) 872-2253

Provides copies of architectural access standards and information about federal compliance requirements.

AT&T Special Needs Center
2001 Route 46, Suite 310
Parsippany, NJ 07054-1315
(800) 233-1222
TDD (800) 833-3232

Information on assistive communication devices.

The Center for Universal Design
School of Design, North Carolina State University
P.O. Box 8613
Raleigh, NC 27695-8613
(919) 515-3082
http://www.design.ncsu.edu/cud
email: cud@ncsu.edu

Has a variety of publications, videos, presentation materials, and product evaluation guides for door hardware, ovens, and other appliances.

Dor-O-Matic
7350 W. Wilson Avenue
Chicago, IL 60656-4786
(800) 543-4635

Automatic door systems with delayed action.

Enerlogic Systems
P.O. Box 3743
Nashua, NH 03061
(603) 880-4066

Home automations system. Uses a home computer and existing wiring.

Essex Electronics, Inc.
1130 Mark Avenue
Carpinteria, CA 93013
(805) 684-7601

Electronic touchpad keyless entry systems.

Grand Traverse Technologies
8130 Lehigh Avenue
Morton Grove, IL 60053
(800) 323-1245

Maker of the Freedom Bath, a tub with a side door that slides down.

Guardian Products/Sunrise Medical
12800 Wentworth Street, Box C-4522
Arleta, CA 91331
(800) 423-8034

Bath lifts, grab bars, and bathing accessories.

Hafele America Co.
3901 Cheyenne Drive
P.O. Box 4000
Archdale, NC 27263
(800) 423-3531

Closet organizing systems and accessories.

L.E. Johnson Products
2100 Sterling Avenue
Elkhart, IN 46516
(800) 837-5664
http://www.johnsonhardware.com

Pocket door kits and hardware.

Paralyzed Veterans of America
National Architecture Program
801 18th Street, N.W.
Washington, D.C. 20006
(202) 416-7645

ProMatura Group
Product Search Services
142 Highway 30
Oxford, MS 38655
(800) 201-1483
http://www.promatura.com

Has a database of products. Provides information for a small fee.

The Ramp Project
Metropolitan Center for Independent Living
1600 University Avenue W., Suite 16
St. Paul, MN 55104
(612) 646-8342
http://www.macil.org/mcil

Ultraflo
P.O. Box 2294
Sandusky, OH 44870
(800) 760-5629
http://www.ultraflo.com

Scald control water distribution system.

U.S. Department of Housing and Urban Development
Office of Fair Housing and Equal Opportunity
451 Seventh Street S.W.
Washington, D.C. 20410
(202) 708-2878

Fair housing accessibility guidelines, Federal Register document Vol. 56, No. 44. March 1991.

X-10 USA, Inc.
P.O. Box 420
Closter, NJ 07624
(800) 442-5138
http://www.x10.com

Carrier current remote control systems.

Sexuality

Able-Together
P.O. Box 460053
San Francisco, CA 94146-0053
(415) 522-9091
http://www.well.com/user/blaine/abletog.html

Information and support specific to gay, lesbian, and bisexual persons with disabilities.

CLEO Living Aids
P.O. Box 1076
White Plains, NY 10602
(800) 321-0595

Adaptive devices for use with sexual products.

PeopleNet
P.O. Box 897
Levittown, NY 11756
(516) 579-4043
http://idt.net/~mauro/

Sexual resources, writings on sexuality and disability, and a meeting service.

Sexuality Reborn: A Video about Sexuality and SCI
Kessler Medical Rehabilitation and Research
1199 Pleasant Valley Way
West Orange, NJ 07052
(800) 248-3221 x6977

Offers a videotape hosted by actor Ben Vereen with interviews of couples with at least one disabled partner.

The Xandria Collection
Special Edition for Disabled People
P.O. Box 31039
San Francisco, CA 94131
(800) 242-2823

Catalog of sexual aids and products.

Parenting resources

Through the Looking Glass
2198 Sixth Street, Suite 100
Berkeley, CA 94710-2204
(800) 644-2666
http://www.lookingglass.org
email: tlg@lookingglass.org

DisAbled Women's Network
From Ontario, Canada: (800) 561-4727
Outside Ontario: (705) 671-0825

Offers the publication, "I want to be a mother. I have a disability: What are my choices?"

Research support organizations

American Paralysis Association
500 Morris Avenue
Springfield, NJ 07081
(201) 379-2690
http://www.apacure.com

The Buoniconti Fund to Cure Paralysis
The Miami Project to Cure Paralysis
1600 N.W. 10th Avenue, R-48
Miami, FL 33136
(305) 243-6001
http://www.miamiproject.miami.edu

Canadian Spinal Research Organization
120 Newkirk Road
Richmond Hill, Ontario, Canada L4C 9S7
(800) 361-4004
http://www.csro.com
email: csro@globalserve.net

The Kent Waldrep National Paralysis Foundation
16415 Addison Road, Suite 550
Addison, TX 75001
(800) 925-2873
http://www.kwnpf.org

People for the Ethical Treatment of Animals (PETA)
501 Front Street
Norfolk, VA 23510
(757) 622-7382
http://www.peta.org

Included here to assist you in addressing the question of the use of animals in research.

PVA Spinal Cord Research Foundation
801 18th Street N.W.
Washington, D.C. 20006
(800) 424-8200 x659
http://www.pva.org

Spinal Cord Society
Wendell Road
Fergus Falls, MN 56537
(218) 739-5252

Adaptive technology

Don Johnston Incorporated
1000 N. Rand Road, Bldg. 115
P.O. Box 639
Wauconda, IL 60084-0639
(800) 999-4660
http://www.donjohnston.com

Software for word prediction, speech synthesis, adaptive keyboards and accessories, educational software.

Dragon Systems
320 Nevada Street
Newton, MA 02460
(800) 437-2466
http://www.dragonsys.com

Voice recognition software.

DynaVox Systems, Inc.
2100 Wharton Street, Suite 400
Pittsburgh, PA 15203
(800) 344-1778
http://www.dynavoxsys.com

Augmentive communication products.

Closing the Gap
P.O. Box 68
Henderson, MN 56044
(507) 248-3294
http://www.closingthegap.com

Bimonthly newsletter, $26 per year.

IBM Independence Series
P.O. Box 1328
Boca Raton, FL 33429-1328
(800) 426-4832
http://www.austin.ibm.com/sns/

Neil Squire Foundation
2250 Boundary Road, Suite 220
Burnaby, British Columbia, Canada V5M 4G5
(604) 473-9363
http://www.neilsquire.ca

Adaptive technology programs, including research and development, consultation, and support for employment using computing.

Trace Research and Development Center
University of Wisconsin-Madison
5901 Research Park Boulevard
Madison, WI 53719-1252
(608) 262-6966
http://www.trace.wisc.edu

Athletics and recreation

American Wheelchair Bowling Association
6264 N. Andrews Avenue
Ft. Lauderdale, FL 33309
(954) 491-2886

Disabled Sports USA
451 Hungerford Drive, Suite 100
Rockville, MD 20850
(301) 217-0960
http://www.dsusa.org/~dsusa/dsusa.html

Handicapped Scuba Association
1104 El Prado
San Clemente, CA 92672-4637
(949) 498-6128

National Wheelchair Basketball Association
Charlotte Institute of Rehabilitation
1100 Blythe Boulevard
Charlotte, NC 28203
(704) 355-1064

National Wheelchair Poolplayers Association
30872 Puritan Street
Livonia, MI 48154-3253
(734) 422-2124
http://www.concentric.net/~nwpa

North American Riding for the Handicapped Association
P.O. Box 33150
Denver, CO 80233
(800) 369-7433
http://www.narha.org

Paralyzed Veterans of America
2111 E. Highland Avenue, Suite 180
Phoenix, AZ 85016-4702
(602) 224-0500
http://www.pva.org

United Cerebral Palsy Athletic Association, Inc.
200 Harrison Avenue
Newport, RI 02840
(401) 848-2460
http://www.uscpaa.org

United States Quad Rugby Association
5861 White Cypress Drive
Lake Worth, FL 33467-6230
(561) 964-1712
http://www.quadrugby.com

Wheelchair Sports USA
3595 Fountain Boulevard, Suite L-1
Colorado Springs, CO 80910
(719) 574-1150
http://www.wsusa.org

Wilderness Inquiry, Inc.
131 Fifth Street, Box 84
Minneapolis, MN 55414-1546
(800) 728-0719
http://www.wildernessinquiry.org

Employment

AgrAbility Project
Breaking New Ground Resource Center
Purdue University
1146 ABE Building
West Lafayette, IN 47907-1146
(800) 825-4264
http://abe.www.ecn.purdue.edu/ABE/Extension/BNG/agrabilityproject

The AgrAbility Project assists agricultural and agribusiness workers who have physical and mental disabilities through education and assistance. Their web site includes links to rural assistive technology information.

Electronic Industries Foundation
2500 Wilson Boulevard
Arlington, VA 22201
(703) 907-7400

Has a program to promote technology training for persons with disability.

Job Accommodation Network
918 Chestnut Ridge Road
P.O. Box 6080
Morgantown, WV 26506-6080
(800) 526-7234
http://www.jan.wvu.edu

The President's Committee on Employment of People with Disabilities
1331 F Street, N.W.
Washington, D.C. 20004-1107
(202) 376-6200
http://www.pcepd.gov

U.S. Small Business Administration
1441 L Street N.W., Room 418
Washington, D.C. 20416
http://www.sbaonline.sba.gov

Loan guarantees under their Handicapped Assistance Loan program. Contact their local office, or see the web site for local resources.

Travel

Access-Able Travel Source, LLC
P.O. Box 1796
Wheat Ridge, CO 80034
(303) 232-2979
http://www.access-able.com

Accessible Vans of America
4 Beryl Road
Paoli, PA 19301
(800) AVA-VANS(282-8267)
http://www.accessiblevans.com

Associated Rollx Vans
6591 W. Highway 13
Savage, MN 55378
(800) 956-6668
http://www.rollxvans.com

Hostelling International—American Youth Hostels
733 15th Street N.W., Suite 840
Washington, D.C. 20005
(202) 783-6161
http://www.hiayh.org

Wheelchair Getaways
(800) 536-5518
http://www.wheelchair-getaways.com

Converted vans available for rental.

Recommended reading

Beyond Ramps: Disability at the End of the Social Contract, by Marta Russell, Common Courage Press.

Cripzen: A Manual for Survival, by Lorenzo W. Milam, Mho & Mho Works. Written with humor and realism, CripZen is a survival text for anyone facing a new world of rehabilitation specialists, nurses, and frightened family members. Milam discusses sex, coping with depression and anger, finding psychological help, and using such spiritual means of survival as meditation.

Don't Worry, He Won't Get Far on Foot, by John F. Callahan, Vintage Books.

Enabling Romance: A Guide to Love, Sex, and Relationships for the Disabled, by Ken Kroll and Erica Levy Klein, Woodbine House.

FDR's Splendid Deception, by Hugh Gregory Gallagher, Vandamere Press.

Fodor's Great American Vacations for Travelers with Disabilities, Fodors Travel Publications.

Living in the State of Stuck: How Technology Impacts the Lives of Persons with Disabilities, by Marcia J. Scherer, Brookline Books.

Moving Violations: War Zones, Wheelchairs, and Declarations of Independence, by John Hockenberry, Hyperion.

No Pity: People with Disabilities Forging a New Civil Rights Movement, by Joseph P. Shapiro, Times Books.

Nothing About Us Without Us: Disability Oppression and Empowerment, by James I. Charlton, University of California Press.

Spinal Network: The Total Wheelchair Book, by Sam Maddox, Spinal Network.

Staring Back: The Disability Experience from the Inside Out, by Kenny Fries (Editor), Plume.

Understanding and Accommodating Physical Disabilities: The Manager's Desk Reference, by Dorothy Stonely Shrout, Quorum Books.

Waist-High in the World: A Life Among the Nondisabled, by Nancy Mairs, Beacon Press.

Women and Disability: The Experience of Physical Disability Among Women, by Susan Lonsdale, St. Martins Press.

Disability publications

Accent On Living
Gillum Road and High Drive
P.O. Box 700
Bloomington, IL 61702
(309) 378-2961
email: acntlvng@aol.com

Enable Magazine
American Association of People with Disabilities
3659 Cortez Road W.
Bradenton, FL 34210
(888) 4-ENABLE (436-2253)
email: readenable@aol.com

Mouth Magazine
61 Brighton Street
Rochester, NY 14607-2656
(716) 442-2916

New Mobility
23815 Stuart Ranch Road
P.O. Box 8987
Malibu, CA 90265
(310) 317-4522
http://www.newmobility.com

Paraplegia News
Published by the Paralyzed Veterans of America
2111 E. Highland Avenue, Suite 180
Phoenix, AZ 85016-4702
(602) 224-0500
email: pvapub@aol.com

The Ragged Edge
P.O. Box 145
Louisville, KY 40201
http://www.ragged-edge-mag.com

Sports 'N Spokes
2111 E. Highland Avenue, Suite 180
Phoenix, AZ 85016-4702
(602) 224-0500
email: pvapub@aol.com

Internet web sites

The following World Wide Web sites have extensive information and links to other sites and sources. Through this list, you should be able to find just about any disability resource you might want.

ABLEDATA
http://www.abledata.com

A large database of disability resources operated by The National Institute on Disability and Rehabilitation Research, U.S. Department of Education.

Amputee Coalition of America
National Limb Loss Information Center
http://www.amputee-coalition.org

disABILITY Information and Resources
http://www.eskimo.com/~jlubin/disabled/all.htm

A huge list of disability-related web sites.

Disability Resources from Evan Kemp Associates
http://www.eka.com

The late Evan Kemp was an attorney and principal figure in the development of the Americans with Disabilities Act (ADA).

Independent Living Research Utilization Program
http://www.bcm.tmc.edu/ilru

Gathers material from Independent Living Centers around the country. They are an information clearinghouse for ILCs, conduct conferences on ILC management, and offer various books, posters, and brochures.

National Rehabilitation Information Center
http://www.cais.net/naric

For twenty years, the staff of NARIC has collected the results of federally funded research projects. NARIC's literature collection, which includes commercially published books, journal articles, and audiovisuals, numbers more than 60,000.

rehabNET—Resource on Disability and Medical Rehabilitation
http://www.rehabnet.com

Sexual Health Network
http://www.sexualhealth.com

The Society for Disability Studies
http://www.wipd.com/sds

Publishes academic studies in the *Disability Studies Quarterly.*

Spinal Cord Injury, Stroke, and Paralysis Resources Guide
http://neurosurgery.mgh.harvard.edu/paral-r.htm

University of Alabama at Birmingham
http://www.spinalcord.uab.edu

UAB is the collector of data from the Model System rehab hospitals. They maintain a comprehensive web site with links to a very wide array of other disability-related sites. It is easily navigated by means of an alphabetized index.

Internet discussion lists

An email address is all it takes to participate in online discussions. Once you have subscribed, all messages in the discussion will be sent to you. You can choose to participate or be a "lurker." Generally, these lists are dedicated to a specific topic, and you should respect the boundaries of the discussion. You will find people very willing and happy to help you address specific needs and questions.

The process of subscription is easy. You simply send a message to a server address, then you will get a response saying that you have been added to the list, or asking you to reply with a confirmation. You will also be sent guidelines and options for the list. It is often possible, for instance, to receive the day's discussion as a single file, rather than having your mailbox fill with each individual message.

List archives at Maelstrom.StJohns.edu
http://maelstrom.stjohns.edu/archives/index.html

This web site provides an index of the many discussion lists hosted by St. John's University. To subscribe to a discussion at St. John's, send email to *listserv@sjuvm.stjohns.edu*, and include the message "subscribe listname." For instance, for the cerebral palsy discussion group, the message should read, "subscribe c-palsy" (without punctuation). The following are a selection of St. John's disability groups:

ADVOCACY: Advocacy for people with disabilities
C-PALSY: Cerebral Palsy
D-SPORT: Sports for persons with disabilities
DIS-SPRT: Disability support for families
MOBILITY: General disabilities discussion
PCA: Personal care assistance
POLIO: Polio and post-polio syndrome
POST-POLIO MED: Q&A about post-polio syndrome
TBI-SPRT: Traumatic brain injury support group

Some other subscriber lists related to disability:

ADA Discussion Group

Send the message "subscribe ada-law" to *ada-law@listserv.nodak.edu*.

HandiRide—A discussion of mobility and transportation issues

Send the message "subscribe handiride-l firstname lastname" to *handiride-lrequest@handinet.org*.

Muscular Dystrophy Discussion Group

Send the message "subscribe" to *md-list-request@basix.com*.

The Parents Chat List—Discussion of parenting with disability

Send the message "subscribe parents chat" to *maiser@hoffman.mgen.pitt.edu*.

Ventilator Users List

Send the message "subscribe" to *vent-users-request@eskimo.com*.

Notes

Chapter 1: *The Disabilities*

1. Cliff Thompson, "Jimmie Heuga: Still Ahead of the Curve," *New Mobility* 8, no. 40 (1997): 49.

2. George H. Kraft, M.D., and Marci Catanzaro, R.N., Ph.D, *Living with Multiple Sclerosis: A Wellness Approach* (New York: Demos Vermande, 1996).

3. S. J. Creange and R. L. Bruno, "Compliance with Treatment for Post-Polio Sequelae: Effect of Type A Behavior, Self-Concept, and Loneliness," *American Journal of Physical Medicine and Rehabilitation* 76 (1997): 378-82.

4. "Vegetarian Diets for Patients with Rheumatoid Arthritis," *American Journal of Natural Medicine* 3, no. 7 (September 1996): 20.

Chapter 2: *Rehabilitation*

1. R. DiFabio, Ph.D., P.T., et al., "Extended Outpatient Rehabilitation: Its Influence on Symptom Frequency, Fatigue, and Functional Status for Persons with Progressive MS," *Archives of Physical Medicine and Rehabilitation* 79, no. 2: 141.

2. Suzanne Nyre and Virginia McKay, "Preadmission Screening and Secondary Transport," in *The Management of High Quadriplegia*, edited by Gale Whiteneck, Ph.D., et al. (New York: Demos Vermande, 1989), 118.

3. Nyre, "Preadmission Screening," 118.

4. "Overview of Spinal Cord Injury Rehabilitation in the Acute Phase, the Rehabilitation Team, and Classification of Spinal Cord Lesion," in *Spinal Cord Injury: Medical Management and Rehabilitation,* edited by Gary M. Yarkony, Rehabilitation Institute of Chicago publication (Gaithersburg, Maryland: Aspen Publishers, 1994), 3.

5. Reynolds Price, *A Whole New Life* (New York: Plume/Penguin Books USA, 1994), 101-2.

6. John Hockenberry, *Moving Violations* (New York: Hyperion, 1995).

7. Jeri Morris, Ph.D., "Spinal Injury and Psychotherapy," in *Spinal Cord Injury: Medical Management and Rehabilitation*, 225.

8. Joan Anderson, "Psychological Issues Related to Ventilator-Dependent Quadriplegia," in *The Management of High Quadriplegia*, 97.

9. Anderson, "Psychological Issues Related to Ventilator-Dependent Quadriplegia," 98

10. Ellen Winchell, Ph.D., *Coping with Limb Loss* (Garden City Park, New York: Avery Publishing Group, 1995), 225-26.

11. Ian Fisher, "Families Struggle to Care for Loved Ones," *New York Times/San Francisco Examiner*, 7 June 1998.

Chapter 3: *Medical Concerns*

1. Peter Risher and Stacey Amorosi, project directors, *The 1998 N.O.D./Harris Survey of Americans with Disabilities*, conducted for The National Organization on Disability (New York: Louis Harris, 1998).

2. Nancy Keene, *Working with Your Doctor: Getting the Healthcare You Deserve* (Cambridge, Massachusetts: O'Reilly & Associates, 1998).

3. *Prevention of Thromboembolism in Spinal Cord Injury, http://www.pva.org/.*

4. *Prevention of Thromboembolism.*

5. The International Association for the Study of Pain, *http://www. halcyon.com/iasp/terms-p.html#Pain.*

6. Elliot J. Roth, M.D., "Pain Management Strategies," in *Spinal Cord Injury: Medical Management and Rehabilitation*, 145.

7. Roth, "Pain Management Strategies," 159.

8. Roth, "Pain Management Strategies," 159.

9. Roth, "Pain Management Strategies," 151.

10. Roth, "Pain Management Strategies," 153.

11. Roth, "Pain Management Strategies," 159.

12. Roth, "Pain Management Strategies," 159.

13. Roth, "Pain Management Strategies," 163.

14. Roth, "Pain Management Strategies," 163.

Chapter 4: *Staying Healthy*

1. S. Kirshblum, M.D., et al., "Bowel Care Practices in Chronic Spinal Cord Injury Patients," *Archives of Physical Medicine and Rehabilitation* 79, no. 1: 20.

2. Kirshblum, "Bowel Care Practices," 20.

3. *Homeopathy web page: http://www.dimensional.com/~stevew/.*

4. G. Whiteneck and R. R. Menter, "Where do we go from here?" in *Aging with Spinal Cord Injury* (New York: Demos Vermande, 1993).

5. R. R. Menter, M.D., et al. "Impairment, Disability, Handicap, and Medical Expenses of Persons Aging with Spinal Cord Injury," *Paraplegia* 29 (1991): 613-19.

6. Annual Report for the Model Spinal Cord Injury Care Systems, National Spinal Cord Injury Statistical Center, University of Alabama at Birmingham, October 1995.

7. K. A. Gerhart, et al., "Long-term Spinal Cord Injury: Functional Changes Over Time," *Archives of Physical Medicine and Rehabilitation* 74 (1993): 1030-34.

8. R. R. Menter, M.D., "Spinal Cord Injury and Aging: Exploring the Unknown," 1993 Heiner Sell Lecture of the ASIA, May 10, 1993, San Diego, California, published in the *Journal of the American Paraplegia Society* 16, no. 4: 179-89.

9. University of Alabama web site: *http://www.spinalcord.uab.edu.*

10. Miriam Braunstein, "Homeward Bound—And Wishing They Weren't," *New Mobility,* September 1997: 32-37.

11. *http://csn.net/rehab/mets/pca.htm.*

Chapter 5: *The Experience of Disability*

1. Irving Kenneth Zola, *Missing Pieces: A Chronicle of Living with a Disability* (Philadelphia: Temple University Press, 1982), 206.

2. Zola, *Missing Pieces,* 219.

3. Zola, *Missing Pieces,* 214.

4. Jen Morris, Ph.D., "Spinal Injury and Psychotherapy," 223-29.

5. Martha Ferguson Gregory, *Sexual Adjustment: A Guide for Spinal Cord Injured* (Bloomington, Illinois: Cheever Publishing, 1974), 20.

6. Zola, *Missing Pieces,* 230.

7. Joseph P. Shapiro, *No Pity: People with Disabilities Forging a New Civil Rights Movement* (New York: Times Books/Random House, 1994), 288.

8. Pema Chödrön, *When Things Fall Apart: Heart Advice for Difficult Times* (Boston/London: Shambhala, 1997), 13.

9. Price, *A Whole New Life,* 55.

10. Zola, *Missing Pieces,* 210.

11. Joan Anderson, "Psychological Issues Related to Ventilator-Dependent Quadriplegia," 107.

12. Zola, *Missing Pieces,* 226.

13. Zola, *Missing Pieces,* 209.

14. Risher, *The 1998 N.O.D./Harris Survey of Americans with Disabilities.*

15. Zola, *Missing Pieces,* 200.

16. Zola, *Missing Pieces,* 235.

Chapter 7: *Home Access*

1. Margaret Wylde, Adrian Baron-Robbins, and Sam Clark, *Building for a Lifetime: The Design and Construction of Fully Accessible Homes* (Newtown, Connecticut: Taunton Press, 1994), 268.

2. Wylde, *Building for a Lifetime,* 167.

Chapter 8: *Intimacy, Sex, and Babies*

1. Margaret A. Nosek, et al., *National Study of Women with Physical Disabilities, Final Report*; Baylor College of Medicine, Center for Research on Women with Physical Disabilities, Department of Physical Medicine and Rehabilitation, Houston, Texas (1997), 3.

2. Marca L. Sipski, M.D., and Craig J. Alexander, Ph.D., "Sexual Activities, Response and Satisfaction in Women Pre- and Post-Spinal Cord Injury," *Archives of Physical Medicine and Rehabilitation* 74 (October 1993).

3. Mitch Tepper, "Love Bites," *New Mobility,* June 1996: 22.

4. Glorya Hale, editor., *The Sourcebook for the Disabled* (New York: Paddington Press, 1979).

5. D. H. Rintala, et al., "Dating issues for women with physical disabilities," *Sexuality and Disability* 15, no. 4 (1997): 219-42.

6. J. Money, "Sexual Problems of the Chronically Ill" in *Sexual Problems: Diagnosis and Treatment in Medical Practice,* edited by C. W. Wahl (New York: The Free Press, 1967).

7. Ken Kroll and Erica Levy Klein, *Enabling Romance, A Guide to Love, Sex, and Relationships for the Disabled* (Woodbine House, 1995), 17.

8. Rintala, "Dating issues for women with physical disabilities," 219-42.

9. Kroll, *Enabling Romance,* 43.

10. A. Frankel, "Sexual Problems in Rehabilitation," *Journal of Rehabilitation* 33, no. 5 (1967): 19-20.

11. *Sexuality Reborn* (video), produced for the Kessler Institute by Marca L. Sipski, M.D., and Craig J. Alexander, Ph.D.

12. Craig J. Alexander, Ph.D., Marca L. Sipski, M.D., and Thomas W. Findley, M.D., Ph.D., "Sexual Activities, Desire, and Satisfaction in Males Pre- and Post-Spinal Cord Injury," *Archives of Sexual Behavior* 22, no. 3 (1993).

13. Rintala, "Dating issues for women with physical disabilities," 219-42.

14. Rintala, "Dating issues for women with physical disabilities," 219-42.

15. *Sexuality Reborn.*

16. Rintala, "Dating issues for women with physical disabilities," 219-42.

17. Kroll, *Enabling Romance,* 28.

18. Helen E. Fisher, Ph.D., *The Anatomy of Love: A Natural History of Mating, Marriage, and Why We Stray* (New York: Fawcett Books, 1995), 26.

19. *Sexuality & Body Image* (video), University of Minnesota.

20. *Sexuality Reborn.*

21. Kevin Robinson, "Caregiver and Spouse: Should the Twain Ever Meet?" *New Mobility,* February 1998: 12.

22. Kroll, *Enabling Romance,* 64.

23. Roberta Travis, "Making Love Like a Woman," *New Mobility,* February 1997: 39.

24. Tepper, "Love Bites," 22.

25. Marca L. Sipski, M.D., Craig J. Alexander, Ph.D., and Raymond C. Rosen, Ph.D., "Orgasm in Women with Spinal Cord Injuries: A Laboratory-Based Assessment," *Archives of Physical Medicine and Rehabilitation* 76 (December 1995): 1097-1102.

26. Tepper, "Love Bites," 22.

27. Rintala, "Dating issues for women with physical disabilities," 219-42.

28. Rintala, "Dating issues for women with physical disabilities," 219-42.

29. Linda Toms-Barker and Vida Maralani, *Challenges and Strategies of Disabled Parents—Findings from a National Survey of Parents with Disabilities*, (Berkeley, California: Berkeley Planning Associates, July 1997).

30. Sam Maddox, *Spinal Network*, (Malibu, California: Miramar Publications, 1994), 354.

31. Nancy L. Brackett, et al., "Endocrine Profiles and Semen Quality of Spinal Cord Injured Men," *The Journal of Urology* 151 (1994): 117.

32. Nancy L. Brackett, M. S. Nash, and C. M. Lynne, "Male Fertility Following Spinal Cord Injury: Facts and Fiction." *Physical Therapy* 76, no. 11 (1996): 1226.

33. Brackett, "Male Fertility Following Spinal Cord Injury," 1225-6.

34. Brackett, "Male Fertility Following Spinal Cord Injury," 1228.

35. Nancy L. Brackett, R. P. Padron, and C. M. Lynne, "Semen Quality of Spinal Cord Injured Men Is Better When Obtained by Vibratory Stimulation Versus Electroejaculation," *The Journal of Urology* 157 (1997): 152-6.

36. Osvaldo F. Padron, et al., "Semen of Spinal Cord Injured Men Freezes Reliably," *Journal of Andrology* 15, no. 13 (1994): 268.

Chapter 9: *Spinal Cord Research*

1. *Mouth, Voice of the Disability Nation,* July/August 1997: 42.

2. *The Project, News from The Miami Project to Cure Paralysis* 11, no. 1 (Spring 1998): 6.

3. Sam Maddox, *The Quest for Cure: Restoring Function After Spinal Cord Injury* (Paralyzed Veterans of America, 1993), 95-96.

4. Gianluca Gallo, Frances B. Lefcort, and Paul C. Letourneau, "The trkA Receptor Mediates Growth Cone Turning Toward a Localized Source of Nerve Growth Factor," *Journal of Neuroscience* 17, no. 14 (15 July 1997): 5445-54.

5. N. Kleitman and R. P. Bunge, "The Schwann Cell: Morphology and Development," in *The Axon*, S. G. Waxman, J. Kocsis, and P. Stys, editors (New York: Rockefeller University Press, 1995), 97-115.

6. X. M. Xu, et al, "A Combination of BDNF and NT-3 Promotes Supraspinal Axonal Regeneration into Schwann Cell Grafts in Adult Rat Thoracic Spinal Cord," *Experimental Neurology* 134: 261-272.

7. Univ. of Florida Brain Institute: *http://www.ufbi.ufl.edu/dept/meeting.html.*

8. Maddox, *The Quest for Cure*, 37.

9. Sygen (GM-1) Use in Spinal Cord Injury: *http://www.chicinn.com/gm1stud2.htm.*

10. From the author's notes, taken at Dr. Geisler's speech.

11. *The Project, News from the Miami Project to Cure Paralysis* 10, no. 3 (Winter 1997): 7.

12. Andrew Blight, Ph.D., "Development of 4-AP for Chronic Spinal Cord Injury," *CSRO Quarterly* 8, no. 2 (Summer 1997). Canadian Spinal Research Organization web site at *http://www.csro.com*.

13. Edward Chaplin, M.D., "Functional Neuromuscular Stimulation for Mobility in People with Spinal Cord Injuries: The Parastep I System," *The Journal of Spinal Cord Medicine* 19, no 2: 99-105.

14. *Sensitive but Sensible: The Absolute Importance of Animal Research for Neurologic Disease*, American Academy of Neurology.

Chapter 10: *Politics and Legislation*

1. Shapiro, *No Pity*, 65.

2. *504 Celebration & Commemoration*, 1997, 42.

3. Shapiro, *No Pity*, 71.

4. "Gina Says," *Mouth Magazine*, February/March 1997: 17.

5. Risher, *The 1998 N.O.D./Harris Survey of Americans with Disabilities*.

6. Shapiro, *No Pity*, 165-6.

7. Risher, *The 1998 N.O.D./Harris Survey of Americans with Disabilities*.

8. Risher, *The 1998 N.O.D./Harris Survey of Americans with Disabilities*.

9. Laura Hershey, "PASS Hits a Wall: But Advocates Are Chipping Away at Work Disincentives," *New Mobility*, April 1998: 31.

10. Braunstein, "Homeward Bound," 32-37.

11. Braunstein, "Homeward Bound," 32-37.

12. Kevin J. Mahoney and Lori Simon-Rusinowitz, "Cash and Counseling Demonstration and Evaluation," *Journal of Case Management* 6, no.1 (1997): 26.

13. Georgea Kovanis, "They Wanted Control of Life: Kevorkian enables people to take final command," *Detroit Free Press*, 5 March 1997.

14. 90-390963-AZ. The People of the State of Michigan *ex rel* Richard Thompson, prosecuting, attorney in and for the County of Oakland, Plaintiff, vs. Jack Kevorkian, Defendant. In a written statement to the court filed August 17, 1991, p. 11.

15. Risher, *The 1998 N.O.D./Harris Survey of Americans with Disabilities*.

16. *Mouth*, September/October 1997: 7.

17. *Mouth*, November/December 1997: 50.

18. Risher, *The 1998 N.O.D./Harris Survey of Americans with Disabilities*.

Chapter 11: *Getting Out There*

1. Risher, *The 1998 N.O.D./Harris Survey of Americans with Disabilities*.

2. Risher, *The 1998 N.O.D./Harris Survey of Americans with Disabilities*.

3. Douglas Kruse and Alan Krueger, *Disability, Employment, and Earnings in the Dawn of the Computer Age—Executive Summary*, Bureau of Economic Research, Rutgers University, October 1995.

4. *Tony Coelho, chairman, opening remarks, President's Committee on Employment of People with Disabilities 51st Annual Conference: http://www50.pcepd.gov/pcepd/ speeches/TCopen98.htm.*

5. "Modern Medics," *Mainstream Magazine,* August 1997, 18-20.

6. Risher, *The 1998 N.O.D./Harris Survey of Americans with Disabilities*.

7. *Tony Coelho's opening remarks.*

8. Kruse, *Disability, Employment, and Earnings.*

9. *Tony Coelho's opening remarks.*

10. Kruse, *Disability, Employment, and Earnings.*

Bibliography

"504 Celebration & Commemoration." Berkeley, California: DREDF, 1997.

Accessible Building Design, and *Planning for Access*. Eastern Paralyzed Veterans Association.

"ADAPT Beats Bad Dog in 44 Cities." *Mouth* 8, no. 3 (1997): 7.

"The Americans with Disabilities Act, Your Personal Guide to the Law," and "The Air Carrier Access Act, Make It Work For You." Paralyzed Veterans of America, Washington, D.C.

Apple, David F., Jr., M.D. *Physical Fitness: A Guide for Individuals with Spinal Cord Injury*. Department of Veterans Affairs, Washington, D.C.

"Autonomic Dysreflexia: A Possible Life Threatening Situation." University of Alabama at Birmingham. *Pushin' On Newsletter* 15, no. 1 (1997).

Axelson, Peter, Jean Minkel, and Denise Chesney. *A Guide to Wheelchair Selection: How to Use the ANSI/RESNA Standards to Buy a Wheelchair*. Washington, D.C.

Bantam Medical Dictionary, Revised edition. New York: Bantam Books, 1990.

Bielunis, Pamela J. *New Horizons in Sexuality After a Spinal Cord Injury*. Bloomington, Illinois: Cheever Publishing, 1995.

Brackett, N. L., et al. "Endocrine Profiles and Semen Quality of Spinal Cord Injured Men." *The Journal of Urology* 151 (1994): 117.

Brackett, N. L., et al. "Male Fertility Following Spinal Cord Injury: Facts and Fiction." *Physical Therapy* 76, no. 11 (1996): 1225-8.

Brackett, N. L., et al. "Semen Quality of Spinal Cord Injured Men Is Better When Obtained by Vibratory Stimulation Versus Electroejaculation." *The Journal of Urology* 157 (1997): 152-6.

Braunstein, Miriam. "Homeward Bound—And Wishing They Weren't." *New Mobility* 8, no. 48 (1997).

Carper, Jean. *Food—Your Miracle Medicine*. New York: HarperCollins, 1993.

Cheever, Raymond, and Betty Garee, editors. *Pressure Sores*. Bloomington, Illinois: Cheever Publishing, 1987.

Chödrön, Pema. *When Things Fall Apart: Heart Advice for Difficult Times*. Boston: Shambhala, 1997.

Complications of SCI. The Rehabilitation Learning Center, Harborview Medical Center, Seattle, Washington.

Davies, Brooks. "Buying a Power Wheelchair." *New Mobility* (February 1997): 64.

DeGraff, Al. *Home Health Aides: How to Manage the People Who Help You*. Fort Collins, Colorado: Saratoga Access Publications, 1988.

Demeter, Stephen, Andersson, Gunnar, and Smith, George, editors. *Disability Evaluation*. St. Louis, Missouri: Mosby-Year Book, 1996.

Facts About Muscular Dystrophy. The Muscular Dystrophy Association, Tucson.

Fisher, Ian. "Families Struggle to Care for Loved Ones." *New York Times/San Francisco Examiner,* June 1998.

Gallagher, Hugh Gregory. *FDR's Splendid Deception.* Vandamere Press, 1994.

Giffels, J. Joseph. *Clinical Trials: What You Should Know Before Volunteering to Be a Research Subject.* New York: Demos Vermande, 1996.

Graham, Judy. *Multiple Sclerosis, A Self-Help Guide to Its Management.* Rochester, Vermont: Healing Arts Press, 1989.

Gregory, Martha Ferguson. *Sexual Adjustment for the Spinal Cord Injured.* Bloomington, Illinois: Cheever Publishing, 1974.

"Greyhound Fails Activists' Test of ADA Compliance." *Ragged Edge* 19, no. 2 (1998): 9.

Gullett, Wayne. "Chair Checkup." *Paraplegia News* 51, no. 5 (1997): 41.

Hockenberry, John. *Moving Violations.* New York: Hyperion Publishers, 1995.

Hollicky, Richard. "Countdown to Comfort." *Paraplegia News* 15, no. 6 (1997): 14.

Holicky, Richard. "Leakproofing: The Joy of Incontinence." *New Mobility* 8, no. 49 (1997).

"How Kansas Got 'Consumer Control' Into the Law." *Ragged Edge* 18, no. 4 (1997): 21.

"How Parents Can Educate Their Neighborhood Schools." *Mouth* 8, no. 4 (1997): 20.

Kantor, Carol. *Standing and Walking with FES for People with Paralysis.* Cleveland: FES Information Center, 1992.

Kirshblum, S., M.D., et al. "Bowel Care Practices in Chronic Spinal Cord Injury Patients." *Archives of Physical Medicine and Rehabilitation* 79, no. 1: 20.

Kirschmann, John D. *The Nutrition Almanac.* New York: McGraw-Hill Paperbacks, 1975.

Kraft, George H., M.D., and Marci Catanzaro, R.N., Ph.D. *Living with Multiple Sclerosis.* New York: Demos Vermande, 1996.

Kroll, Ken, and Erica Levy Klein. *Enabling Romance: A Guide to Love, Sex, and Relationships for the Disabled.* Bethseda, Maryland: Woodbine House, 1992.

Kruse, Douglas, and Alan Krueger. *Disability, Employment, and Earnings in the Dawn of the Computer Age — Executive Summary.* Bureau of Economic Research, Rutgers University. October 1995.

Linville, Brian T., Dean A. Brusinghan, and William E. Field. *Plowshares #9.* Breaking New Ground Resource Center. Purdue University, 1990.

Maddox, Sam. *Spinal Network.* Malibu, California: Miramar Publishing, 1994.

Maddox, Sam. "Front- and Mid-Wheel Drive: A New Era Arrives for Power Chairs." *New Mobility* (January 1998).

Maddox, Sam, editor. *Spinal Network, The Total Wheelchair Book.* Malibu, California: Miramar Publishing, 1994.

Mahoney, Kevin J., and Lori Simon-Rusinowitz. "Cash and Counseling Demonstration and Evaluation." *Journal of Case Management* 6, no. 1 (1997).

McCourt, A. E., editor. *The Specialty Practice of Rehabilitation Nursing: A Core Curriculum.* Skokie, Illinois: Rehabilitation Nursing Foundation, 1993.

McMullin-Powell, Daniese. "Riding the Dog." *Ragged Edge* 19, no. 1 (1998): 9.

Menter, Robert, M.D. "Spinal Cord Injury and Aging: Exploring the Unknown." *Journal of the American Paraplegia Society* 16, no. 4 (1993).

Menter, Robert, M.D., et al. "Bowel Management Outcomes in Individuals with Long Term Spinal Cord Injury." *Archives of Physical Medicine and Rehabilitation* 78, no. 9: 608.

Messina, Virginia, R.D., and Mark Messina, Ph.D. *The Vegetarian Way*. New York: Crown Trade Paperbacks, 1996.

"Modern Medics." *Mainstream Magazine* 21, no. 10 (1997): 18-20.

Morris, Jeri. "Spinal Injury and Psychotherapy: A Treatment Philosophy." *Spinal Cord Injury, Medical Management and Rehabilitation*. Gaithersburg, Maryland: Aspen Publishers, 1994.

Moyers, Bill. *Healing and the Mind*. New York: Doubleday, 1993.

Nyre, Suzanne, and Virginia McKay. "Preadmission Screening and Secondary Transport," in *The Management of High Quadriplegia*, edited by Gale Whiteneck, Ph.D., et al. New York: Demos Vermande, 1989.

Padron, O. F. et al. "Semen of Spinal Cord Injured Men Freezes Reliably." *Journal of Andrology* 15, no. 13 (1994): 268.

"Personal Care Assistants: How to Find, Hire, and Keep Them." *Paraplegia News* 49, no. 1 (1997): 16-17.

Price, Reynolds. *A Whole New Life*. New York: Plume/Penguin Books USA, 1994.

Progress in Research, Newsletters of The American Paralysis Association.

The Project, News from the Miami Project to Cure Paralysis 10, no. 3 (1997): 7.

The Project, News from The Miami Project to Cure Paralysis 11, no. 1 (1998): 6.

"Protest Halts Service at S.F. Bus Terminal." *San Francisco Chronicle*, 9 August 1997.

Ready, Willing & Available: A Business Guide for Hiring People with Disabilities. President's Committee on Employment of People with Disabilities, 1993.

Reagan, Jan, and Ronald Mace, FAIA. *Bathing Beauties: Creating Safer and More Usable Bathrooms*. Center for Universal Design. North Carolina State University.

Residential Remodeling and Universal Design. U.S. Department of Housing and Urban Development, 1996.

"Resource Guide to Seating and Positioning." *Mainstream Magazine* (November 1996).

Robbins-Roth, Cynthia, Ph.D. "Bringing Biology to Bear on the Nervous System." *Bioventure News* 10, no. 6 (1995).

Robinson, Kevin. "Caregiver and Spouse: Should the Twain Ever Meet?" *New Mobility* (February 1998).

Rosner, Louis J., M.D., and Shelly Ross. *Multiple Sclerosis*. New York: Simon & Schuster, 1992.

Roth, Elliot, M.D. "Practical Pain Management Strategies," and "Pain in Spinal Cord Injury." *Spinal Cord Injury: Medical Management and Rehabilitation*. Gaithersburg, Maryland: Aspen Publishers, 1994.

Schapiro, Randall, M.D. "The Rehabilitation of Progressive Multiple Sclerosis." *MS Management* 3, no. 1 (1996).

Shapiro, Joseph P. *No Pity: People with Disabilities Forging a New Civil Rights Movement*. New York: Times Books/Random House, 1994.

Shield, L., M.D. *Scoliosis*. Royal Children's Hospital. Melbourne, Australia.

Shrout, Richard Neil. *Resource Directory for the Disabled*. Facts on File, New York, 1991.

Smith, Douglas. "Returning to Work? How Social Security Can Help." *Paraplegia News* 52, no. 2 (1998).

Spinal Cord Injury: Patient Education Manual. Gaithersburg, Maryland: Aspen Publishers, 1995.

Sternfeld, Leon, M.D. *Cerebral Palsy, Health, and Medical Horizons*. New York: Macmillan Educational Company, 1991.

Sunderlin, Ann. "Ready, Set, Roll." *Sports 'N Spokes* 23, no. 6 (1997): 68-73.

Tepper, Mitchell, M.P.H., "Possible Effects of SCI on Sexual Function." Sexual Health Network.

Tepper, Mitchell, M.P.H., "Sexual Pleasure: What About Me?" *New Mobility* (June 1996).

Thompson, Cliff. "Jimmie Heuga: Still Ahead of the Curve." *New Mobility* 8, no. 40 (1997): 49.

Vogel, Bob. "Powering Your Chair: Battery Basics." *New Mobility* (September 1996): 59.

Walsh, Alison, Jodi Abbott, and Peg Smith, editors. *Able to Travel: A Rough Guide Special*. England: Rough Guides Ltd., 1994.

Winchell, Ellen, Ph.D. *Coping with Limb Loss*. Garden City Park, New York: Avery Publishing Group, 1995.

Wylde, Margaret, Adrian Baron-Robbins, and Sam Clark. *Building for a Lifetime: The Design and Construction of Fully Accessible Homes*. Newtown, CT: Taunton Press, 1994.

X Paralympics Commemorative Issue. The Paralyzed Veterans of America. *Sports 'N Spokes* 22, no. 6 (1996).

Yarkony, Gary, M.D., editor. *Spinal Cord Injury: Medical Management and Rehabilitation*. Gaithersburg, Maryland: Aspen Publishers, 1994.

Young, Wise, M.D., Ph.D. *Pain in Spinal Cord Injury*. Canadian Spinal Research Organization, 1997.

Zola, Irving Kenneth. *Missing Pieces: A Chronicle of Living with A Disability*. Philadelphia: Temple University Press, 1982.

Index

emotions (*continued*)

anger, as response to disability, 175–178

denial, 172–174

depression, 178–182

humor, as means of coping, 186–187

responses to disability, many possible, 64

suicide, consideration of, 64, 182–184

support, ongoing need for, 187–189

employment

computers, made possible by, 485–487

Job Accommodation Network, 484–485

President's Committee on Employment of People with Disabilities, 483–484

resources, 519–520

right to work, 488

starting a business, 487

temporary work, 487–488

unemployment, factors influencing, 481–483

volunteering/advocacy, 488–489

end of rehab, adjustment to, 72–78

ErgoDynamic Seating System, 245

ergonomics, 476–478

ethics in research

of animal use, 412–414

of fetal cell use, 390–391

exacerbations

causes of in multiple sclerosis patients, 6

multiple sclerosis, symptoms of, 5–6

exercise, 114–120

See also sports

F

family and friends

as personal assistant, 154

caregivers, after rehab, 75–76

counseling for, 69–70

parents, dependency on, 196

role in rehab process, 46–47

sharers of disability, 192–196

Feldenkrais method, 140–142

FES (functional electrical stimulation), 55, 403–409, 508

See also walking

fetal cell research, 389–391

finding an accessible home, 312–314

Fisher, Helen

walking, as cue to attract mate, 333

Fleming, Ann Marie

adjustment begins at end of denial, 173

adjustment more difficult with age, 191

grief and loss, 174

helplessness, feelings of, by family, 69

letting go, 194

self-destructive behavior may lessen with disability, 191

FNS (functional neuromuscular stimulation), 403–409

See also walking

footrests, 253–255

Frankel, A.

disability may reveal sexual conflict, 323

Freehand System (of hand grip/ release), 407–409

Friedreich's ataxia (FA), 4

friends. *See* family and friends

funding of wheelchair, 211–215

G

gait training, 53–56
  See also walking
Gill, Carol
  adjusting to disability, 162, 164,
    167, 170, 192
  asking for help, consequences of,
    200
  family member/partner as
    personal assistant,
    difficult for relationship,
    195
  pride, role in public image, 210
  public attitude/prejudice toward
    disability, 206, 208, 209
  responses to disability, emotional,
    171, 175, 176
Ginns, Sheldon
  chair riders, access to campus as
    factor in increased
    number of, 479
Gittler, Michelle
  patient endorsement of Viagra,
    355
Greenhalgh, Jody
  insurance, issues with managed
    care, 33
  need for referral to rehab center
    from acute care, 26, 27
  occupational vs. physical therapy,
    56
  rehab team, role of members in,
    39
  transition of children with
    disabilities to adulthood,
    31
  wheelchair, care in selection
    important, 213–214,
    218
Gregory, Martha
  future as tragic, view of
    nondisabled person,
    171–172
grief and loss, coping with feelings of,
  174–175

H

Hale, Glorya
  orgasm not essential to
    satisfaction, 319
Hall, Bob
  posture, importance of in
    prevention of physical
    problems, 242
  wheelchair, dealer choice of may
    be inappropriate, 219–
    220
hand grip and release system, 407–
  409
Hatch, Bill
  homebound status, Medicare
    payment for support
    services and, 434
health maintenance
  methods of, 114–144
  sexual activity, importance to,
    342
help, 199–205
  See also dependency
heterotopic ossification, 87–88
home access, 262–315
  adapting existing home, 262,
    268–269
  bathroom, 297–304
  bedroom, 310–311
  behavioral changes and, 314–315
  features effecting, 275–297
  finding an accessible home, 312–
    314
  kitchen, 304–309
  Lifespan model used to maximize
    quality of life, 262–263
  mobile/modular homes, 314
  needs met by, 263
  outdoor spaces, 312
  planning, 269–275
  resources, 511–514
  storage and utilities, 311–312
  Universal Design, 263–265
homebound, legal definition of, 433
homeopathy, 144

muscular dystrophy (MD), 6–7
myasthenia gravis (MG), 7–8
myelin, 5, 375–387
myotonic dystrophy, 7

N

O

P

About the Author

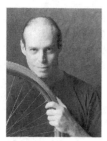 In 1973, when he was 18, Gary Karp fell out of a tree, injuring his spinal cord at mid-back and becoming paraplegic. After his accident, Gary graduated from college with degrees in architecture, and then worked in the presentation graphics field as a designer and manager, specializing in computer graphics. In that field, he pioneered a desktop services division, conducted training, and was a highly regarded public speaker.

In 1992, Gary developed a repetitive strain injury as a result of computer work. After taking a year off from work to recover, he switched careers and established Onsight, an ergonomics consulting business which provides training and individual workstation consultation services to a range of clients in the San Francisco Bay Area.

Outside work, Gary has been performing music—playing guitar, piano, and singing—in local cafes and coffeehouses since he was a teenager, and has recorded a CD of original guitar music.

In 1988, a friend introduced him to juggling, and Gary has been hooked ever since. He enjoys the juggling community, where he has learned about the value of making mistakes, the Zen experience of staying in the moment, and juggling with others in club passing patterns. He discovered through juggling—as with his disability—that his limits are much further out than he'd realized. He has also produced, performed, and emceed at fundraisers and juggling festivals across the country.

Gary's first book, *Choosing a Wheelchair: A Guide for Optimal Independence*, was published in the summer of 1998. Through his writing, Gary is interested in helping people with disabilities adapt as effectively as possible so that they can reach their optimal quality of life.

Colophon

Patient-Centered Guides are about the experience of illness. They contain personal stories as well as a combination of practical and medical information. The faces on the covers of our Guides reflect the human side of the information we offer.

Edie Freedman designed the cover of *Life on Wheels: For the Active Wheelchair User,* using Adobe Photoshop 5.0 and QuarkXPress 3.32 with Onyx BT and Berkeley fonts from Bitstream. All cover photos are used with permission. Mike Siegel shot the photograph of Jim Lubin, a vent-using quadriplegic who is a hard-core computer user. Jim was named person of the year by *New Mobility* magazine for his development and maintenance of a comprehensive web site. The women's tennis photo was taken by

Curt Beamer, © 1997 Sports 'N Spokes/Paralyzed Veterans of America. The photograph of the student with the backpack is from Photodisc. The cover mechanical was prepared by Kathleen Wilson. The interior layout for the book was designed by Nancy Priest, Edie Freedman, and Alicia Cech. The interior fonts are Berkeley and Franklin Gothic. The text was prepared by Mike Sierra using FrameMaker 5.5. The text was copyedited by Lunaea Hougland and proofread by Kim Brown. Jeff Liggett, Colleen Gorman, and Jane Ellin conducted quality assurance reviews. The index was written by Katherine J. Wilkinson. The illustrations that appear in this book were produced by Robert Romano and Rhon Porter using Macromedia Freehand 8 and Adobe Photoshop 5. Interior composition was done by Claire Cloutier LeBlanc, Sebastian Banker, and Susan Reinbold. Whenever possible, our books use RepKover™ lay-flat binding. If the page count exceeds the limit for lay-flat binding, perfect binding is used.

The photo of the author used in this colophon was taken by Katya Kallsen. The photos of the Quickie 2 manual folding chair (Figure 6-2) and Shadow Heat sport chair (Figure 6-3) were taken by Keith Seaman of Camerad and are reprinted with his permission. The photos of the Action A-4™ rigid-frame manual wheelchair (Figure 6-1) and the Action Power 9000™ Storm Series® wheelchair (Figure 6-4) are reprinted with permission from Invacare. The photo of the Chairman front-wheel drive power chair (Figure 6-5) is reprinted with permission from Goran Udden, president of Permobil. The illustrations in Chapter 7, *Home Access*, are reprinted from *Building for a Lifetime: The Design and Construction of Fully Accessible Homes* by Margaret Wylde, Adrian Baron-Robbins, and Sam Clarke, copyright 1994, by permission of the publisher, the Taunton Press. The photo of the Freedom Bath side-entrance bathtub is reprinted with permission of ARJO, photo provided courtesy of the Taunton Press. The photo of the van with a ramp is reprinted with permission of the Braun Corporation. The photo of the joystick driving control is reprinted with permission of Ahnafield Corporation. The photo of the men's field club-throwing event was taken by Curt Beamer, © 1997 Sports 'N Spokes/Paralyzed Veterans of America and is reprinted with their permission. The photo of men's basketball was taken by Curt Beamer, © 1993 Sports 'N Spokes/Paralyzed Veterans of America and is reprinted with their permission. The photos of the wheelchair back with tension-adjustable straps, using a grabber arm in the kitchen, and the wheelie technique were taken by Larry Watson of O'Reilly & Associates, Inc.

Patient-Centered Guides™

Questions Answered
Experiences Shared

*We are committed to empowering individuals to evolve
into informed consumers armed with the latest information and
heartfelt support for their journey.*

When your life is turned upside down, your need for information is great. You have
to make critical medical decisions, often with what seems little to go on. Plus you
have to break the news to family, quiet your own fears, cope with symptoms or
treatment side effects, figure out how you're going to pay for things, and sometimes
still get to work or get dinner on the table.

Patient-Centered Guides provide authoritative information for intelligent
information seekers who want to become advocates of their own health. They
cover the whole impact of illness on your life. In each book, there's a mix of:

- **Medical background for treatment decisions**
  We can give you information that can help you to intelligently work with
  your doctor to come to a decision. We start from the viewpoint that modern
  medicine has much to offer and also discuss complementary treatments.
  Where there are treatment controversies we present differing points of view.

- **Practical information**
  Once you've decided what to do about your illness, you still have to deal with
  treatments and changes to your life. We cover day-to-day practicalities, such as
  those you'd hear from a good nurse or a knowledgeable support group.

- **Emotional support**
  It's normal to have strong reactions to a condition that threatens your life or
  changes how you live. It's normal that the whole family is affected. We cover
  issues like the shock of diagnosis, living with uncertainty, and communicating
  with loved ones.

Each book also contains stories from both patients and doctors — medical
"frequent fliers" who share, in their own words, the lessons and strategies they
have learned when maneuvering through the often complicated maze of medical
information that's available.

We provide information online, including updated listings of the resources that
appear in this book. This is freely available for you to print out and copy to
share with others, as long as you retain the copyright notice on the print-outs.

http://www.patientcenters.com

Other Books in the Series

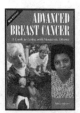

Advanced Breast Cancer
A Guide to Living with Metastatic Disease
By Musa Mayer
ISBN 1-56592-522-X, Paperback 6" x 9", 542 pages, $19.95

"An excellent book...if knowledge is power, this book will be good medicine."
—David Spiegel, M.D.
Stanford University,
Author, *Living Beyond Limits*

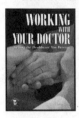

Working with Your Doctor
Getting the Healthcare You Deserve
By Nancy Keene
ISBN 1-56592-273-5, Paperback, 6" x 9", 382 pages, $15.95

"Working with Your Doctor fills a genuine need for patients and their family members caught up in this new and intimidating age of impersonal, economically-driven health care delivery."
—James Dougherty, M.D.
Emeritus Professor of Surgery,
Albany Medical College

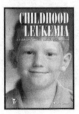

Childhood Leukemia
A Guide for Families, Friends & Caregivers
By Nancy Keene
ISBN 1-56592-191-7, Paperback, 6" x 9", 566 pages, $24.95

"What's so compelling about Childhood Leukemia *is the amount of useful medical information and practical advice it contains. Keene avoids jargon and lays out what's needed to deal with the medical system."*
—The Washington Post

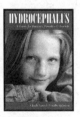

Hydrocephalus
A Guide for Patients, Families & Friends
By Chuck Toporek and Kellie Robinson
ISBN 1-56592-410-X, Paperback, 6" x 9", 384 pages, $19.95

"In this book, the authors have provided a wonderful entry into the world of hydrocephalus to begin to remedy the neglect of this important condition. We are immensely grateful to them for their groundbreaking effort."
—Peter M. Black, M.D., Ph.D.
Franc D. Ingraham Professor of Neurosurgery,
Harvard Medical School
Neurosurgeon-in-Chief,
Brigham and Women's Hospital, Children's Hospital,
Boston, Massachusetts

Patient-Centered Guides
Published by O'Reilly & Associates, Inc.
Our products are available at a bookstore near you.
For information: **800-998-9938** • **707-829-0515** • **info@oreilly.com**
101 Morris Street • Sebastopol • CA • 95472-9902

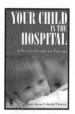

Your Child in the Hospital
A Practical Guide for Parents
By Nancy Keene and Rachel Prentice
ISBN 1-56592-346-4, Paperback, 5" x 8", 136 pages, $9.95

"When your child is ill or injured, the hospital setting can be overwhelming. Here is a terrific 'road map' to help keep families 'on track.'"
—James B. Fahner, M.D.
Division Chief, Pediatric Hematology/Oncology
DeVos Children's Hospital, Grand Rapids, Michigan

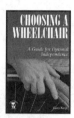

Choosing a Wheelchair
A Guide for Optimal Independence
By Gary Karp
ISBN 1-56592-411-8, Paperback, 5" x 8", 192 pages, $9.95

"I love the idea of putting knowledge often possessed only by professionals into the hands of new consumers. Gary Karp has done it. This book will empower people with disabilities to make informed equipment choices."
—Barry Corbet
Editor, *New Mobility Magazine*

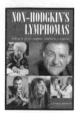

Non-Hodgkin's Lymphomas
Making Sense of Diagnosis, Treatment & Options
By Lorraine Johnston
ISBN 1-56592-444-4, Paperback, 6" x 9", 584 pages, $24.95

"When I gave this book to one of our patients, there was an instant, electric connection. A sense of enlightenment came over her while she absorbed the information. It was thrilling to see her so sparked with new energy and focus."
—Susan Weisberg, LCSW
Clinical Social Worker,
Stanford University Medical Center

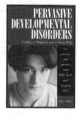

Pervasive Developmental Disorders
Finding a Diagnosis and Getting Help
By Mitzi Waltz
ISBN 1-56592-530-0, Paperback, 6" x 9", 592 pages, $24.95

"Mitzi Waltz's book provides clear, informative, and comprehensive information on every relevant aspect of PDD. Her in-depth discussion will help parents and professionals develop a clear understanding of the issues and, consequently, they will be able to make informed decisions about various interventions. A job well done!"
—Dr. Stephen M. Edelson
Director, Center for the Study of Autism,
Salem, Oregon

Patient-Centered Guides
Published by O'Reilly & Associates, Inc.
Our products are available at a bookstore near you.
For information: **800-998-9938** • **707-829-0515** • **info@oreilly.com**
101 Morris Street • Sebastopol • CA • 95472-9902